KAPLAN) MEDICAL

Anatomy Coloring Book

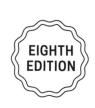

EIGHTH EDITION

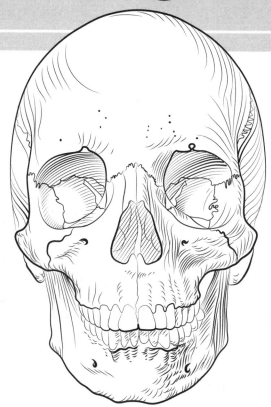

The Easiest Way to Learn Human Anatomy

Illustrations by Stephanie McCann, MA

Text by Eric Wise, MA

© 2021 Stephanie McCann and Eric Wise

Published by Kaplan Publishing, a division of Kaplan, Inc.
750 Third Avenue
New York, NY 10017

10 9 8 7 6 5 4 3 2

ISBN-13: 978-1-5062-7640-3

Kaplan Publishing books are available at special quantity discounts to use for sales promotions, employee premiums, or educational purposes. For more information or to purchase books, please call the Simon & Schuster special sales department at 866-506-1949.

▪ Table of Contents

kaptest.com/retail-book-corrections-and-updates

The material in the book is current at the time of publication. If there are any important changes or corrections to this book, we will post that information at kaptest.com/retail-book-corrections-and-updates.

■ About the Authors

Stephanie Paulnock McCann is a medical illustrator and fine artist with a studio in Tacoma, Washington. She holds a BA in Fine Art from the University of California at Santa Cruz and an MA in Medical and Biological Illustration from The Johns Hopkins University.

Ms. McCann specializes in work that depicts the amazing beauty of the anatomy of the human body in both traditional and digital media.

Before retiring, McCann was chief of the Medical Illustration Department at Letterman Army Medical Center in San Francisco and, later, instructor of Biological Illustration and Digital Drawing at Santa Barbara City College. She and her SBCC students exhibited their work at the Santa Barbara Museum of Natural History and the Step One Gallery in Carpinteria, California. Ms. McCann's work has also been exhibited at the Society of Illustrators in New York. Her medical illustrations have appeared in textbooks, journals, product advertising, training manuals, and legal presentations. Her 3D texture painting for Santa Barbara Studios can be seen in the films *Star Trek: Insurrection* and *Paulie: A Parrot's Tale*. She currently focuses on her fine art painting.

You can see her artwork at www.stephaniemccann.com.

Eric Wise has been teaching biology for over 30 years at colleges and universities in California. He has taught human anatomy at California State University, California community colleges, and the University of California systems. He received BA degrees in biology, botany, and French from Humboldt State University in Northern California and an MA in biology from California Polytechnic State University, San Luis Obispo. He initiated a cadaver program at Yuba College and has taught a diverse course load from marine biology to plant taxonomy.

Mr. Wise is currently an instructor at Santa Barbara City College, where he has taught various classes since 1990, including anatomy and physiology, ecology, physical anthropology, and botany. Mr. Wise is the author of three laboratory manuals in anatomy and physiology and enjoys gardening, swimming, music, and teaching.

Contributing editor **David Seiden** is professor of neuroscience and cell biology at the University of Medicine and Dentistry of New Jersey—Robert Wood Johnson Medical School; he also served as an assistant professor and associate professor of anatomy at that institution. Dr. Seiden was visiting associate professor of anatomy and cell biology at Harvard Medical School and is co-author of *USMLE Step 1: Anatomy*, published by Kaplan Medical. Dr. Seiden received his BS from The City College of New York and his PhD from Temple University.

■ Dedications

From Stephanie McCann

...to my daughter, Natalie, for living through the creation of this book with me.

...to my teachers, Ranice Crosby, director emerita, and Gary Lees, chairman and director, Department of Art as Applied to Medicine, The Johns Hopkins University, for giving me my start in this wonderful career.

From Eric Wise

...to my three brothers, Steve, Mike, and Phil, for their love during good times and bad.

...to Ashley for her love and support.

▪ Introduction

People have been involved with learning anatomy since prehistoric times. Paintings in Stone Age caves 18,000 years ago show evidence of anatomical structures in animals and, in some cases, humans. In ancient Greece, Aristotle wrote extensively about the natural world, and human structure was part of that writing. The Roman physician Galen was perhaps the most influential anatomist of ancient times. His works were used as the primary source of anatomical knowledge for about 1,500 years.

A major change in the science of anatomy came with the Renaissance. Instead of relying on the texts of the ancient Greeks or Romans, scholars used a new sense of inquiry and investigation. Andreas Vesalius, an anatomist teaching in Italy, did detailed studies and drawings of the human body. Leonardo da Vinci's anatomical studies were not only great works of art, but were also a means of scientific exploration.

Today there are many anatomical resources available in books and on the Internet. Technologies for medical imaging, such as CT scans and MRI images, give detailed understanding of the relationship of structures in the human body. On the Web, you can find anatomy course outlines, images of the 1918 edition of *Gray's Anatomy*, cadaver photographs, and photomicrographs of microscopic anatomy. These different views and new technologies have deepened our knowledge of human anatomy.

We have designed this coloring book in appreciation of the incredible beauty of the human body, hoping to inspire you in your studies of anatomy. The connection of the eye and the hand in coloring the anatomical structures and filling in the names of these structures will be a valuable learning experience for you. Here's how to get the best results from your experience.

HOW TO USE THIS BOOK

This book is primarily arranged by human organ system. Thus, all of the bones that make up the skeletal system are covered in one chapter, while the heart and blood vessels that make up the cardiovascular system are covered in another. In the Muscular System chapter is a **special flashcard section**, which you can color and carry with you. (See page 109 for tips on how to get the most from the muscle flashcards.) Also included in the book are **Learning Hints**, new in this edition, which are boxed side notes with word associations and other mnemonics to help you remember the material.

This book is meant to be handled, colored, written on, and even torn apart in the case of the muscle flashcards. There is no single way to use the coloring book, so choose the method that suits you best. Here are a couple of possibilities:

- **Write and learn.** You can learn anatomical features by looking at the key on the facing page, finding the corresponding letter on the illustration, and writing in the term next to the letter before coloring the anatomical feature. This is a great learn-by-doing technique.

- **Test yourself.** Another way to use the book is as a review of anatomical features or as a self-test tool. In this method, examine the illustrations, fill in the appropriate blank in pencil, and then look at the key at the bottom of the facing page. Correct your errors and then color in the illustration as a way to cement your knowledge.

COLORING TOOLS AND TECHNIQUES

Tools

The preferred medium for this book is colored pencils. Colored ball-point pens or felt-tipped markers will give you brighter color saturation but will permit less control in shading your illustrations. If you do use felt-tipped markers, be sure to put one or two sheets of paper under the page you are drawing on to absorb any ink that might bleed through the paper.

Although you can use any of a variety of brands of colored pencils, be sure to buy a good-quality set such as Prismacolor, Faber-Castel, Prang, or Crayola. The investment that you make by purchasing more expensive colored pencils is usually justified with superior results—and you will be using them a lot. Options for colored pencils include boxed sets of preselected colors as well as stand-alone colors that you select and purchase individually. You should select at least 12 to 15 colors for illustrating this book, most of which should be bright colors. Include white for highlights, and also include gray and black for shadows or lines.

Look over each page before you begin coloring so that you can color related structures in context with each other. For the best learning experience, use the same color for the same structures. If there is a bone in three illustrations on one page, for example, color that bone the same color in all three illustrations. That way, you will not only find that bone easily, but also you will reinforce your knowledge of that structure in three ways at once: by name, shape, and color.

Color Guides

Each two-page spread throughout the *Anatomy Coloring Book* provides a Color Guide section making specific recommendations for coloring the material. You should read the Color Guide before you start coloring the page. Of course, you are free to use whatever color scheme you want to further your goal of learning the structures better.

Be aware that there are standardized colors for most anatomy drawings. For instance, blood vessels carrying oxygenated blood are colored red, and those that carry deoxygenated blood are colored blue. The lymphatic system is conventionally colored in green, nerves in yellow, and the digestive organs in pink. The muscles, by convention, are also colored red, but since this is a coloring book you will probably want to select an individual color for each muscle. If you are coloring arteries or veins, you may want to use different colors for these vessels found in different areas.

Techniques

This book is designed for you to use single, bold colors for each structure, but layering one color on top of another can be used to blend colors together if desired. Keep bits of colored lead off the paper to avoid streaking stray colors across the page as your hand brushes over the paper. If you are right-handed, it is beneficial to color on the left side of the paper first. If you are left-handed, then it is helpful to start on the right, to avoid smearing the color with your hand.

When you color, you will typically want to follow the length of the figure to be illustrated, going along the contours of the illustration. When you have selected a direction, keep the colored pencil in that orientation as you color in the entire object (muscle, bone, stomach). As a general rule, you should make the edges of the object darker than the center, as this is how light plays on an object. Begin using light pressure when you color. You can always go back and deepen the color as you work on the drawings.

▪ Welcome

Welcome to Kaplan Medical's *Anatomy Coloring Book*, Eighth Edition. We hope you like exploring and using the book. This unique resource is approachable and informative, and provides an enjoyable way to learn human anatomy.

- In this edition, our new **Learning Hint** feature presents word associations and other mnemonics to help you remember the material. Each of these useful tips appears in a box accompanying the related anatomy discussion.

- Our **exclusive muscle flashcards** appear in the Muscular System chapter. This section has 96 images printed on durable card stock; flip over to see the muscle's name, origin, insertion, action, and related nerve. Use the flashcards to test yourself on the go. Simply color the muscle structures, tear along the perforations, and carry the cards with you.

- Our **expansive page design** with larger images and more space than in past editions offers greater ease of coloring.

- The optimized page layouts also help **avoid bleed-through** from one image to another, because all descriptive text is placed on the left-hand page and all illustrations for coloring on the right. There are no back-to-back images.

Whatever reason you have for studying anatomy, this book will help you deepen your enjoyment and learning. We would love to hear about your experiences, so feel free to contact us at **book.support@kaplan.com**. Thanks and happy coloring!

■ Chapter One: **Introduction**

ANATOMICAL POSITION AND TERMS OF DIRECTION

When studying the human body, it is important to place the body in anatomical position. **Anatomical position** is described as the body facing you, feet placed together and flat on the floor. The head is held erect, arms straight by the side with palms facing forward. All references to the body are made as if the body is in this position, so when you describe something as being above something else, it is always with respect to the body being in anatomical position.

The relative positions of the parts of the human body have specific terms. **Superior** means above while **inferior** means below. **Medial** refers to being close to the midline while **lateral** means to the side. **Anterior** or **ventral** is to the front while **posterior** or **dorsal** is to the back. **Superficial** is near the surface while **deep** means to the core of the body. When working with the limbs, **proximal** means closer to the trunk while **distal** is toward the ends of the limbs. Write the directional terms in the spaces provided, and color in the arrows in reference to these terms. Note that these terms are somewhat different for four-legged animals.

Answer Key

a. Superior
b. Inferior
c. Lateral
d. Medial
e. Proximal
f. Distal
g. Anatomical position
h. Posterior
i. Anterior
j. Dorsal
k. Ventral

LEARNING HINT

When you read **proximal**, think of *approximate* (meaning "close") in relation to the trunk, whereas **distal** is *distant* from the trunk.

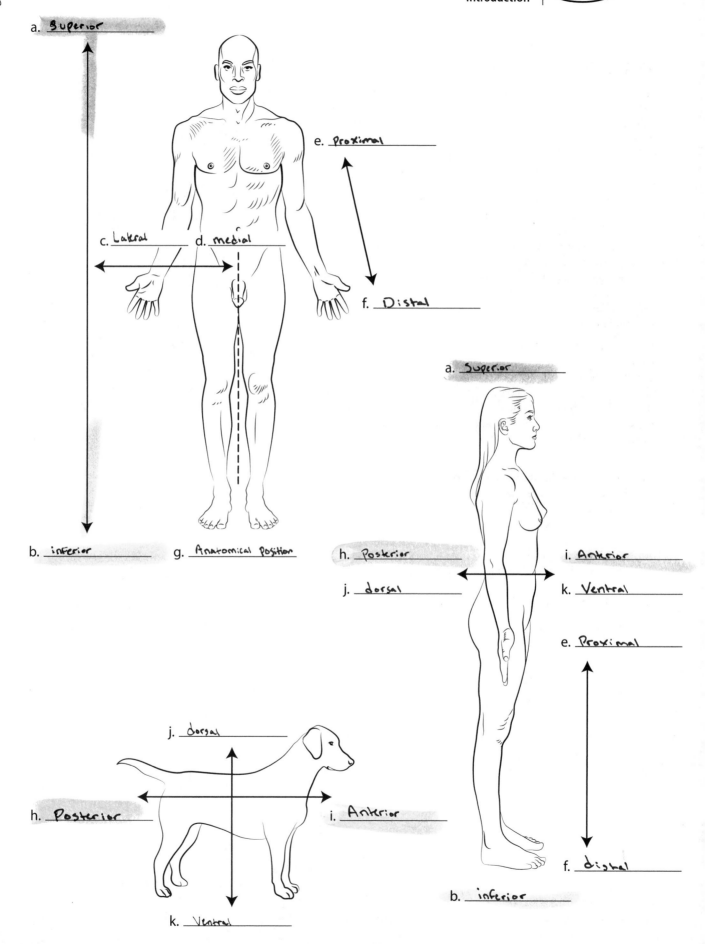

a. Superior

b. inferior

c. Lateral

d. medial

e. Proximal

f. Distal

g. Anatomical Position

h. Posterior

i. Anterior

j. dorsal

k. Ventral

a. Superior

e. Proximal

f. distal

b. inferior

j. dorsal

h. Posterior

i. Anterior

k. Ventral

ANATOMICAL PLANES OF THE BODY

Many specimens in anatomy are sectioned so that the interior of the organ or region can be examined. It is important that the direction of the cut is known so that the proper orientation of the specimen is known. A heart looks very different if it is cut along its length as opposed to horizontally. A horizontal cut is known as a **transverse section** or a **cross section**. A cut that divides the body or an organ into anterior and posterior parts is a **coronal section** or **frontal section**. One that divides the structure into left and right parts is a **sagittal section**. If the body is divided directly down the middle, the section is known as a **midsagittal section**. A midsagittal section is reserved for dividing the body into equal left and right parts. If an organ (such as the eye) is sectioned into two equal parts such that there is a left and right half, then this is known as a **median section**.

There are three figures at the bottom of the page showing the sections of the brain. In each figure, the first illustration indicates how the sectioning plane passes through the brain. The second shows what the sectioning plane looks like removed from the organ. The third shows a rotated view of the sectioning plane, positioned so that it is facing you.

Color Guide: Label the illustration, and color in the appropriate planes. Use yellow for the coronal section, which is represented by the letter "a" in both the full-body illustration and the section of the brain. Use blue to color the transverse section represented by "b," and lightly color over the yellow to produce a green color where the two planes intersect. Use red to color the midsagittal section at "c." Use purple to color in the parts of the illustration that have not been sectioned.

Answer Key

a. Frontal (coronal) plane
b. Transverse (cross section) plane
c. Median (midsagittal) plane

LEARNING HINT

Corona means "crown." In Roman times, crowns were worn more vertically.

Sagittal refers to an arrow, as if an arrow struck the body from the front, dividing it into left and right planes.

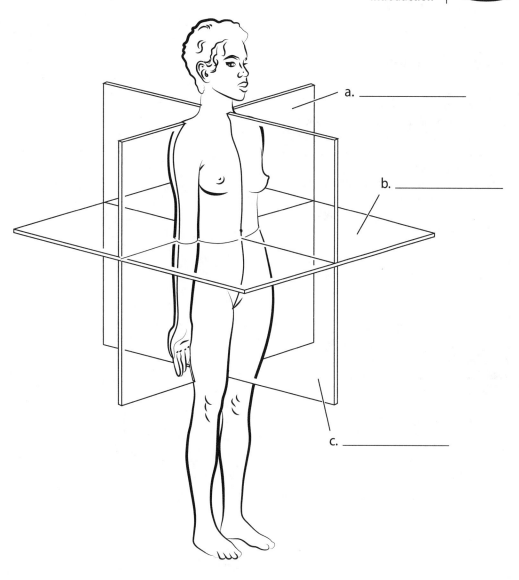

a. _____

b. _____

c. _____

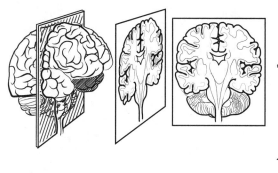

a. _____

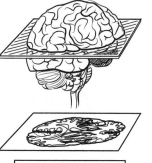

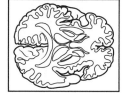

b. _____

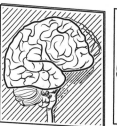

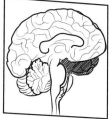

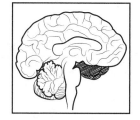

c. _____

HIERARCHY OF THE BODY

The human body can be studied at different levels. Organs such as the stomach can be grouped into organ systems (digestive system) or can be studied on a smaller scale like the cellular level. The ranking of these levels is called a **hierarchy**. The smallest organizational unit is the **atom**. Individual atoms are grouped into larger structures called **molecules**. These in turn make up **organelles**, which are part of larger, more complicated systems called **cells**. Cells are the structural and functional units of life. Cells are clustered into **tissues**, which are aggregations of cells that have a common function. **Organs** are discrete units made up of two or more tissues, and organs are grouped into **organ systems** that compose the **organism**.

Color Guide: Label the levels of the hierarchy, and color each item a different color. Use flesh tones for the skin in "a" and blue for the running suit. Color the lungs pink in both "b" and "c." In "d," the small structures in the cells are nuclei; color these purple. Use gray to color larger, stippled mucous cells, and color the rest of the illustration pink. Color "f" a medium gray. In "g," color the large center red, and use blue for the smaller spheres.

Answer Key

a. Organism (human)
b. Organ system (respiratory system)
c. Organ (lung)
d. Tissue (epithelium)
e. Cells
f. Organelle (cilia)
g. Molecule
h. Atom

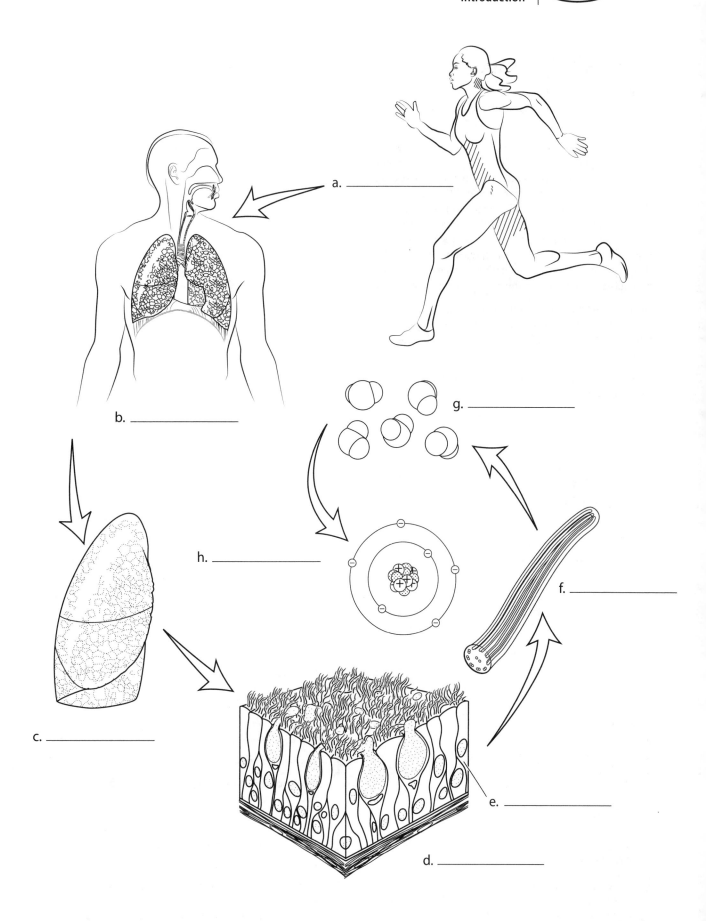

a. _____

b. _____

c. _____

d. _____

e. _____

f. _____

g. _____

h. _____

REGIONS OF THE ABDOMEN

Anatomists divide the abdomen into nine regions.
Write the names of the regions in the spaces indicated.

Color Guide: Color both the left and right **hypochondriac** regions in light blue. Inferior to the hypochondriac regions are the **lumbar** or **lateral abdominal** regions. These are commonly known as the "love handles." Use yellow for these regions. Below the lumbar regions are the **inguinal** or **iliac** regions. You should color these green. In the middle of the abdomen is the **umbilical** region. Color this region red. Above this is the **epigastric** region. Color this region purple. Below the umbilical region is the **hypogastric** region. Color this region a darker blue.

In clinical settings, a quadrant approach is used. Color the **right upper quadrant** red, the **right lower quadrant** blue, the **left upper quadrant** yellow, and the **left lower quadrant** brown.

Finish by coloring the bones pale yellow and the skin a shade of your choice.

Answer Key

a. Right hypochondriac
b. Right lumbar (lateral abdominal)
c. Umbilical
d. Right inguinal or iliac
e. Epigastric
f. Left hypochondriac
g. Left lumbar (lateral abdominal)
h. Left inguinal or iliac
i. Hypogastric
j. Left upper quadrant
k. Right upper quadrant
l. Left lower quadrant
m. Right lower quadrant

LEARNING HINT

Hypochondriac means "below the cartilage." The common use of the word (someone who frequently thinks they are sick) reflects the Greek origin of the word, as the ancient Greeks considered the region to be the center of sadness.

The prefix **epi-** refers to "above" and the root **gastric** means "stomach," while the prefix **hypo-** means "below."

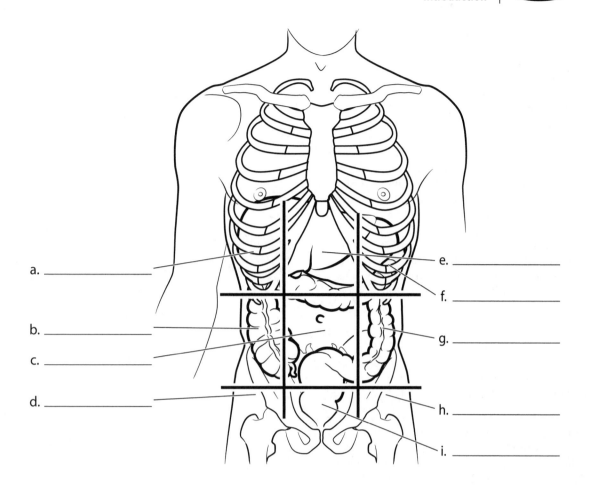

a. _____

b. _____

c. _____

d. _____

e. _____

f. _____

g. _____

h. _____

i. _____

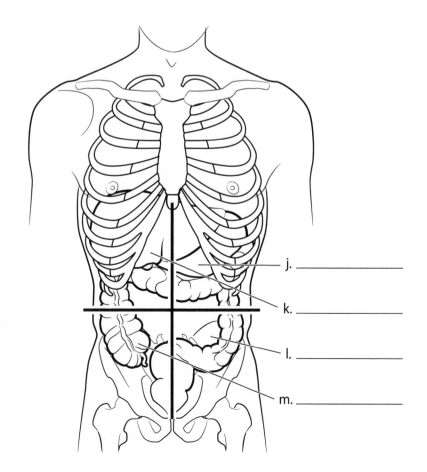

j. _____

k. _____

l. _____

m. _____

ORGAN SYSTEMS

The human body is either studied by regions or by organ systems. This book uses the organ system approach in which individual organs (such as bones) are grouped into the larger organ system (e.g., the skeletal system). Typically, 11 organ systems are described. The **skeletal system** consists of all of the bones of the body. Examples are the **femur** and the **humerus**. The **nervous system** consists of the **nerves**, **spinal cord**, and **brain** while the **lymphatic system** consists of **lymph glands**, conducting tubes called **lymphatics**, and organs such as the **spleen**. The term immune system is more of a functional classification and will not be treated as a separate system here. The **muscular system** consists of individual skeletal muscles such as the **pectoralis major** and **deltoid**. Label the organ systems underneath each illustration, and label the selected organs by using the terms available.

Organ System	Organ	Organ	Organ
Skeletal system	Femur	Humerus	
Nervous system	Nerves	Spinal cord	Brain
Lymphatic system	Lymph nodes	Spleen	
Muscular system	Pectoralis major	Deltoid	

Color Guide: In the top left figure, color the bones light gray, and shade in the rest of the body pink. At top right, color the brain yellow and the rest of the body pink. At bottom left, color the spleen brown and the rest of the body pink. (Most of the lymphatic system is very small, so do not color the lymph glands here.) At bottom right, color the muscles red. Leave the tendons and other connective tissue white (such as the areas near the knees and belly).

Answer Key

a. Humerus
b. Femur
c. Skeletal
d. Brain
e. Spinal cord
f. Nerves
g. Nervous
h. Spleen
i. Lymph nodes
j. Lymphatic
k. Deltoid
l. Pectoralis major
m. Muscular

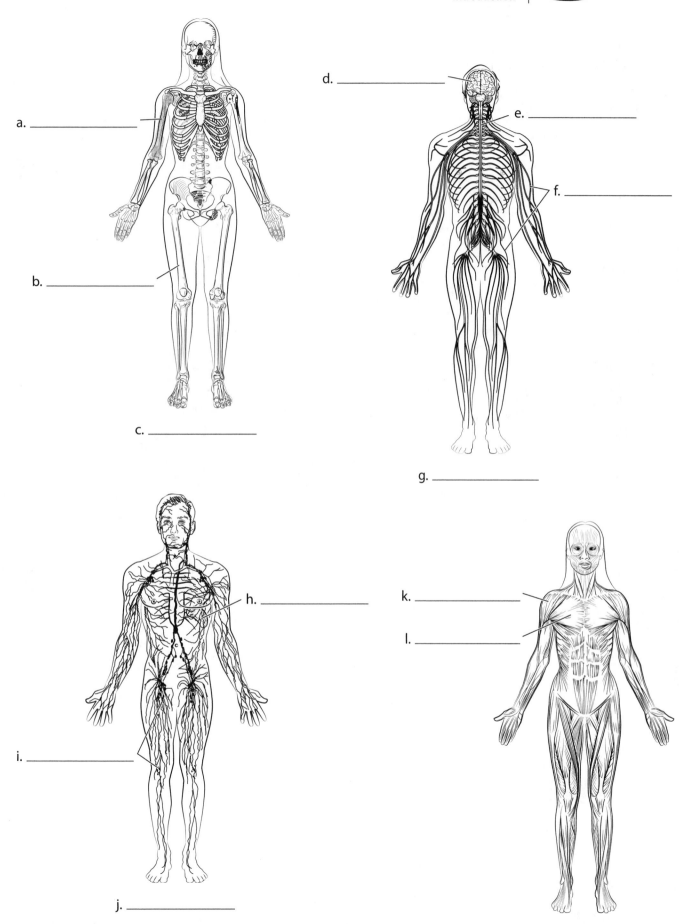

a. _____

b. _____

c. _____

d. _____

e. _____

f. _____

g. _____

h. _____

i. _____

j. _____

k. _____

l. _____

m. _____

ORGAN SYSTEMS *(continued)*

The **skin** and other structures are in the **integumentary system**, and the **digestive system** involves the breakdown and absorption of food with organs such as the **esophagus** and **stomach**. The **endocrine system** is made of the glands, such as the **thyroid gland** and the **adrenal glands**, that secrete hormones. The **respiratory system** involves the transfer of oxygen and carbon dioxide between the air and the blood. The respiratory system consists of organs such as the **trachea** and **lungs**. Label the organ systems underneath each illustration, and label the selected organs by using the terms available.

Organ System	Organ	Organ
Integumentary system	Skin	
Digestive system	Esophagus	Stomach
Endocrine system	Thyroid gland	Adrenal glands
Respiratory system	Trachea	Lungs

Color Guide: Select any color for the skin. Color the esophagus, stomach, and intestines pink, and use brown for the liver. Color the thyroid gland brown and the adrenal glands yellow. Use a different shade of pink for the trachea and lungs.

Answer Key

a. Skin
b. Integumentary
c. Esophagus
d. Stomach
e. Digestive
f. Thyroid gland
g. Adrenal gland
h. Endocrine
i. Trachea
j. Lung
k. Respiratory

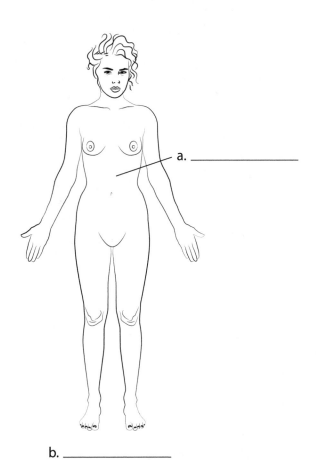

a. _____

b. _____

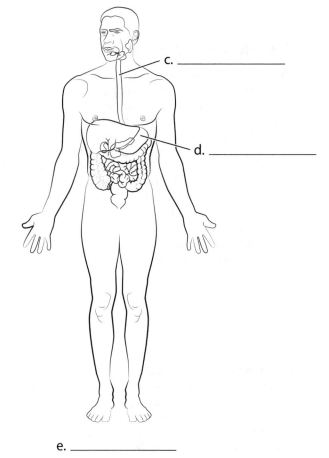

c. _____

d. _____

e. _____

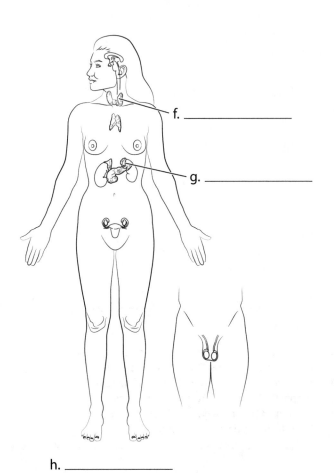

f. _____

g. _____

h. _____

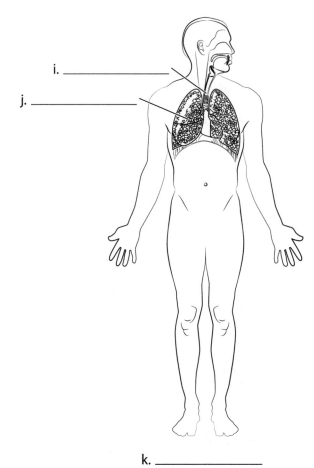

i. _____

j. _____

k. _____

ORGAN SYSTEMS *(continued)*

The **heart** and associated **blood vessels** compose the
cardiovascular system, which circulates blood throughout
the body. The **urinary system** filters, stores, and conducts
some wastes from the body. The **bladder** and **urethra** are
part of the **urinary system**. The **testes** and **ovaries** are part
of the **reproductive system**, which perpetuates the species.
The differentiation of male and female systems makes this
organ system unique among the other systems. The 11
organ systems can be remembered by the memory clue
"LN Cries Drum." Each letter represents the first letter
of a name of an organ system. Label the organ systems
underneath each illustration, and label the selected organs
by using the terms available.

Organ System	Organ	Organ
Cardiovascular system	Heart	Blood vessels
Urinary system	Bladder	Urethra
Reproductive system	Testes	Ovaries

Color Guide: Color the heart red, and use purple for the
rest of the blood vessels. Use dark brown for the kidneys
(the uppermost structures) and lighter brown for the
rest of the urinary system. Color the female reproductive
system pink and the male reproductive system brown.
Select any color for the skin tones.

Answer Key

a. Heart
b. Blood vessels
c. Cardiovascular
d. Bladder
e. Urethra
f. Urinary
g. Ovary
h. Testis
i. Reproductive

LEARNING HINT

The **11 organ systems** can be remembered by the
memory clue "LN Cries Drum," where each letter
represents the initial letter of an organ system:
Lymphatic, Nervous, Cardiovascular, Respiratory,
Integumentary, Endocrine, Skeletal, Digestive,
Reproductive, Urinary, and Muscular.

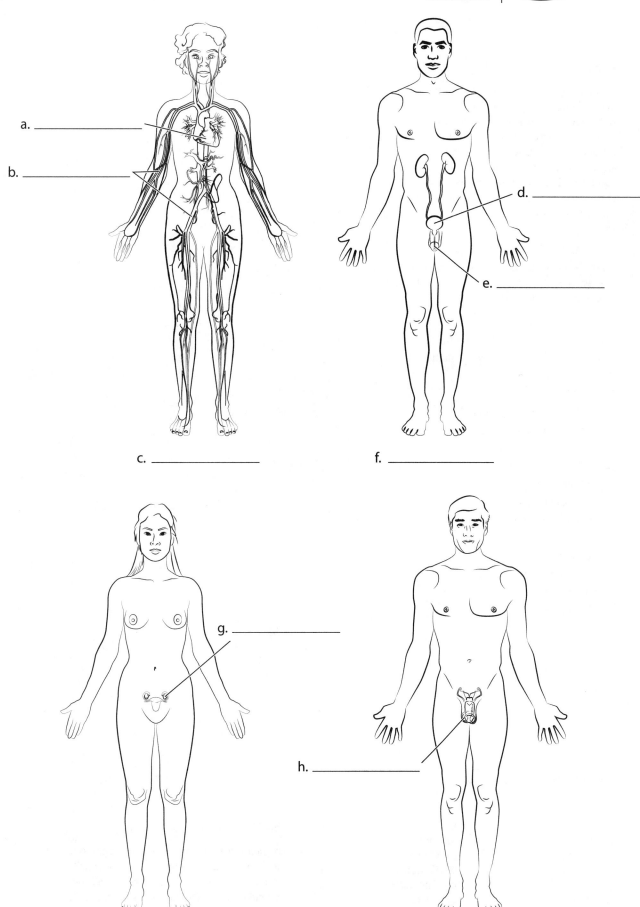

a. _____

b. _____

c. _____

d. _____

e. _____

f. _____

g. _____

h. _____

i. _____

BODY REGIONS (ANTERIOR)

There are specific anatomical terms for regions of the body. These areas or regions frequently have Greek or Latin names because early Western studies in anatomy occurred in Greece and Rome. During the Renaissance, European scholars studied anatomy and applied the ancient names to the structures. Label the various regions of the anterior side of body using the following alphabetical list of terms. The anatomical names are given first with the common names in parentheses. Check your work by using the key at the bottom of the page.

Color Guide: Color in the anterior regions of the body. Suggested colors are given below, but feel free to use whatever color you wish.

Abdominal (belly): blue

Antebrachial (forearm): light green

Antecubital (front of elbow): medium green

Brachial (arm): dark green

Cervical (neck): red

Coxal (hip, trochanteric): dark blue

Cranial (head): orange

Crural (leg): yellow

Deltoid (shoulder): yellow

Digital (fingers): purple

Femoral (thigh): brown

Genicular (knee): orange

Genital (sex organ): pink

Inguinal (groin): dark red

Palmar (palm): yellow green

Pectoral (chest): light blue

Pedal (foot): red

Sternal (center of chest): dark blue

Answer Key

a.	Cranial	j.	Coxal
b.	Cervical	k.	Palmar
c.	Deltoid	l.	Digital
d.	Sternal	m.	Inguinal
e.	Pectoral	n.	Genital
f.	Brachial	o.	Femoral
g.	Antecubital	p.	Genicular
h.	Abdominal	q.	Crural
i.	Antebrachial	r.	Pedal

LEARNING HINT

The prefix **ante-** means "before." **Deltoid** is named for a muscle that is triangular, like a river delta. **Femoral** is named after the femur bone, and **geniculate** means "to kneel" (as in *genuflect*).

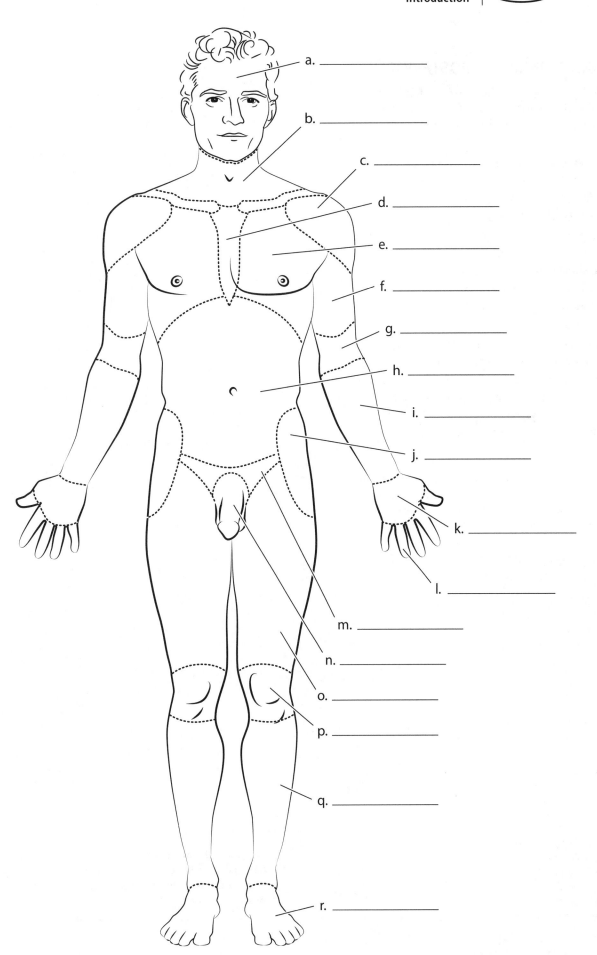

a. _____

b. _____

c. _____

d. _____

e. _____

f. _____

g. _____

h. _____

i. _____

j. _____

k. _____

l. _____

m. _____

n. _____

o. _____

p. _____

q. _____

r. _____

BODY REGIONS (POSTERIOR)

Label the regions of the posterior side of body using the following alphabetical list of terms. The anatomical names are given first with the common names in parentheses.

Color Guide: Color in the posterior regions of the body. Suggested colors are given below, but feel free to use whatever color you wish.

Antebrachial (forearm): light green
Brachial (arm): dark green
Calcaneal (heel): red
Cranial (head): orange
Cervical (neck): red
Femoral (thigh): brown
Gluteal (buttocks): blue
Lumbar (love handles): purple
Olecranon (elbow): medium green
Popliteal (back of knee): orange
Scapular (shoulder blade): pink
Sural (calf): yellow
Vertebral (backbone): yellow

Answer Key

a. Cranial
b. Cervical
c. Scapular
d. Brachial
e. Vertebral
f. Olecranon
g. Lumbar
h. Antebrachial
i. Gluteal
j. Femoral
k. Popliteal
l. Sural
m. Calcaneal

LEARNING HINT

In anatomy, the **brachium**, or arm, is the region from the shoulder to the elbow, and the **leg** is from the knee to the ankle. The term **calcaneal** refers to the calcaneus, or "heel bone."

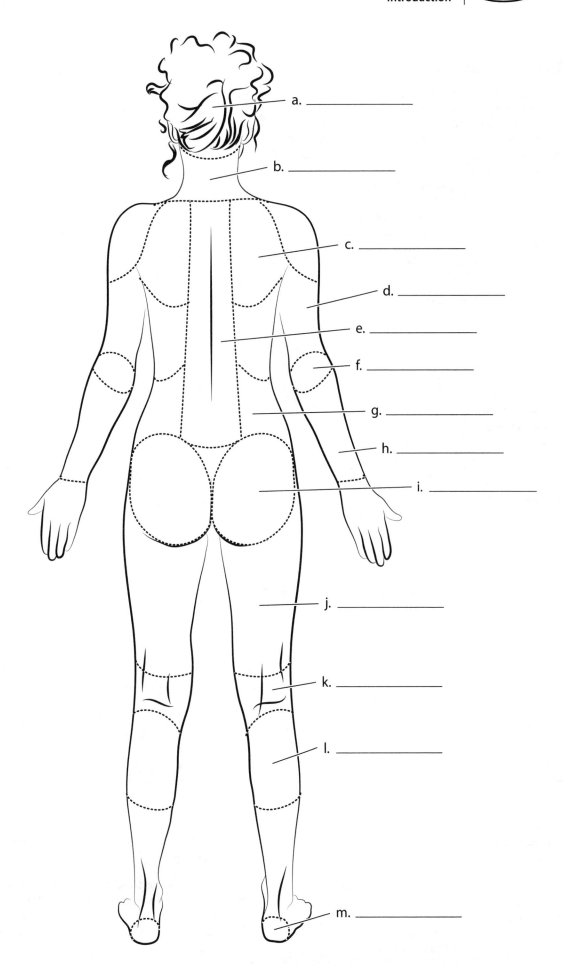

a. _____

b. _____

c. _____

d. _____

e. _____

f. _____

g. _____

h. _____

i. _____

j. _____

k. _____

l. _____

m. _____

BODY CAVITIES

The organs of the body are frequently found in body cavities. The **cranial cavity** houses the brain, and the **spinal canal** surrounds the spinal cord. The upper **thoracic cavity** is subdivided into the **pleural cavities**, housing the lungs, and the **mediastinum**. The mediastinum contains the heart in the **pericardial cavity** as well as the major vessels near the heart, nerves, and esophagus. Below the thoracic cavity is the **abdominopelvic cavity**, which contains the upper **abdominal cavity**, housing the digestive organs, and the inferior **pelvic cavity**, which holds the uterus and rectum in females or just the rectum in males. Label the specific cavities of the body using the list below.

Color Guide: There is no standard color scheme for the body cavities, so use either the suggested colors or any that you choose.

Cranial cavity: purple
Spinal canal: red
Thoracic cavity: blue
Pleural cavities: pink
Mediastinum: yellow
Pericardial cavity: orange
Abdominopelvic cavity: yellow
Abdominal cavity: dark brown
Pelvic cavity: light brown

Answer Key

a. Cranial cavity
b. Spinal canal
c. Thoracic cavity
d. Mediastinum
e. Pericardial cavity
f. Pleural cavity
g. Abdominopelvic cavity
h. Abdominal cavity
i. Pelvic cavity

LEARNING HINT

The **thorax** is the chest, and **pleura** is another word for the lungs. Pleurisy is an inflammation of the lungs.

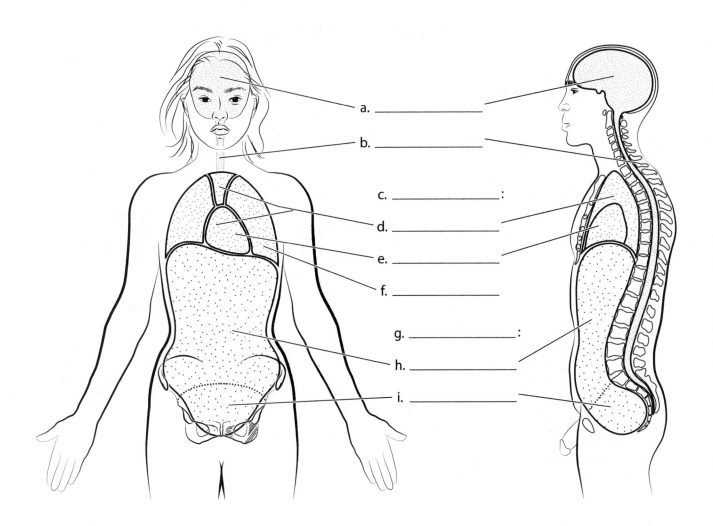

a. _____

b. _____

c. _____ :

d. _____

e. _____

f. _____

g. _____ :

h. _____

i. _____

Chapter Two: **Cells, Tissues, and Integument**

OVERVIEW OF CELL AND PLASMA MEMBRANE

Cells consist of an enclosing **plasma membrane**, an inner **cytoplasm** with numerous **organelles**, and other cellular structures. The fluid portion of the cell is called the **cytosol**. One of the major structures in the cell is the **nucleus**. It is the genetic center of the cell and consists of fluid **karyoplasm**, **chromatin** (containing DNA), and the **nucleolus**.

The **cytoskeleton** consists of microtubules, intermediate filaments, and microfilaments. It is involved in maintaining cell shape, fixing organelles, and directing some cellular activity.

Label the organelles of the cell. The **mitochondria** are the energy-producing structures of the cell while the **Golgi apparatus** assembles complex biomolecules and transports them out of the cell. Proteins are made in the cell by ribosomes. If the ribosomes are found by themselves in the cytoplasm, they are called **free ribosomes**. If they are attached to the **rough endoplasmic reticulum**, they are called **bound ribosomes**. The **smooth endoplasmic reticulum** manufactures lipids and helps in breaking down toxic materials in the cell. Other structures in the cell are **vesicles** (sacs that hold liquids). **Phagocytic vesicles** ingest material into the cell. **Lysosomes** contain digestive enzymes while **peroxisomes** degrade toxic hydrogen peroxide in the cell. **Centrioles** are microtubules grouped together and are involved in cell division.

Color Guide: In the upper illustration, color the nucleus purple and the nucleolus dark blue. Choose different dark colors for the rest of the organelles. Use a light color, such as light blue or yellow, for the cytosol. Use another light color to shade in the outer surface of the plasma membrane seen at the bottom of the cell.

The **plasma membrane** is composed of a **phospholipid bilayer** consisting of **phosphate molecules** on the outside and inside of the membrane and a **lipid layer** in between. **Cholesterol molecules** occur in the membrane and, depending on their concentration, can make the membrane stiff or more fluid. Proteins that are found on the outside of the membrane are called **peripheral proteins** while proteins that pass through the membrane are called **integral proteins**. Frequently, these make up gates or channels that allow material to pass through the membrane. Attached to proteins on the cell membrane are **carbohydrate chains**. These provide cellular identity. Label and color the cell membrane structures.

Color Guide: In the lower illustration, color the phosphate molecules on the outside and inside of the membrane one color and the lipid layer a contrasting color. Use a light color for the integral proteins and a darker color for the peripheral proteins. Use dark colors for the carbohydrate chains.

Answer Key

a. Golgi apparatus
b. Lysosome
c. Peroxisome
d. Phagocytic vesicle
e. Nucleus
f. Nucleolus
g. Chromatin
h. Karyoplasm
i. Cytoskeleton
j. Centrioles
k. Plasma membrane
l. Cytoplasm
m. Rough endoplasmic reticulum
n. Smooth endoplasmic reticulum
o. Mitochondrion
p. Free ribosomes
q. Phospholipid bilayer
r. Integral protein
s. Carbohydrate chain
t. Peripheral protein
u. Phosphate molecule
v. Lipid layer
w. Cholesterol molecule

LEARNING HINT

Karyoplasm is named for the Greek *karyon*, meaning "kernel" or "nut." Microscopically, the nucleus of a cell looks like the kernel in a fruit.

The term **endoplasmic reticulum** literally means "the little net inside the goo."

a. _____

b. _____

c. _____

d. _____

e. _____

f. _____

g. _____

h. _____

i. _____

j. _____

k. _____

l. _____

m. _____

n. _____

o. _____

p. _____

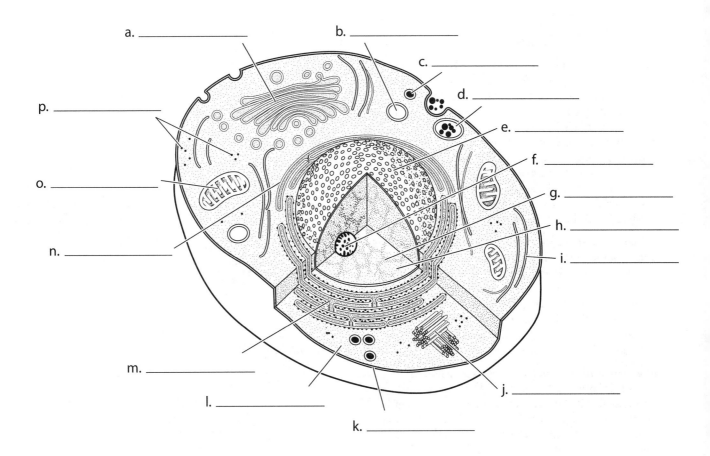

q. _____

r. _____

s. _____

t. _____

u. _____

v. _____

w. _____

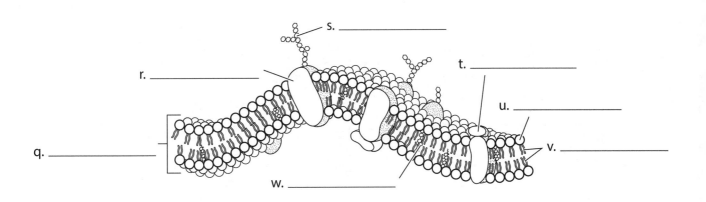

SIMPLE EPITHELIA

As noted earlier in the Hierarchy of the Body section, tissues are collections of cells that have a common function. There are four types of tissues in humans, and these make up all of the organs and binding material in the body. **Epithelial tissue** makes up the linings of the body. In many cases, where there is exposure (outside, such as the skin, or inside, such as in blood vessels), epithelium is the tissue found. It is named according to its layers and the shape of cells (such as cuboidal). Simple epithelium is made of one layer of cells, while stratified epithelium is made up of many layers of cells.

Simple squamous epithelium is a single layer of flattened cells. **Simple cuboidal epithelium** is also a single layer of cells, but the cells are in the shape of cubes. **Simple columnar epithelium** is a single layer of long columnar cells. The **basement membrane** is the noncellular layer that attaches the epithelium to lower layers. Label the nuclei, basement membrane, cell membrane, and cilia in this tissue.

Pseudostratified ciliated columnar epithelium is in a single layer of cells, but it looks stratified on first appearance. All of the cells are attached to the basement membrane. However, not all of the cells reach the surface of the tissue. Label the **nuclei**, **basement membrane**, **cell membrane**, and **cilia** in this tissue.

Color Guide: Color the basement membrane red. Color the nuclei purple, the cytoplasm blue, and the cilia pink.

Answer Key

a. Simple squamous epithelium
b. Simple cuboidal epithelium
c. Simple columnar epithelium
d. Cilia
e. Cell membrane
f. Nuclei
g. Basement membrane
h. Pseudostratified ciliated columnar epithelium

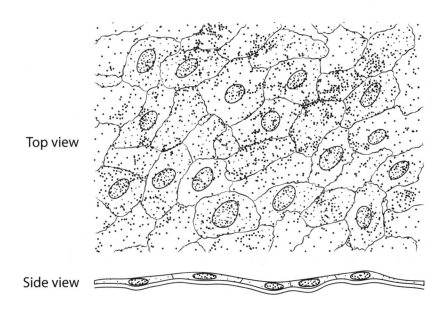

Top view

Side view

a. _____

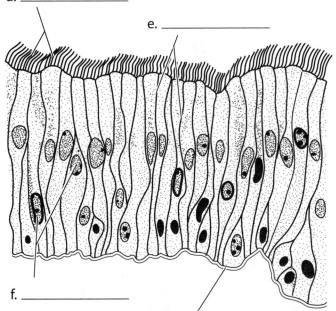

b. _____

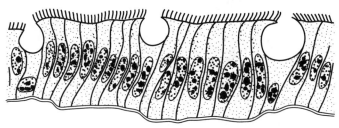

c. _____

d. _____

e. _____

f. _____

g. _____

h. _____

STRATIFIED EPITHELIA

There are two common epithelial tissues that are many-layered. **Stratified squamous epithelium** is many layers of flattened cells. There are two major subtypes of stratified squamous epithelium. **Keratinized epithelium** is found on the skin and is toughened by the protein keratin. **Nonkeratinized stratified squamous epithelium** is found in the oral cavity and vagina and is a mucous membrane.

The other main type of layered epithelial tissue is **transitional epithelium**. This is tissue that lines part of the urinary tract including the bladder. When the bladder is empty, the cells bunch up on one another and the tissue is thick. When the bladder is full, the cells stretch out into a few layers. Label the cell types for each picture.

Color Guide: Color the basement membrane red, the cytoplasm blue, and the nuclei purple.

LEARNING HINT

The word **keratin** is derived from *keratos*, which is Greek for "horn," as in the horns of an animal. Keratin is the protein that gives toughness to the skin, nails, and hair, as well as some animal horns. Keratin prevents the secretion of mucus, so some locations of the body, such as the mouth and vagina, lack this hard protein even though the epithelium is multilayered.

Answer Key
a. Stratified squamous epithelium
b. Transitional epithelium

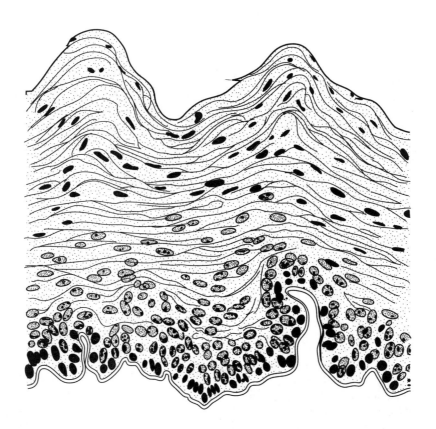

a. _____

Stretched

Relaxed

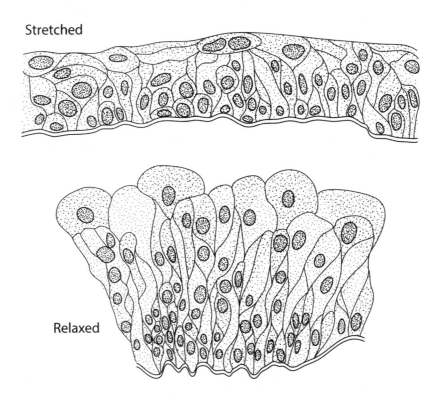

b. _____

GLANDS

Glands develop embryologically from epithelial tissue, which is why they are covered in this section. There are several types of glands in the human body. Some of these glands secrete their products into tubes or ducts. These are known as **exocrine** glands. Other glands secrete their products into the spaces between cells where they are picked up by the blood or lymph system. These are the **endocrine** glands. Endocrine glands secrete hormones that have an impact on target tissues of the body.

Glands can be unicellular or multicellular. Glands that consist of just one cell are called **goblet cells**. They secrete mucus, which is a lubricant. There are many types of multicellular glands. They are classified by how they secrete their products. Some glands secrete products from **vesicles** pinched off from the cell. These are called **merocrine** glands. In these glands, no cellular material is lost in the secretion of material. An example of a merocrine gland is a sweat gland. Some cells squeeze parts of the cell off to secrete cellular products. These are known as **apocrine** glands. The lactiferous glands that produce milk are apocrine glands. Some secretions occur by the entire cell rupturing. These are called **holocrine** glands. Oil glands of the skin are holocrine glands. Label the glands in the figures.

Color Guide: Color the nuclei purple and the cytoplasm light blue. Use yellow for the goblet cell.

Answer Key
a. Exocrine gland
b. Endocrine gland
c. Goblet cell
d. Merocrine glands
e. Vesicles
f. Apocrine glands
g. Holocrine glands

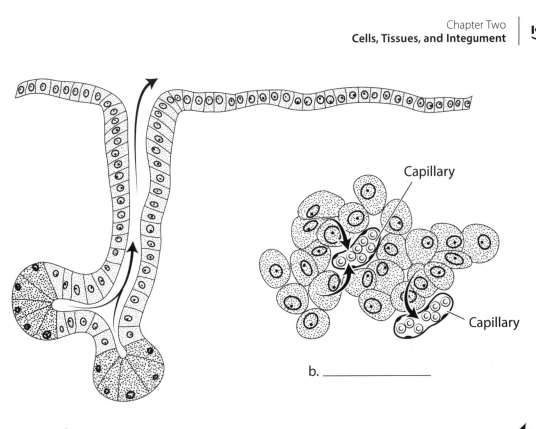

a. _____

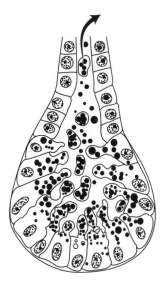

Capillary

Capillary

b. _____

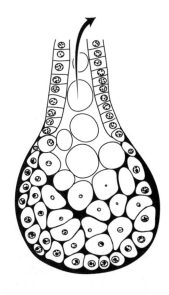

c. _____

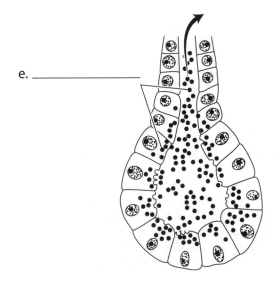

e. _____

d. _____

f. _____

g. _____

CONNECTIVE TISSUE

Another of the four tissues of the human body is connective tissue. **Connective tissue** is a varied group of associated tissues, all of which are derived from an embryonic tissue known as **mesenchyme**. Connective tissue not only has cells, as do all of the other tissues, but it also has **fibers** and a large amount of background substance called **matrix**. There are many specific tissues that belong to connective tissue. **Loose connective tissue** is found wrapping around organs or under the epidermis and is composed of **collagenous fibers**, **elastic fibers**, and **reticular fibers**; a liquid matrix; and numerous cells, many of which have an immune function. **Dense regular connective tissue** has a few cells called **fibrocytes** and a small amount of matrix with most of the tissue composed of a regular arrangement of **collagenous fibers**. This specific tissue makes up tendons and ligaments. If the fibers are not in an orderly arrangement, then the tissue is called **dense irregular connective tissue**. This tissue is found in places like the white of the eye.

An analogy for connective tissue from the construction industry is reinforced concrete. In this example, the cement is the matrix, the steel rebar pieces are the fibers, and the rocks in the concrete are the cells. What makes connective tissue variable is the nature of the matrix and the fibers. Matrix can be pliable to produce rubbery tissue (e.g., cartilage at the end of the nose), fluid (blood), or hard (bone). Likewise, the fibers of connective tissue vary; they can be tough, like those found in tendons or bone, or elastic, such as those in the external ear. Label the connective tissues in the figures.

Color Guide: Use pink for the collagenous fibers. Color the nucleus purple, and leave the elastic fibers black.

Answer Key

a. Matrix
b. Fibrocyte
c. Collagenous fiber
d. Elastic fiber
e. Loose connective tissue
f. Dense regular connective tissue
g. Dense irregular connective tissue

LEARNING HINT

Collagenous fibers come from the Greek *kolla*, meaning "glue." Animal glues are obtained by processing collagenous fibers. To remember collagen, think of the word *collage*, which is paper glued down into a design. **Reticular fibers** are named for the Latin word *rete*, meaning "net." These fibers form a net or meshwork that commonly occurs as an internal framework for soft organs like the spleen.

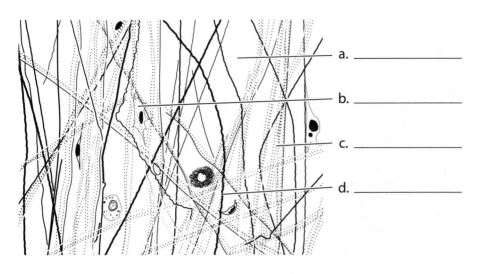

a. _____

b. _____

c. _____

d. _____

e. _____

c. _____

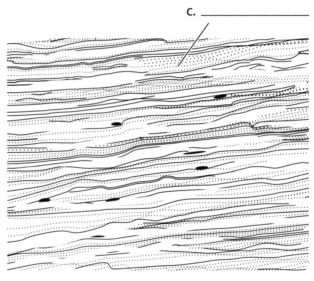

f. _____

c. _____

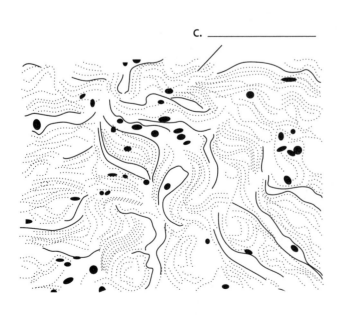

g. _____

CONNECTIVE TISSUE *(continued)*

Elastic connective tissue contains **elastic fibers** and is found in areas that recoil when stretched such as in the walls of arteries. **Reticular connective tissue** consists of **reticular fibers** that form an internal support in soft organs such as the liver and spleen. **Adipose tissue** consists of specialized fat-storing cells called **adipocytes**. Adipose tissue is a little different from the other connective tissues in that it consists mostly of cells, with very few fibers and little matrix. In other connective tissues, the fibers and matrix usually make up most of the tissue. Label the components of these connective tissues.

Color Guide: Use pink for the collagenous fibers, and leave the elastic fibers black.

Answer Key

a. Collagenous fibers
b. Elastic fibers
c. Elastic connective tissue
d. Reticular fibers
e. Reticular connective tissue
f. Adipocyte
g. Adipose tissue

a. _____   b. _____

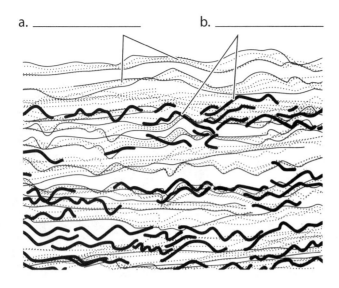

c. _____

d. _____

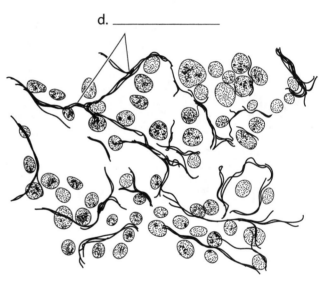

e. _____

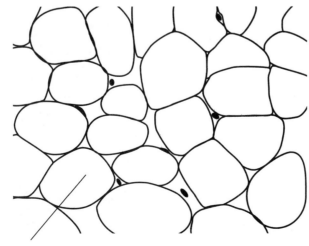

f. _____

g. _____

CONNECTIVE TISSUE *(continued)*

Cartilage

Cartilage is another form of connective tissue. The most common kind of cartilage is **hyaline cartilage**. It contains a semisolid **matrix**, **collagenous fibers**, and **chondrocytes** (cartilage cells). The end of the nose is pliable due to hyaline cartilage. **Fibrocartilage** is similar to hyaline cartilage, having the same components, but there are more collagenous fibers in fibrocartilage. It is found in areas where there is more stress, such as the joint between the bones of the thigh and leg. **Elastic cartilage** has a matrix, chondrocytes, and **elastic fibers**. These fibers make the cartilage more bendable than hyaline cartilage. Label the cells and fibers of cartilage.

Color Guide: Color the cell nuclei dark purple, the cytoplasm light purple, and the fibers of cartilage red or dark pink. Use pale pink to shade the matrix.

Answer Key

a. Matrix
b. Chondrocytes
c. Hyaline cartilage
d. Collagenous fibers
e. Fibrocartilage
f. Elastic fibers
g. Elastic cartilage

a. _____   b. _____

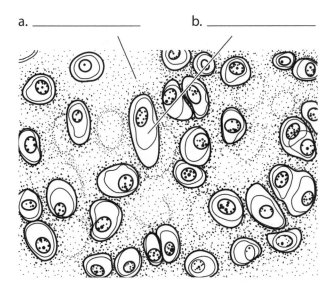

c. _____

b. _____   d. _____

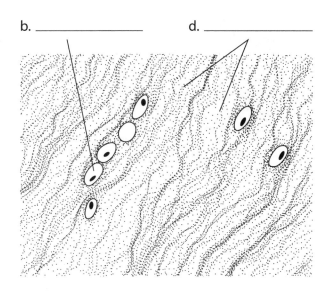

e. _____

a. _____   b. _____

f. _____

g. _____

CONNECTIVE TISSUE *(continued)*

Bone and Blood

Bone cells are **osteocytes**, and the fibers are collagenous fibers enclosed in a hard matrix of bone salts. You will not see the fibers in the illustration because they are covered by the dense matrix. Label the osteocytes and matrix of bone.

Blood is another kind of connective tissue. The matrix in blood is the **plasma**, and the cells are **erythrocytes** (red blood cells) and **leukocytes** (white blood cells). **Platelets** are small fragments in the blood that aid in clotting.

Color Guide: Color the matrix of bone yellow. Color the erythrocytes red, and use pale blue for the cytoplasm of the leukocytes. Shade the plasma around the red blood cells a pale yellow.

Answer Key

a. Matrix
b. Osteocyte
c. Bone
d. Erythrocyte
e. Platelet
f. Leukocytes
g. Plasma
h. Blood

a. _____

b. _____

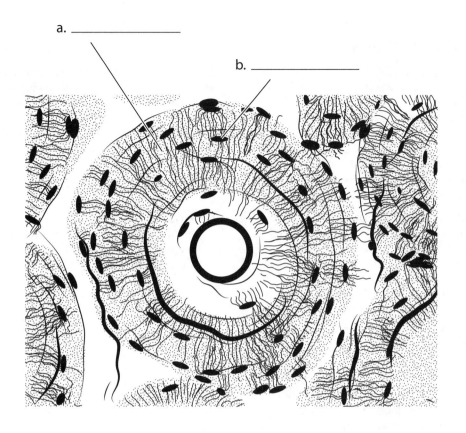

c. _____

d. _____   e. _____

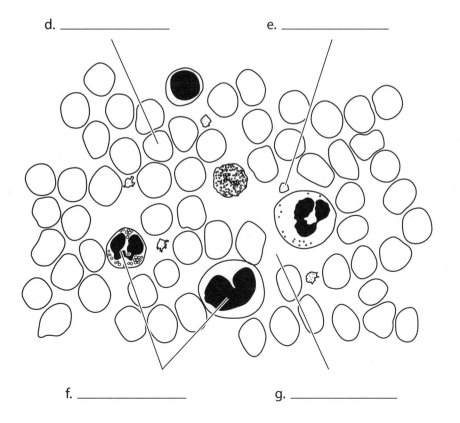

f. _____   g. _____

h. _____

MUSCLE AND NERVOUS TISSUE

Muscular tissue is composed of specialized cells involved in contraction. **Skeletal muscle** makes up body muscles and represents around 40 percent of the body mass. Skeletal muscle is striated, and the fusion of individual cells produces longer mature cells that are multinucleate. These nuclei are found on the edges of the cells. Skeletal muscle can be consciously controlled and is called **voluntary muscle**. Label the **striations** of the skeletal muscle cells, the **nuclei**, and individual **cells**.

Cardiac muscle is also **striated**, but the striations are not as obvious as in skeletal muscle. This muscle is found in the heart and is involuntary. It does not involve conscious control. Cardiac muscle typically has only one centrally located nucleus per cell, and the cells themselves are branched. They attach to other cells by **intercalated discs**, which allow communication between cells for the conduction of impulses during the cardiac cycle. Label these features on the illustration.

Smooth muscle is not striated and is involuntary. The cells are slender and have one nucleus located in the center of the cell. It is widely distributed in the body, making up, among other things, part of the digestive system, reproductive system, and integumentary system. Smooth muscle is found in glands and other areas not under conscious control. Label the nucleus and cell of smooth muscle.

Nervous tissue consists of the **neuron** and associated **glial cells**. Neurons have numerous branched extensions called **dendrites**, a central **nerve cell body** (**soma**) that houses the nucleus, and a long extension called an **axon**. The glial cells, also known as **neuroglia**, have many functions. Some of these are supportive of the neuron, and some may involve processing of neural information. Label the parts of the neuron and the glial cells.

Color Guide: Color the muscle cells dark red and the muscle fibers light red. Use dark purple for the nucleus of the nerve cell body, lighter purple for the cytoplasm, and light blue for the background.

Answer Key

a. Striations
b. Nuclei
c. Cell
d. Skeletal muscle
e. Intercalated disc
f. Cardiac muscle
g. Smooth muscle
h. Nerve cell body
i. Glial cells (neuroglia)
j. Dendrites
k. Axon
l. Nervous tissue

a. _____   b. _____

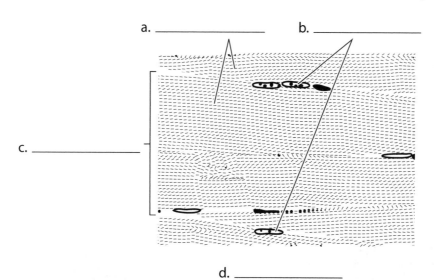

c. _____

d. _____

b. _____   e. _____

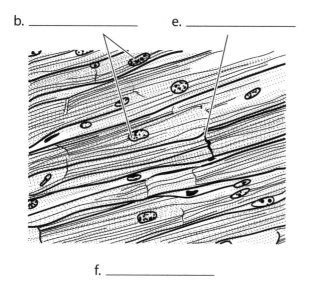

f. _____

b. _____   c. _____

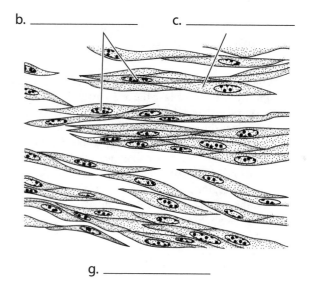

g. _____

h. _____   i. _____

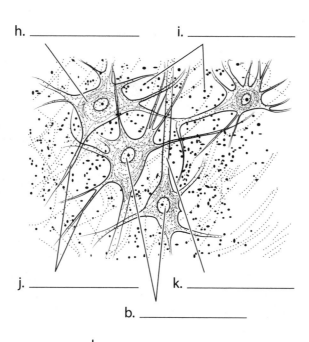

j. _____   k. _____

b. _____

l. _____

INTEGUMENTARY SYSTEM

The most superficial layer of the skin is the epidermis, which consists of five layers as shown in the upper illustration. The deepest layer is the **stratum basale**, and there are specific cells called **melanocytes** that secrete the brown pigment **melanin**. Locate the **stratum spinosum**. The **stratum granulosum** is superficial to the stratum spinosum. The **stratum lucidum** (found only in thick skin) is a thin layer. The most superficial (or topmost) layer is the **stratum corneum**.

In the lower illustration, the **epidermis** is a thin layer. The **dermis** consists of two layers, an upper **papillary layer** and a deeper **reticular layer**. **Sweat glands** are also found in the dermis. The **hypodermis** is not a part of the integument; it contains a significant amount of fat. Two types of touch receptors can easily be seen in microscopic sections. These are the **Meissner corpuscles** and the **Pacinian corpuscles** (lamellar corpuscles).

Color Guide: Color the five layers of the epidermis in the upper illustration. Make the majority of the stratum basale pink, the melanocytes brown, and the stratum spinosum light blue. The stratum granulosum has purple granules in it, so color that layer using purple dots. Use light yellow for the stratum lucidum and orange for the stratum corneum. In the lower illustration, color the epidermis red-orange, the papillary layer of the dermis light pink, and the reticular layer a darker pink. Use purple for the sweat glands. Shade the hypodermis yellow to represent the fat found there, and color the Pacinian corpuscle light pink. Leave the Meissner corpuscle uncolored.

Answer Key

a. Stratum corneum
b. Stratum lucidum
c. Stratum granulosum
d. Stratum spinosum
e. Stratum basale
f. Melanocyte
g. Epidermis
h. Papillary layer
i. Reticular layer
j. Dermis
k. Hypodermis
l. Sweat gland
m. Pacinian corpuscle
n. Meissner corpuscle

LEARNING HINT

The word **stratum** comes from Latin and means "layer," as in *stratus clouds*, the type of clouds that form a flat sheet.

The root *derma* comes from the Greek word meaning "leather." To produce leather goods, such as a purse or belt, leather makers remove both the **epidermis** (*epi* = "on top") from the surface of the **dermis** and the **hypodermis** (*hypo* = "below"), which is the layer beneath the dermis.

The name of the **papillary layer** of the dermis comes from the Latin word *papilla*, which means a "nipple" or "bump."

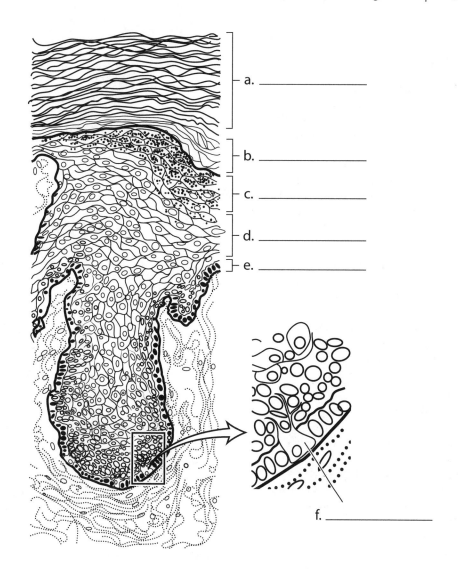

a. _____

b. _____

c. _____

d. _____

e. _____

f. _____

Epidermis magnified

l. _____

n. _____

g. _____

h. _____

i. _____

j. _____

k. _____

m. _____

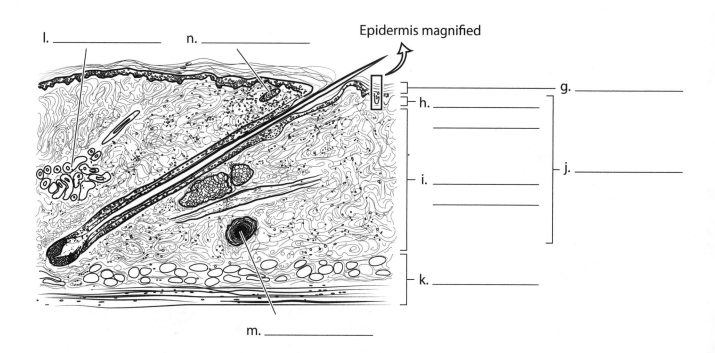

HAIR AND NAILS

Hair originates from the **dermal papilla**, which contains capillaries and nerves and is part of the **hair bulb**. Superficial to the hair bulb is the **hair root**, which is the part of the hair that is in the skin. The hair is enclosed by the **hair follicle**. Associated with the hair is the **arrector pili**, a bundle of smooth muscle that causes the hair to "stand on end" and also causes secretion of the **sebaceous glands** in an association known as the pilosebaceous unit. Once the hair erupts from the skin, it is known as the **hair shaft**, which consists of layers of dead keratinized cells.

Fingernails and toenails are considered accessory structures of the integument. Label the diagram noting the **nail proper**, the **free edge** (the part that you cut with clippers), the **nail fold** (**paronychium**), and the **nail groove**. At the base of the nail is the **lunule**, the **eponychium** (cuticle), and the **nail root**. Note also the **hyponychium**, the **germinal matrix**, and the **nail bed**, which contributes cells that make up the nail proper.

Color Guide: In the upper illustration, use red for the arrector pili muscle, medium purple for the hair follicle, and your choice of color for the hair root and shaft. Color the sebaceous gland pale gray and the matrix dark purple. Save the dermis for last, and color it pink. In the lower illustration, use yellow for the bones, pale gray for the nail plate, and purple for the hyponychium and germinal matrix. Select colors of your choice for the other structures.

Answer Key

a. Bulb
b. Hair follicle
c. Hair root
d. Hair shaft
e. Sebaceous gland
f. Arrector pili muscle
g. Papilla
h. Matrix
i. Nail plate
j. Nail fold (paronychium)
k. Lunule
l. Eponychium
m. Nail root
n. Germinal matrix
o. Nail bed
p. Hyponychium
q. Free edge

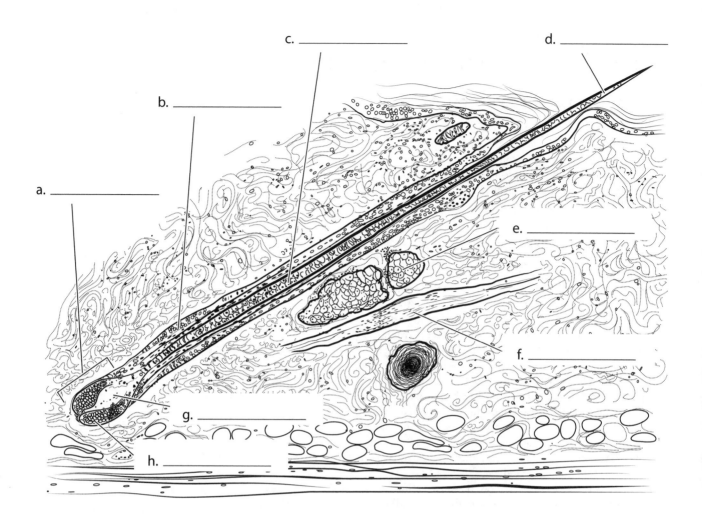

c. _____

d. _____

b. _____

a. _____

e. _____

f. _____

g. _____

h. _____

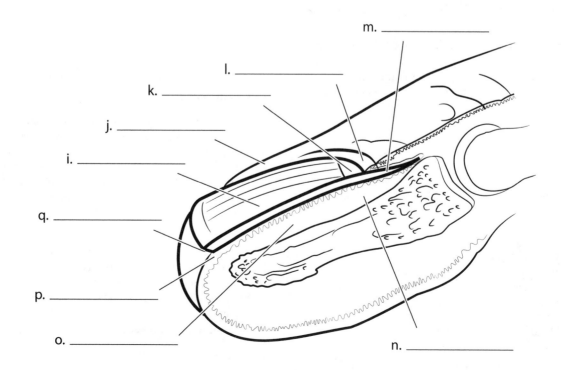

m. _____

l. _____

k. _____

j. _____

i. _____

q. _____

p. _____

o. _____

n. _____

Chapter Three: **Skeletal System**

OVERVIEW OF THE SKELETAL SYSTEM

The skeletal system consists of two main groups of bones: those of the axial skeleton and those of the appendicular skeleton. The axial skeleton consists of the skull and vertebral column, and the appendicular skeleton consists of the bones of the pectoral girdle, the upper limb bones, the pelvic girdle or hip bones, and the lower limb bones.

FRONTAL ASPECT OF THE SKULL

The skull is a complex structure. There are 8 cranial bones and 14 facial bones in the skull. From the anterior view, most of the facial bones can be seen, and some of the cranial bones are visible, too. The bone that makes up the forehead and extends beyond the eyebrows is the **frontal bone**. This bone forms the upper rim of the **orbit**, which is a socket that encloses the eye. In the back of the orbit is the **sphenoid bone**, and the lateral walls of the orbit are composed of the **zygomatic bones**. The bridge of the nose consists of the paired **nasal bones**, and just lateral to them are the two **maxillae**. These bones hold the upper teeth. The lower teeth are held by the **mandible**. Inside the nasal cavity, two projections can be seen. These are the **inferior nasal conchae**. The wall that divides the nasal cavity is the **nasal septum**, and it consists of two bones, the **ethmoid bone** and the **vomer**. Along the side of the skull are the **temporal bones**, located posterior to the zygomatic bones; these bones will be illustrated and described in the next few pages. Inside the skull are the small ear ossicles; these will be covered along with the ear, in the chapter on sense organs. Label the major bones of the skull.

Color Guide: Use darker colors for the bones inside the eye sockets. As you color in the skull, use the same color for the same bone on different pages. This will help you associate each bone with a color in the various views.

Answer Key
a. Orbit
b. Frontal bone
c. Temporal bone
d. Sphenoid bone
e. Nasal bone
f. Zygomatic bone
g. Nasal septum
h. Maxilla
i. Mandible

LEARNING HINT

Use this mnemonic to remember the **14 facial bones**: "In New Zealand, very many people love mandarins." Each word in the sentence represents the first letter of a facial bone: Inferior nasal conchae, Nasal, Zygomatic, Vomer, Maxilla, Palatine, Lacrimal, Mandible. (All of these except the mandible and vomer are pairs of bones.)

For the **8 cranial bones**, this memory device may be useful: "Time passes on for everyone somehow." The first letter of each word represents a cranial bone: Temporal, Parietal, Occipital, Frontal, Ethmoid, Sphenoid. (Both temporal and parietal are pairs of bones.)

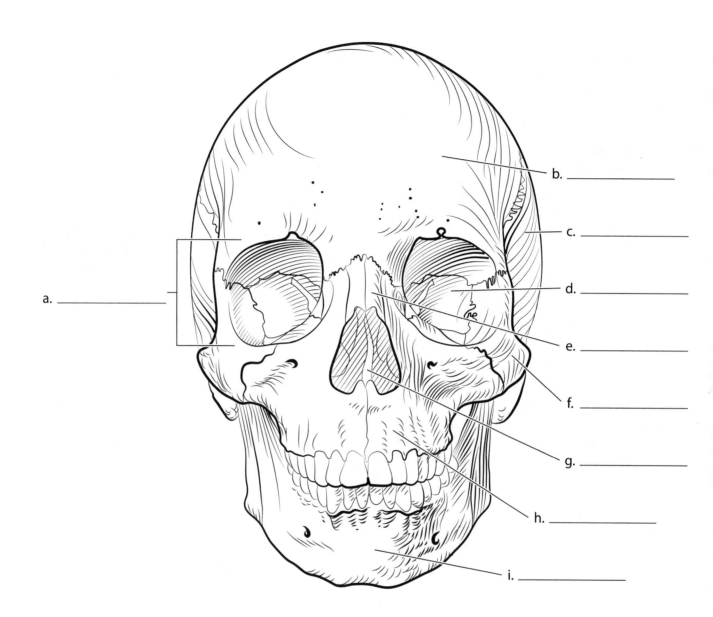

a. _____

b. _____

c. _____

d. _____

e. _____

f. _____

g. _____

h. _____

i. _____

LATERAL VIEW OF THE SKULL

Many bones seen from the anterior view can also be seen from the lateral view. The **frontal bone** is joined to the **parietal bones** by the **coronal suture**. The parietal bones span much of the cranium and articulate with the **occipital bone** at the **lambdoid suture**. There is a posterior extension of the **occipital bone** known as the **external occipital protuberance**. The exterior aspect of the **temporal bone** is seen from the lateral view, and many of the significant features such as the **mastoid process**, **external acoustic meatus**, and **styloid process** are visible. On the side is the elongated **zygomatic arch**. The zygomatic arch consists of part of the **zygomatic bone** and the zygomatic process of the temporal bone. The temporal bone articulates with other cranial bones by the **squamous suture**. The bone anterior to the temporal bone is the **sphenoid bone**. It is a bone that is found in the middle of the skull. The **nasal bone** is visible from the lateral view, and its relationship with the **maxilla** can be seen here. Behind the maxilla is the **lacrimal bone**, which houses the nasolacrimal canaliculus, a duct that drains tears from the eye into the nose. The **mandible** articulates with the rest of the skull at the **mandibular condyle**. A depression anterior to the condyle is the **mandibular notch**, and the section of bone anterior to the mandibular notch is the **coronoid process**. Label the major features of the skull seen in lateral view.

Details of the mandible can be seen in the isolated bone. In addition to the features of the mandible just listed, find the **mandibular foramen** and the **mental foramen** of the mandible. These are holes for the passage of nerves and blood vessels. The main portion of the mandible is the **body**, and the upright part is the **ramus**. The **angle** is the posterior junction of these two parts. The teeth are located in alveoli, and the small segments of bone between the teeth are the alveolar processes. Label the features of the mandible.

Color Guide: Use the same colors for the bones as you did in the previous illustration, and color the shaded areas thoroughly to produce a deep tone. In the lower figure, use darker colors to shade in "s," "v," and "x" to distinguish these specific parts of the mandible.

Answer Key

a. Coronal suture
b. Parietal bones
c. Zygomatic arch
d. Temporal bone
e. Squamous suture
f. Lambdoid suture
g. External occipital protuberance
h. Occipital bone
i. Mastoid process
j. External acoustic meatus
k. Styloid process
l. Mandible
m. Maxilla

n. Zygomatic bone
o. Nasal bone
p. Lacrimal bone
q. Sphenoid bone
r. Frontal bone
s. Coronoid process
t. Mandibular foramen
u. Mandibular notch
v. Mandibular condyle
w. Ramus
x. Angle
y. Body
z. Mental foramen

LEARNING HINT

The **zygomatic bone** comes from the Greek word *zygoma*, meaning "yoke." Like a yoke that holds a pair of oxen together, this structure connects the temporal bone to the maxilla. The word *temporal* refers to "time," and the **temporal bone** is so named because it is located where many people first get gray hair as they grow older.

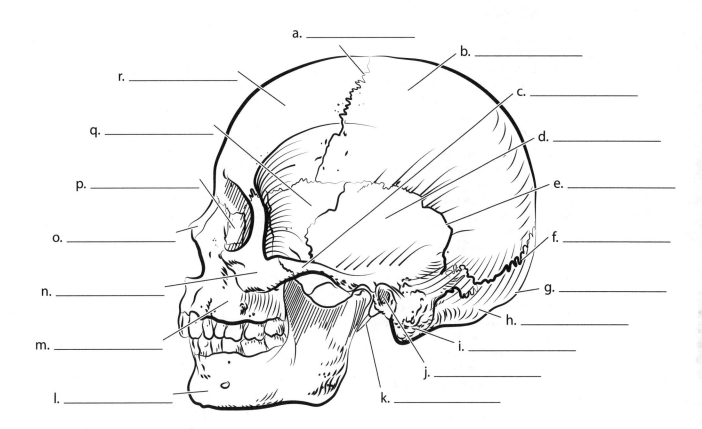

a. _____
b. _____
r. _____
c. _____
q. _____
d. _____
p. _____
e. _____
o. _____
f. _____
n. _____
g. _____
m. _____
h. _____
l. _____
i. _____
j. _____
k. _____

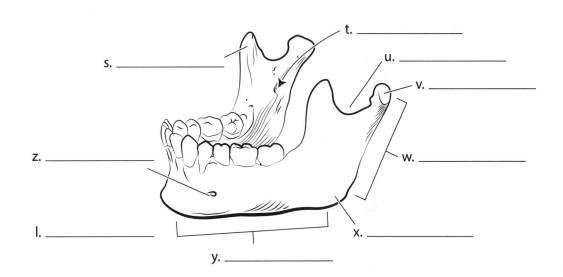

t. _____
s. _____
u. _____
v. _____
z. _____
w. _____
l. _____
x. _____
y. _____

SKULL—TOP AND BOTTOM VIEWS

The superior aspect of the skull consists of few bones and few sutures. The **frontal bone** is the most anterior bone with the **parietal bones** directly posterior to it. The **coronal suture** separates the two, and the **sagittal suture** separates the parietal bones. The **lambdoid suture** separates the parietal bone from the **occipital bone**. Label the bones and sutures in the illustrations.

The inferior aspect of the skull is more complex than the superior view. In the inferior view, the mandible has been removed so some of the underlying structures can be seen. The large opening in the occipital bone is the **foramen magnum**. The two bumps lateral to the foramen magnum are the **occipital condyles**, and the raised bump at the posterior part of the skull is the **external occipital protuberance**. The bone more anterior and lateral to the occipital bone is the temporal bone. The **jugular foramen** is located between the occipital and temporal bone. Another opening nearby is the **carotid canal**. Lateral to this is the **styloid process**, an attachment point for muscles. Lateral to this is a depression called the **mandibular fossa**. It is here that the mandible articulates with the temporal bone. The **foramen lacerum** and **foramen ovale** are medial to the mandibular fossa. The **sphenoid bone** spans the skull, and the major features seen from the inferior view are the **greater wing** and the **lateral** and **medial pterygoid plates**. The hard palate is made of the **palatine process of the maxilla** and the **palatine bones**. The bone that opens into the nasal cavity is the **vomer**. Label these features of the skull.

Color Guide: Use the same colors that you used for the same bones in previous illustrations of the skull. Color the shaded areas more heavily to produce deep colors in these regions.

Answer Key

a. Frontal bone
b. Maxilla
c. Coronal suture
d. Palatine bone
e. Vomer
f. Parietal bone
g. Sphenoid bone
h. Sagittal suture
i. Temporal bone
j. Lambdoid suture
k. Occipital bone
l. Palatine process of maxilla

m. Greater wing of sphenoid bone
n. Lateral pterygoid plate of sphenoid bone
o. Medial pterygoid plate of sphenoid bone
p. Foramen ovale
q. Foramen lacerum
r. Mandibular fossa
s. Styloid process
t. Carotid canal
u. Jugular foramen
v. Occipital condyle
w. Foramen magnum
x. External occipital protuberance

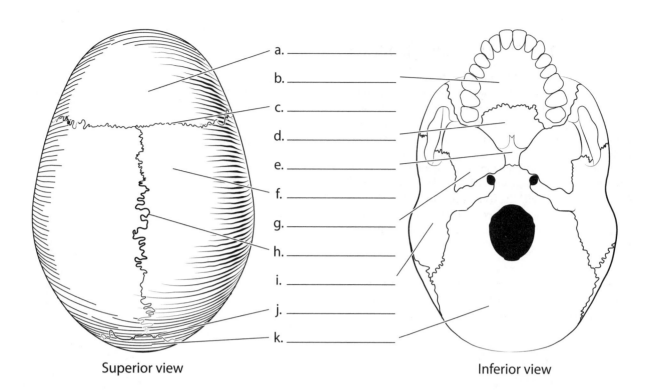

a. _____

b. _____

c. _____

d. _____

e. _____

f. _____

g. _____

h. _____

i. _____

j. _____

k. _____

Superior view   Inferior view

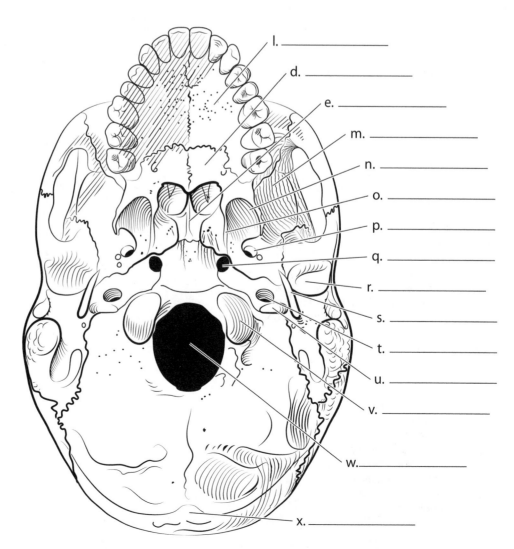

l. _____

d. _____

e. _____

m. _____

n. _____

o. _____

p. _____

q. _____

r. _____

s. _____

t. _____

u. _____

v. _____

w. _____

x. _____

MIDSAGITTAL SECTION OF THE SKULL

Several features of the skull can be seen when it is sectioned in the midsagittal plane. Locate the major bones of the skull and the features seen in this section. The nasal septum consists of two bony structures, the **perpendicular plate of the ethmoid bone** and the **vomer**. The **crista galli** extends superiorly from the **cribriform plate of the ethmoid bone**. The junction of the **maxilla** and the **palatine bone** that make up the hard palate can be seen from this view as well. The **frontal sinus** and the **sphenoid sinus** are two cavities seen here. Label the bones and the major features of the midsagittal section of the skull using the terms provided.

Color Guide: Use the same colors that you used for the same bones in previous illustrations of the skull. Color the sinuses in a darker shade of the color used for the specific bones that hold the sinuses.

Answer Key

a. Frontal bone
b. Frontal sinus
c. Crista galli
d. Nasal bone
e. Cribriform plate of the ethmoid bone
f. Perpendicular plate of the ethmoid bone
g. Vomer
h. Maxilla
i. Palatine bone
j. Mandible
k. Coronal suture
l. Squamosal suture
m. Parietal bone
n. Temporal bone
o. Sella turcica (pituitary fossa)
p. Occipital bone
q. Internal acoustic meatus
r. Sphenoid bone
s. Sphenoid sinus

a. _____

b. _____

c. _____

d. _____

e. _____

f. _____

g. _____

h. _____

i. _____

j. _____

k. _____

l. _____

m. _____

n. _____

o. _____

p. _____

q. _____

r. _____

s. _____

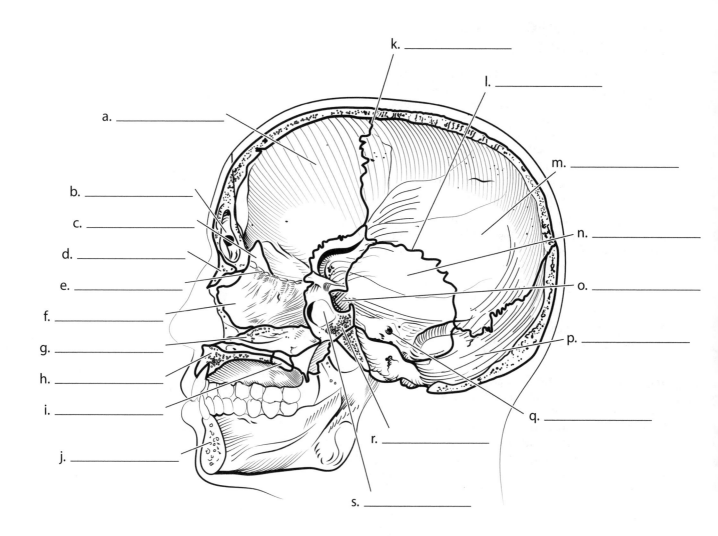

SPHENOID, TEMPORAL, AND ETHMOID BONES

A few bones of the skull are frequently studied as separate bones. The **sphenoid bone** has a superficial resemblance to a bat or butterfly. There are the **lesser wings**, the **greater wings**, and the **pterygoid plates**, all of which resemble wings. The **dorsum sellae** is the posterior part of the **sella turcica** (a depression that holds the pituitary gland). Locate the **foramen rotundum**, **foramen ovale**, **optic canal**, and **foramen spinosum** on the sphenoid bone. These holes enclose parts of the trigeminal nerve.

The temporal bone has a flat **squamous part** and a denser **petrous part**. The **mandibular fossa** is a depression where the mandible articulates. The section of the temporal bone that connects to the zygomatic bone is the **zygomatic process**. There are two significant canals or meatuses for hearing. These are the **external acoustic meatus** and the **internal acoustic meatus**. The **mastoid process** is a large bump that can be palpated directly posterior to the ear. The **styloid process** anchors a number of small hyoid muscles.

The **ethmoid bone** is located just posterior to the nose and is best seen isolated from the rest of the skull bones. The **cribriform plate** of the ethmoid has small holes in it called **olfactory foramina**. Locate the **crista galli** and the **perpendicular plate**. The ethmoid has four curved structures lateral to the perpendicular plate. These are the two **superior nasal conchae** and the two **middle nasal conchae**. The **ethmoid sinuses** are numerous small holes in the bone. Locate the structures of these skull bones, and label them in the illustration.

Color Guide: Color the features of the bones using the same color for each bone as you did in previous illustrations.

Answer Key

(Sphenoid features)
a. Sella turcica (pituitary fossa, hypophyseal fossa)
b. Optic canal
c. Lesser wing
d. Greater wing
e. Foramen spinosum
f. Pterygoid hamulus
g. Dorsum sellae
h. Foramen ovale
i. Foramen rotundum
j. Anterior clinoid process

(Temporal features)
k. Squamous part
l. Zygomatic process
m. Mandibular fossa
n. External acoustic meatus
o. Styloid process
p. Mastoid process

(Ethmoid features)
q. Crista galli
r. Middle nasal concha
s. Perpendicular plate
t. Superior nasal concha

LEARNING HINT

The **sphenoid bone** gets its name from a Greek word meaning "wedge" because it appears to wedge into the bottom part of the skull. The Latin word *concha*, meaning "seashell," was applied to the nasal **conchae** because they look like small shells inside the nose. **Ethmoid** comes from the Greek word for "sieve," because this bone is full of holes.

Sphenoid bone

b. _____

a. _____ c. _____

j. _____

i. _____

h. _____

g. _____ f. _____

d. _____

e. _____

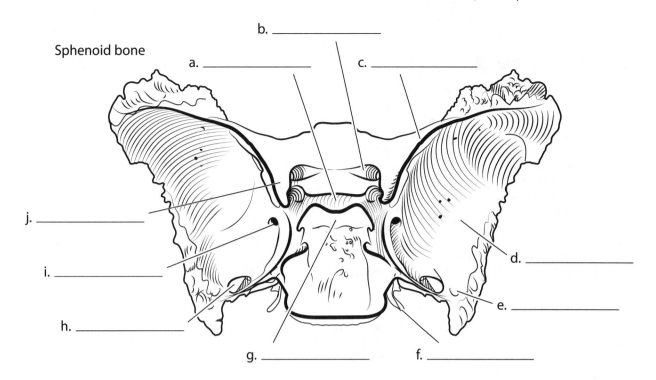

Temporal bone

k. _____

l. _____

m. _____

n. _____

o. _____

p. _____

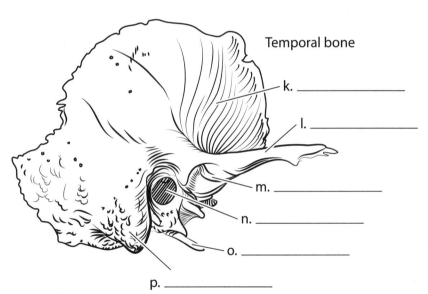

Ethmoid bone

q. _____

t. _____ r. _____

s. _____

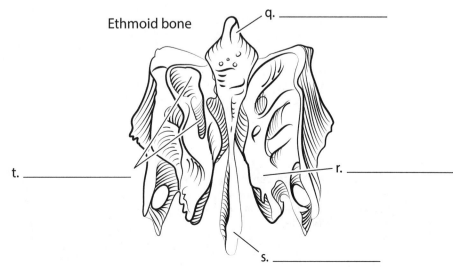

VERTEBRAL COLUMN

We are unique as animals because of our upright posture. The vertical position of the spine is reflected in the increase in size of the vertebra from superior to inferior. The vertebral column is divided into five major regions. There are 7 **cervical** (neck) **vertebrae** and 12 **thoracic vertebrae** that articulate with ribs. The 5 **lumbar vertebrae** are found in the lower back, and the **sacrum** consists of 5 fused **sacral vertebrae**. The **coccyx** is the terminal portion of the vertebral column consisting of 4 **coccygeal vertebrae**. The vertebral column in the adult has curves. The uppermost is the **cervical curvature**, and the lower ones are the **thoracic**, **lumbar**, and **pelvic curvatures**. Label the illustration with the regions and the curvatures.

Color Guide: Color each region of the vertebral column ("a" through "e") a different color of your choosing. Color along the curved arrows to highlight the spinal curvatures.

Answer Key

a. Cervical vertebrae (cervical curvature)
b. Thoracic vertebrae (thoracic curvature)
c. Lumbar vertebrae (lumbar curvature)
d. Sacrum (pelvic curvature)
e. Coccyx

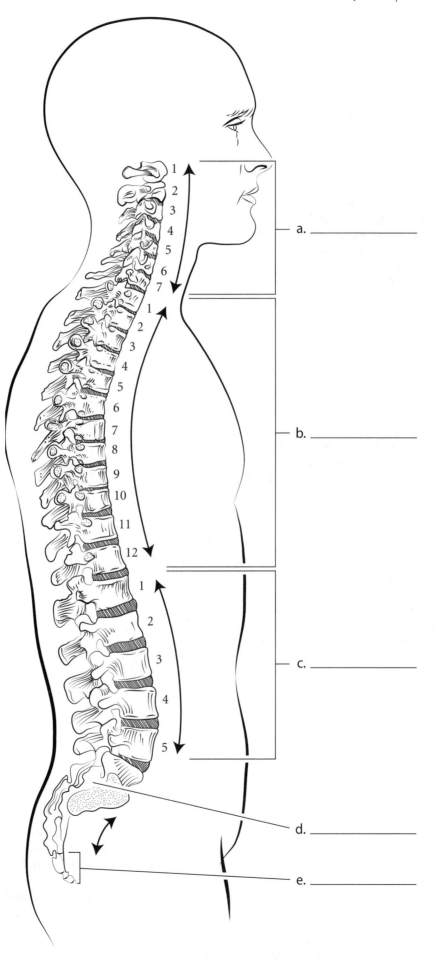

a. _____

b. _____

c. _____

d. _____

e. _____

ATLAS

The **atlas** is the first cervical vertebra. It is called C1. It is unique among the vertebrae because it has no body. Label the **vertebral foramen**, **superior articular facet**, **transverse foramen**, and **lateral masses**.

AXIS

The **axis** is the second cervical vertebra (C2), and it has a **body** with a projection that arises from the body known as the **odontoid process** or **dens**. Label the axis with the bold print terms in this section, including the **superior articular facets**, the **transverse foramen**, the **spinous process**, and the **vertebral foramen**.

ATLAS AND AXIS

Here are the **atlas** and **axis** together.

HYOID

The hyoid bone is a floating bone, which means that it has no hard attachments to other bones. The main part of the hyoid is the **body**, and the two pairs of horns that arise from the hyoid are the **greater horns** (greater cornua) and the **lesser horns** (lesser cornua). Label these parts of the bone.

Color Guide: In the top two illustrations, color "c" black and leave "a" uncolored. Use different shades of one color for the other parts of the atlas, and select a different color for the remaining parts of the axis, making the shaded areas of the illustration darker. In the third illustration, use the same two colors that you used for the atlas and axis in the upper illustrations. In the bottom illustration, color each labeled part of the hyoid a separate color, making the shaded areas darker.

Answer Key

a. Vertebral foramen
b. Lateral masses
c. Transverse foramen
d. Superior articular facet
e. Spinous process
f. Body
g. Odontoid process (dens)
h. Axis
i. Atlas
j. Lesser cornu
k. Greater cornu
l. Body

LEARNING HINT

The **atlas**, which supports the head, is named for the Greek mythological figure who held up the heavens. The **axis** functions like the axle of a car: The atlas rotates around the axis. The **hyoid** is so named because it is U-shaped, like the Greek letter upsilon.

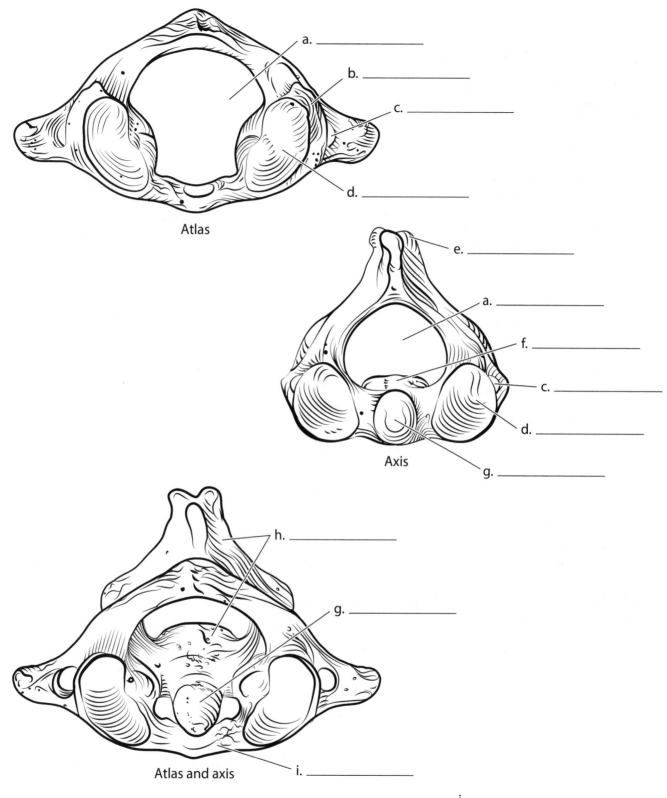

a. _____

b. _____

c. _____

d. _____

Atlas

e. _____

a. _____

f. _____

c. _____

d. _____

g. _____

Axis

h. _____

g. _____

i. _____

Atlas and axis

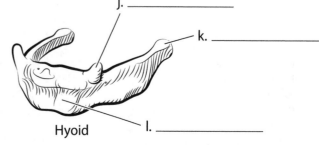

j. _____

k. _____

l. _____

Hyoid

CERVICAL, THORACIC, AND LUMBAR VERTEBRAE

Features Common to Vertebrae

The opening where the spinal cord passes through the vertebra is known as the **vertebral foramen**. The **body** of the vertebra is the weight-bearing part of the vertebra and the **spinous process** is the part that extends posteriorly. This process is an extension from the **vertebral arch** that curves from the body enclosing the vertebral foramen. This arch is composed of the two **pedicles** and the two **laminae**. The **superior articular process** and the **superior articular facet** (the flat surface on the process) are the parts that join with the vertebra above. The **inferior articular process** and the **inferior articular facet** are the parts of the vertebra that join with the vertebra below.

Typical Cervical Vertebrae, Superior and Lateral Views

Cervical vertebrae are distinct from all other vertebrae by having two **transverse foramina**. These house blood vessels. Another characteristic of the cervical vertebrae is that several of them have a **bifid spinous process**.

Typical Thoracic Vertebrae, Superior and Lateral Views

The thoracic vertebrae typically have longer **spinous processes** than cervical vertebrae, and many of them point in an inferior direction. The **body** is larger in thoracic vertebrae, and they are the only bones with **costal facets**, which are attachment points for the ribs. The **transverse processes** can be seen along with the **transverse costal facets**.

Typical Lumbar Vertebrae, Superior and Lateral Views

The lumbar vertebrae have larger bodies because they support more weight. The **spinous process** is shorter and more horizontal in lumbar vertebrae than in thoracic vertebrae. There are no costal facets and no transverse foramina. Label the parts of the vertebrae in the illustration.

Color Guide: Color each labeled part of the vertebrae a different color, using the same color for the same structure in all drawings on this page. For example, color the transverse process the same color in all of the figures in which it appears. Leave the foramina uncolored, as these are open spaces.

Answer Key

a. Bifid spinous process
b. Spinous process
c. Vertebral foramen
d. Lamina of vertebral arch
e. Pedicle of vertebral arch
f. Superior articular process
g. Transverse process
h. Body

i. Inferior articular process
j. Transverse foramen
k. Uncas of vertebral body
l. Superior costal facet
m. Inferior costal facet
n. Costal facet of
   transverse process

Cervical vertebra

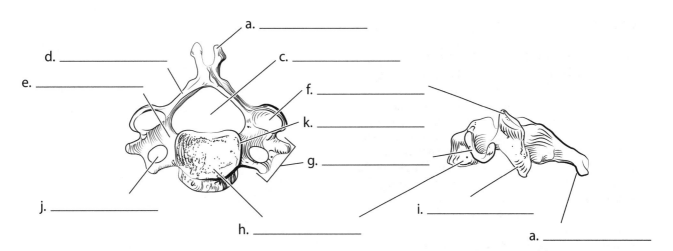

a. _____

d. _____

e. _____

c. _____

f. _____

k. _____

g. _____

j. _____

h. _____

i. _____

a. _____

Thoracic vertebra

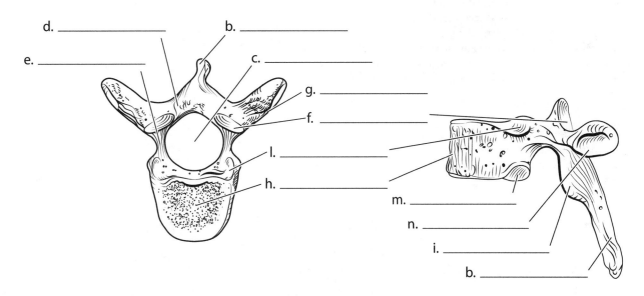

d. _____

e. _____

b. _____

c. _____

g. _____

f. _____

l. _____

h. _____

m. _____

n. _____

i. _____

b. _____

Lumbar vertebra

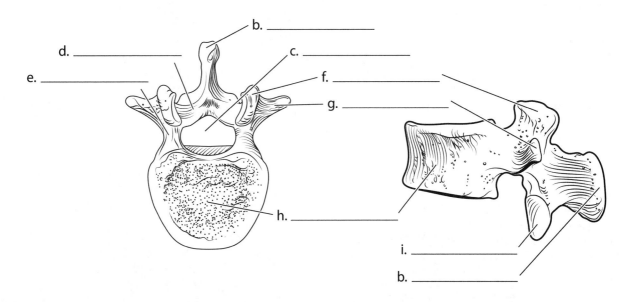

b. _____

d. _____

e. _____

c. _____

f. _____

g. _____

h. _____

i. _____

b. _____

SACRUM AND COCCYX

Sacrum and Coccyx, Anterior View

The terminal portion of the vertebral column consists of two structures that are fused bones. The **sacrum** is five fused vertebrae, and the **coccyx** is composed of three to five vertebrae. The top rim is the **sacral promontory**, and the winglike expansion where the ilium attaches is the **ala**. The area where the vertebrae join are the **transverse lines**. The holes running down each side are the **anterior sacral foramina**. At the top of the sacrum are the **superior articular processes**, and they attach to the lumbar vertebra. Label the parts of the sacrum and the coccyx.

Sacrum and Coccyx, Posterior View

From the posterior view, the **median sacral crest** results from the fusion of the spinous processes of the sacral vertebrae. The **posterior sacral foramina** are on each side of the crest, and the **lateral sacral crests** are lateral to the foramina. The **superior articular processes** can be seen from this view, as well as the **auricular surface**, which forms part of the sacroiliac joint. (The word *auricular* means "ear shaped.") Label the features of the sacrum and the coccyx.

Color Guide: Color the sacrum one color and the coccyx another, using a different shading (or color) for individual parts of the bones. Use black for "e" and "j," which are spaces.

Answer Key

a. Superior articular process
b. Lateral mass (ala)
c. Sacral promontory
d. Transverse lines
e. Anterior sacral foramina
f. Coccyx
g. Auricular surface
h. Lateral sacral crest
i. Median sacral crest
j. Posterior sacral foramina

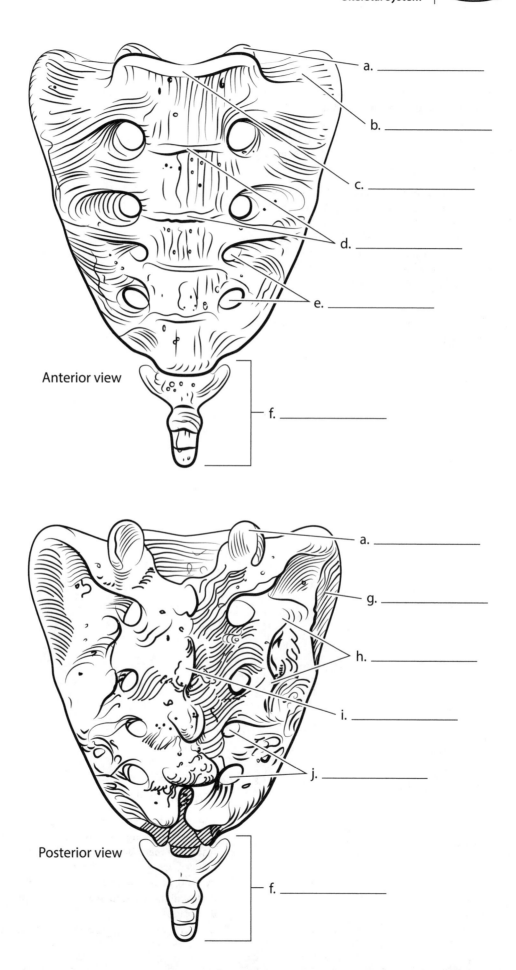

a. _____

b. _____

c. _____

d. _____

e. _____

Anterior view

f. _____

a. _____

g. _____

h. _____

i. _____

j. _____

Posterior view

f. _____

STERNUM AND RIBS

The **sternum** is commonly known as the breastbone and is divided into three areas: the upper **manubrium** with the **suprasternal notch** and the **clavicular notches**, the **body** with the **costal notches** (where the ribs attach), and the **xiphoid process**. Between the manubrium and the body is the **sternal angle**. Label these features on the illustration.

For ribs, you will find the terminal portion of the rib is an expanded **head**. The constricted region below that is the **neck**. The **tubercle** of the rib is a bump that attaches to the transverse process of the vertebra. The bend in the rib is known as the **angle**, and the depressed area of the rib where nerves and blood vessels are found is the **costal groove**. Label the various parts of the ribs.

Color Guide: Color the individual parts of a rib, and the rib as it joins with a vertebra, in colors of your choosing.

Answer Key

a. Suprasternal notch
b. Clavicular notch
c. Manubrium
d. Sternal angle
e. Costal notches
f. Body
g. Xiphoid process
h. Head
i. Tubercle
j. Neck
k. Angle of rib
l. Costal groove

LEARNING HINT

The parts of the sternum are named after the parts of a sword—though this "sword" has a very short blade. The **manubrium** is the butt-end of the handle; *manus* (Latin for "hand") refers to work done by hand, as in *manual labor*. The **body** is the handle itself, and the **xiphoid process** (Latin *xiphoeidus*) is the "blade."

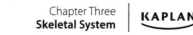

a. _____

b. _____

c. _____

d. _____

e. _____

f. _____

g. _____

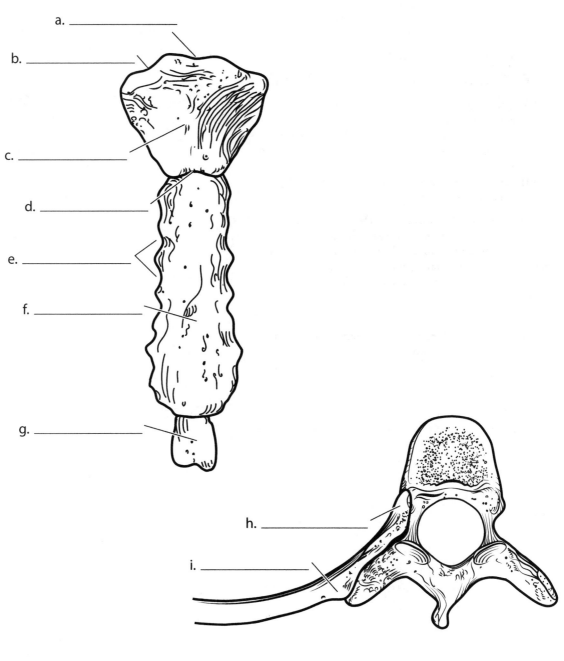

h. _____

i. _____

h. _____

k. _____

j. _____

i. _____

l. _____

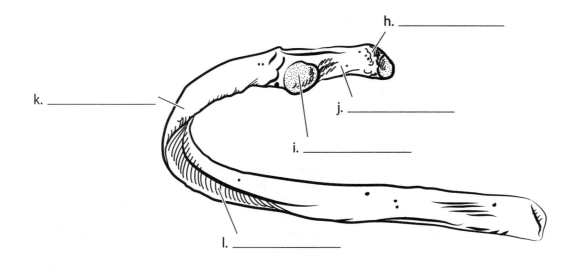

APPENDICULAR SKELETON— PECTORAL GIRDLE AND UPPER LIMB

The appendicular skeleton is so named because it is appended (added on) to the axial skeleton. The pectoral girdle is located in the chest and upper back region, and the upper limb bones are attached to the pectoral girdle by the humerus. Attached to the sacrum of the axial skeleton is the pelvic girdle (hip bones), and the lower limb bones are connected to the hip by the femur.

The pectoral girdle is made of the **clavicles** and the **scapulae**. The upper limb consists of the **humerus** of the arm; the **radius** and **ulna** of the forearm; and the **carpals**, **metacarpals**, and **phalanges** of the hand. Locate these major regions of the upper limb, and label them on the diagram.

Color Guide: Color the bones and groups of bones in the illustration in different colors.

Answer Key

a. Clavicle
b. Humerus
c. Scapula
d. Radius
e. Ulna
f. Carpals
g. Metacarpals
h. Phalanges

LEARNING HINT

The **radius** is on the lateral side of the forearm (the thumb side). If you extend your thumb like a hitchhiker and rotate your forearm and hand, you will see that the thumb forms the radius of a circle.

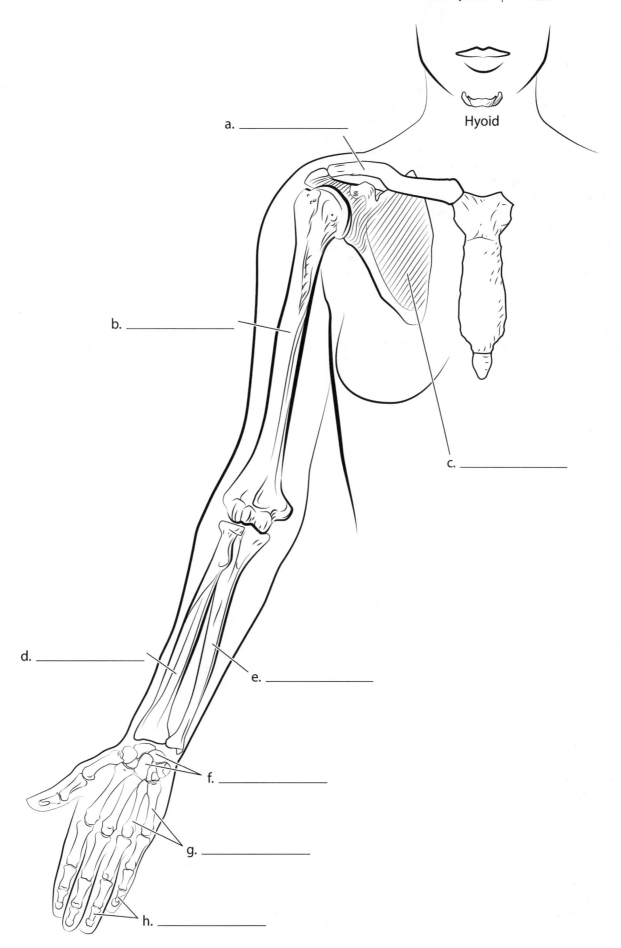

Hyoid

a. _____

b. _____

c. _____

d. _____

e. _____

f. _____

g. _____

h. _____

SCAPULA

Each scapula is a triangular bone, and the three edges are known as the **superior border**, the **lateral border**, and the **medial border**. The **scapular spine** is on the posterior surface, and it expands into a terminal process known as the **acromion**. Above the spine is the **supraspinous fossa**. Below the spine is the **infraspinous fossa**, and on the anterior side of the scapula are the **subscapular fossa** and the **coracoid process**. The **inferior angle** of the scapula is at the junction of the medial and lateral borders. Inferior to the acromion is the **glenoid cavity (fossa)**. This is a depression where the head of the humerus articulates with the scapula. Label the various features of the scapula. Locate as many of the features as possible from the various angles presented.

Color Guide: Color in the regions of the bone with different colors, using the same color for the same region in each of the various views seen on this page.

Answer Key

a. Acromion
b. Superior border
c. Coracoid process
d. Glenoid cavity
e. Subscapular fossa
f. Lateral border
g. Medial border
h. Inferior angle
i. Supraspinous fossa
j. Scapular spine
k. Infraspinous fossa

LEARNING HINT

The term **acromion** is a combination of two Greek words that identify its location, *acros* for "tip" and *omos* for "shoulder." The acromion forms the tip of the shoulder.

The **coracoid process** comes from the Greek *corax*, meaning "crow," as this process looks a little like a crow's beak.

Anterior view

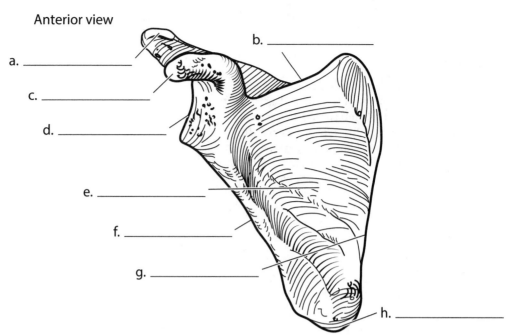

a. _____

b. _____

c. _____

d. _____

e. _____

f. _____

g. _____

h. _____

Posterior view

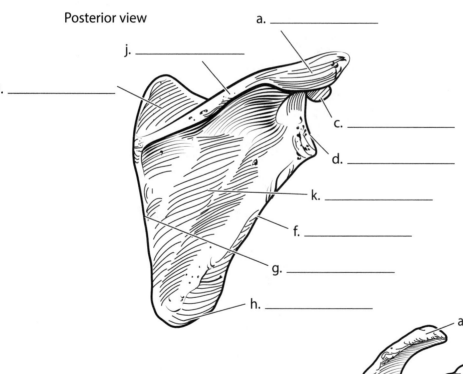

a. _____

j. _____

i. _____

c. _____

d. _____

k. _____

f. _____

g. _____

h. _____

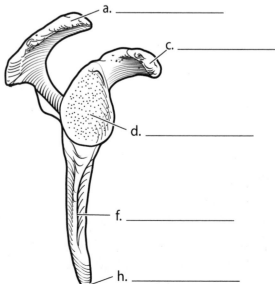

a. _____

c. _____

d. _____

f. _____

h. _____

CLAVICLE

The clavicle is a thin bone that stabilizes the shoulder joint in a lateral position. It has a blunt end that articulates with the sternum (the **sternal end**) and a flattened end that joins with the acromion process of the scapula. This is called the **acromial end**. A small bump on the inferior part of the clavicle has a ligament that attaches to the coracoid process of the scapula. This bump is called the **conoid tubercle**. The clavicle attaches to the sternum superior to the **first rib**, which is itself attached to the **first thoracic vertebra**. Label the clavicle and the ends of the bone.

Color Guide: Color the acromial end of the clavicle one color and the sternal end another color. Select a third color for the conoid tubercle.

Answer Key

a. First thoracic vertebra
b. First rib
c. Scapula
d. Acromial end of clavicle
e. Sternal end of clavicle
f. Sternum
g. Conoid tubercle

Superior view

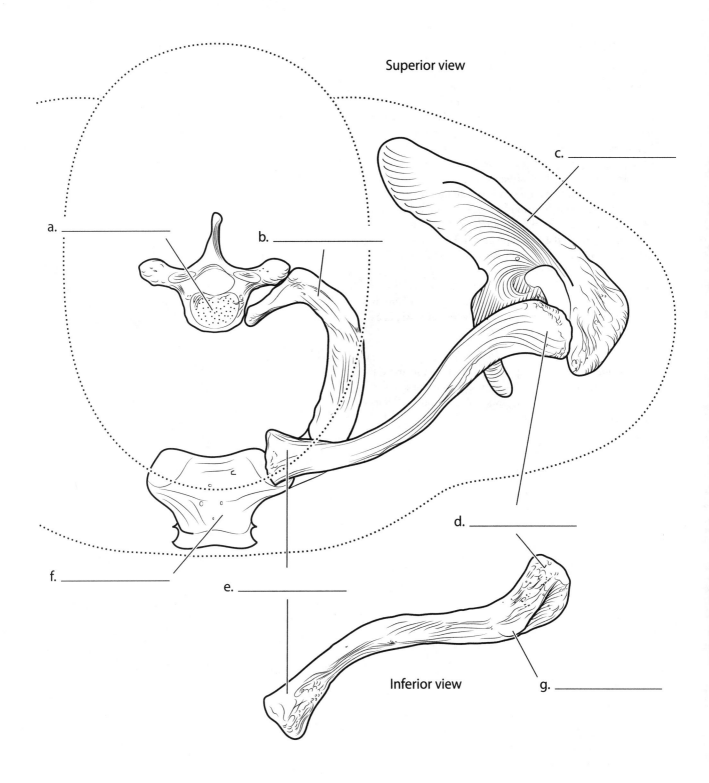

a.

b.

c.

d.

e.

f.

g.

Inferior view

HUMERUS

The humerus has a proximal **head** that fits into the glenoid fossa of the scapula. Just at the edge of the head is a rim known as the **anatomical neck**. Below this neck are the **greater tubercle** and **lesser tubercle**, and the depression between the two is the **intertubercular groove (sulcus)**. Below these is the **surgical neck** of the humerus. (It is called the "surgical neck" of the humerus because that is the part of the bone that is frequently broken.) The deltoid muscle attaches to the humerus at the **deltoid tuberosity**, and the two expanded, winglike processes at the distal end of the humerus are the **supracondylar ridges**. Inferior to these are the **medial** and **lateral epicondyles**, and at the articulating ends of the humerus are the lateral **capitulum** and the medial **trochlea**. The depression on the anterior surface of the humerus into which the ulna fits is called the **coronoid fossa**, and the posterior depression where the elbow locks into the humerus is the **olecranon fossa**. Label these features in the figure.

Color Guide: Color in the specific parts of the illustration with different colors, using the same color for the same area of the humerus in both views (anterior and posterior) seen on the page.

Answer Key

a. Greater tubercle
b. Head
c. Anatomical neck
d. Lesser tubercle
e. Intertubercular groove
f. Surgical neck
g. Deltoid tuberosity
h. Supracondylar ridges
i. Lateral epicondyle
j. Coronoid fossa
k. Olecranon fossa
l. Medial epicondyle
m. Capitulum
n. Trochlea

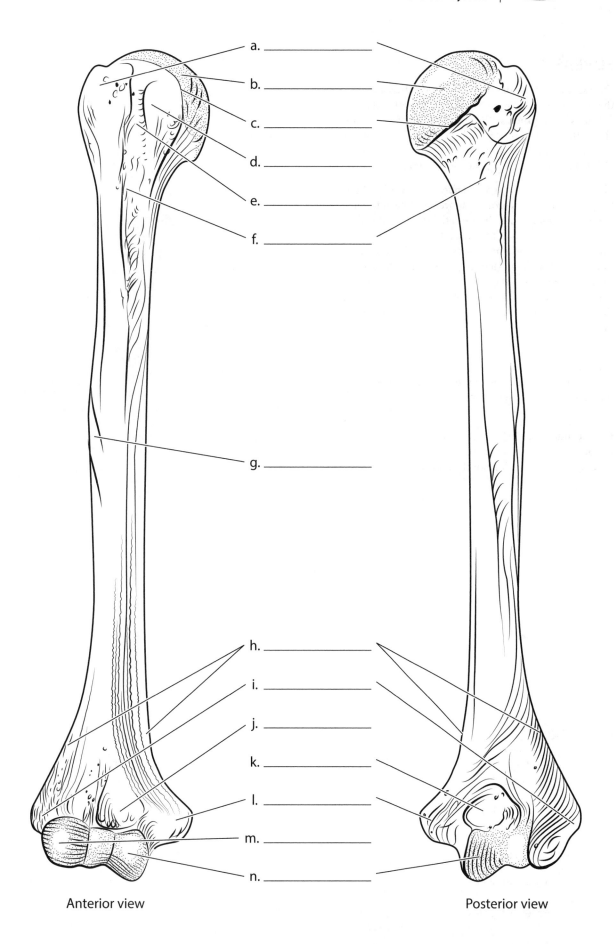

a. _____

b. _____

c. _____

d. _____

e. _____

f. _____

g. _____

h. _____

i. _____

j. _____

k. _____

l. _____

m. _____

n. _____

Anterior view   Posterior view

FOREARM BONES

The radius has a circular **head**, a **radial tuberosity** on the shaft (where the biceps brachii muscle attaches), and a distal **styloid process**. The circular head of the radius allows this bone to rotate. At the distal end of the radius, there is a depression where the ulna joins with the radius. This is known as the **ulnar notch** of the radius.

The ulna has a proximal **olecranon process** (elbow) on the posterior side, a **coronoid process** on the anterior side, and the **trochlear notch** between the two. Just distal to the coronoid process of the ulna is the **tuberosity of the ulna**, a projection where muscles attach. The **head** of the ulna is distal, and an extended part of the distal ulna is the **styloid process**. At the proximal portion of the ulna is a depression where the head of the radius articulates with the ulna. This depression is known as the **radial notch** of the ulna.

When the two bones are joined, you can see where each fits into the other. On the edge of each bone is the **interosseous margin**. This is a ridge where the interosseous membrane connects the bones.

Color Guide: Use the same colors for the specific parts of the ulna in both views (lateral and anterior) seen on the page. Use different colors for the radius.

Answer Key

a. Olecranon process
b. Trochlear notch
c. Coronoid process
d. Radial notch
e. Tuberosity of the ulna
f. Head of radius
g. Radial tuberosity
h. Interosseous margin
i. Head of ulna
j. Styloid process of ulna
k. Ulnar notch
l. Styloid process of radius

Ulna, lateral view

Ulna and radius, anterior view

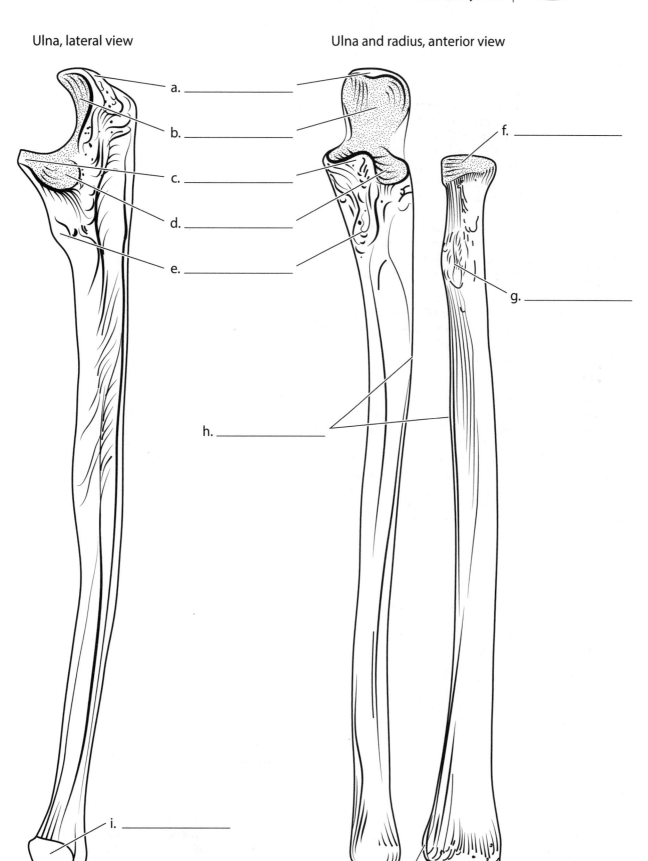

a. _____

b. _____

c. _____

d. _____

e. _____

f. _____

g. _____

h. _____

i. _____

j. _____

k. _____

l. _____

HAND BONES

The hand consists of 27 bones divided into three groups: the **carpals**, the **metacarpals**, and the **phalanges**. The thumb is known as the **pollex** and is listed as the first digit of the hand. The index finger is the second digit, and the fingers are listed sequentially with the little finger being the fifth digit. The bones of the fingers are known as **phalanges**, and they are named according to what digit they belong to and for their position relative to the point of origin: proximal, middle, or distal. Therefore, the bony tip of the little finger is the distal phalanx of the fifth digit while the bone in the place where you would normally wear a wedding ring is the proximal phalanx of the fourth digit. Each phalanx has a **proximal base**, a **shaft**, and a **distal head**.

The **metacarpals** are the bones of the palm of the hand. Each metacarpal also has a proximal base, a shaft, and a distal head. There are five metacarpals, and they are named for the phalanges that extend from them. The first metacarpal articulates with the thumb.

The carpals are the bones of the wrist. There are eight carpal bones in two rows. The bone under the thumb is the **trapezium**. The one medial to it is the **trapezoid**. The **capitate** is found under the third metacarpal, and the **hamate** finishes that row. Proximal to the trapezium is the **scaphoid**, which joins with the radius. The next bone in line is the **lunate**, followed by the **triquetrum**, and finally the little **pisiform** bone. If you memorize the bones in this sequence, you can use the following mnemonic device to remember them: "The Tom Cat Has Shaken Loose To Prowl." The first letter of the mnemonic represents the first letter of the carpal bone. Label the illustration.

Color Guide: Color all of the phalanges one color. Color the metacarpals another color, and color the carpal bones individual colors. Use the same color scheme for the bones across the various illustrations of the hand.

Answer Key

a. Phalanges
b. Head
c. Shaft
d. Base
e. Hamate
f. Capitate
g. Triquetrum
h. Lunate
i. Metacarpal
j. Trapezoid
k. Trapezium
l. Scaphoid
m. Pisiform

LEARNING HINT

The carpal bones are best understood by shape. **Capitate** means "head" (as in *decapitate*), and **triquetrum** derives from the Latin word for "triangular." Both **trapezoid** and **trapezium** are 4-sided shapes, while the **scaphoid** (from the Greek for "boat") is shaped like a little boat. The **pisiform** is shaped like a green pea, the **lunate** like the moon, and the **hamate** (like its Latin namesake) has a hook.

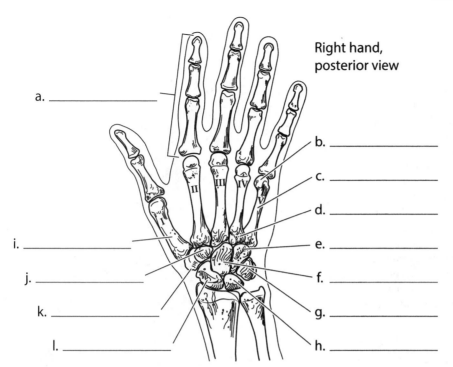

Right hand,
posterior view

a. _____

b. _____

c. _____

d. _____

e. _____

f. _____

g. _____

h. _____

i. _____

j. _____

k. _____

l. _____

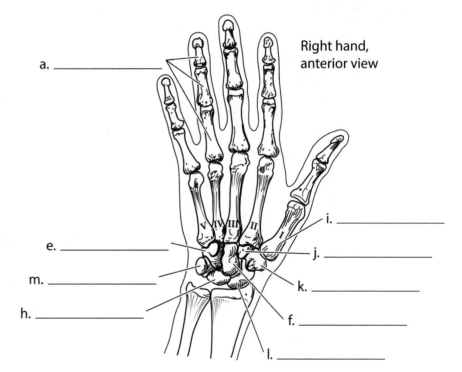

Right hand,
anterior view

a. _____

e. _____

m. _____

h. _____

i. _____

j. _____

k. _____

f. _____

l. _____

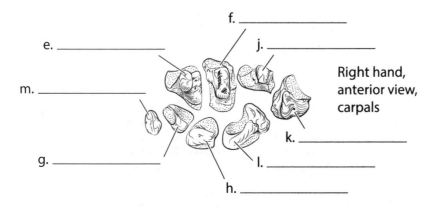

Right hand,
anterior view,
carpals

f. _____

j. _____

e. _____

m. _____

g. _____

k. _____

l. _____

h. _____

HIP

Each **coxal bone** (hip bone) is a result of the fusion of three bones: the **ilium**, the **ischium** (pronounced ISS-kee-um), and the **pubis**. The two coxal bones, when joined together by the **pubic symphysis**, form the pelvis, which can be divided into an upper **false pelvis** and a lower **true pelvis** separated by the pelvic brim. The **anterior superior iliac spine** and the **anterior inferior iliac spine** can be seen from the front. The top ridge of the pelvis is the **iliac crest**. The large inferior hole is the **obturator foramen**, and the depression superior to it is the **acetabulum**, where the femur joins the hip. Note the junction of the sacrum and the ilium that forms the **sacroiliac joint**. The **ischial tuberosity** is a large process that you can feel as you sit on a hard surface such as a bench. Label the features of the hip, sacrum, and coccyx.

Color Guide: Use a different color for each specific part of the hip. In the bottom illustration, use a different color for each of the fused bones.

Answer Key

a. Iliac crest
b. Sacroiliac joint
c. Greater sciatic notch
d. Anterior superior iliac spine
e. Anterior inferior iliac spine
f. Acetabulum
g. Obturator foramen
h. Pubic symphysis
i. False pelvis
j. True pelvis
k. Ilium
l. Ischium
m. Pubis

LEARNING HINT

There are two funny names for structures in the hip. The **obturator foramen** comes from the word *obturate*, which means "to block up." It is so named because the foramen is covered with fibrous tissue. The **acetabulum** is a Latin word meaning "vinegar cup." This structure is shaped like a shallow bowl.

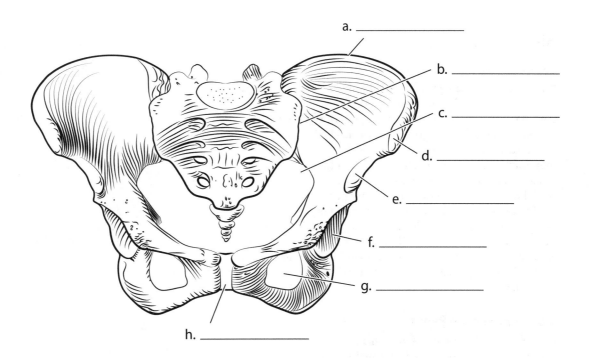

a. _____

b. _____

c. _____

d. _____

e. _____

f. _____

g. _____

h. _____

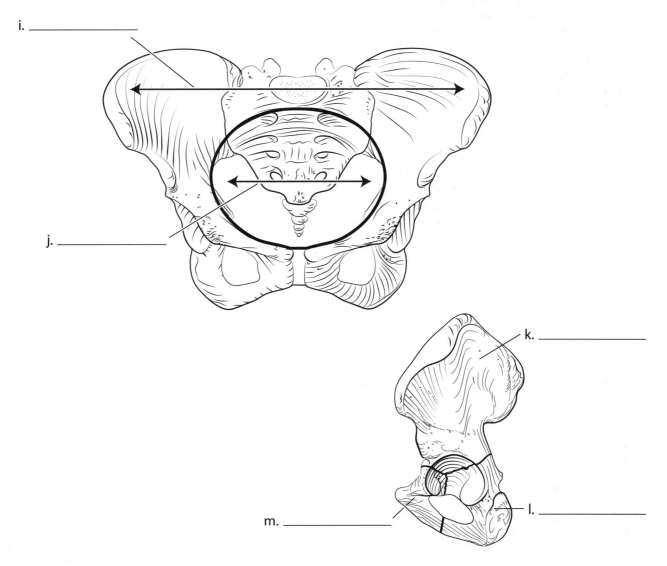

i. _____

j. _____

k. _____

l. _____

m. _____

HIP (continued)

Lateral View

When seen from a lateral view, several features are apparent in the coxal bone. Locate the iliac crest, the **posterior superior iliac spine**, and the **posterior inferior iliac spine** along with the **greater sciatic notch**, the **spine of the ischium**, and the **lesser sciatic notch**. The **ischial tuberosity** is at the posterior, inferior edge of the ischium. Just anterior to the tuberosity is a strip of bone called the **ischial ramus** that attaches to the **inferior pubic ramus**. The body of the pubis is the most anterior part of the pubis, and the **superior pubic ramus** is the portion that forms part of the acetabulum. The **ala** is the expanded blade of the ilium. The **obturator foramen** is an opening covered by a membrane. Label these features on the illustration.

Male and Female Pelvis

Differences can be seen between the male and female pelvis. The **subpubic angle** in males is less than 90 degrees, and the female angle is greater than 90 degrees. The ilium in males is typically more vertical than in individuals who have had children. A further distinction is seen in the side view of a pelvis in which thesciatic notch in the female pelvis has a much wider angle than in the male pelvis. Color in the upper portion of the ilium.

Color Guide: In the upper illustration, lightly color the three fused bones using the same color scheme as in the previous illustration. Use different colors for the various regions represented, such as the posterior inferior iliac spine. In the lower illustrations, color in the upper portion of the ilium with the same color you used for the ilium in previous illustrations, and lightly color the other bones.

Answer Key

a. Iliac crest
b. Posterior superior iliac spine
c. Posterior inferior iliac spine
d. Greater sciatic notch
e. Ischial spine
f. Lesser sciatic notch
g. Ischial tuberosity
h. Ischial ramus
i. Anterior superior iliac spine
j. Anterior inferior iliac spine
k. Superior pubic ramus

l. Inferior pubic ramus
m. Obturator foramen
n. Acetabulum
o. Wing (ala) of ilium
p. True pelvis
   (male: narrower and heart-shaped, female: wider and oval)
q. Subpubic angle
r. Male
s. Female

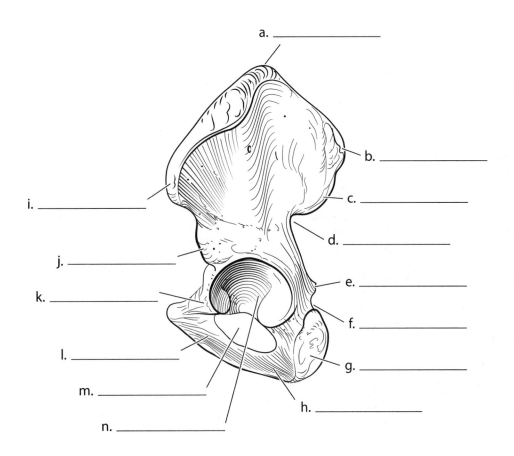

a. _____

b. _____

c. _____

d. _____

e. _____

f. _____

g. _____

h. _____

i. _____

j. _____

k. _____

l. _____

m. _____

n. _____

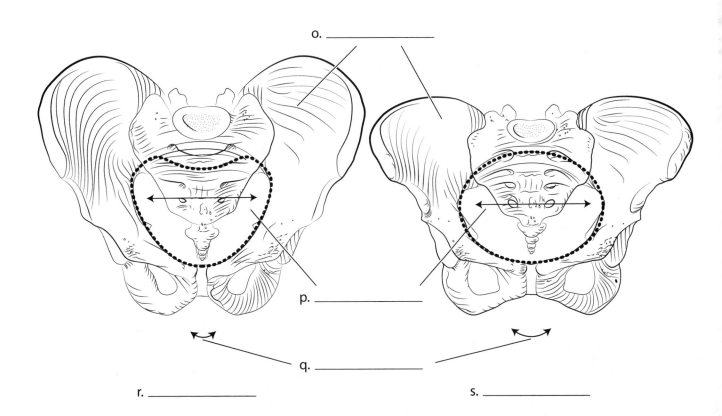

o. _____

p. _____

q. _____

r. _____

s. _____

LOWER LIMB—FEMUR AND PATELLA

The lower limb consists of the **femur** of the thigh; the **tibia** and **fibula** of the leg; and the **tarsals**, **metatarsals**, and **phalanges** of the foot. Locate these major regions of the lower limb and label them on the diagram.

The femur seen from the anterior view shows a proximal **head** and a constricted **neck**. Two large processes are distal to the neck. These are the **greater trochanter** and the **lesser trochanter**. There is a raised section of bone between them called the **intertrochanteric line**. The main part of the bone is the shaft, and the **lateral epicondyle** and **medial epicondyle** are the distal expansions of the bone. The posterior view of the femur has additional features such as the **intertrochanteric ridge**, the **linea aspera**, the **lateral condyle**, and the **medial condyle**. The femur is bowed, and this can be seen from a lateral view; the placement of the **patella** can also be seen from a lateral view. The **base** of the patella is superior, and the **apex** is inferior. Label the features of the femur and patella.

Color Guide: Color in each anatomical area in the figure with a different color, using the same color for the same area seen in both anterior and posterior views on this page.

Answer Key

a. Femur
b. Patella
c. Tibia
d. Fibula
e. Tarsals
f. Metatarsals
g. Phalanges
h. Greater trochanter
i. Head
j. Neck
k. Intertrochanteric line
l. Intertrochanteric ridge
m. Lesser trochanter
n. Linea aspera
o. Lateral epicondyle
p. Lateral condyle
q. Medial epicondyle
r. Medial condyle
s. Base of patella
t. Apex of patella

LEARNING HINT

Condyles are bumps, and **epicondyles** are bumps on top of bumps. The **intertrochanteric ridge** is a posterior, raised section of bone between the two trochanters, while the **intertrochanteric line** is an anterior, smaller raised section of bone.

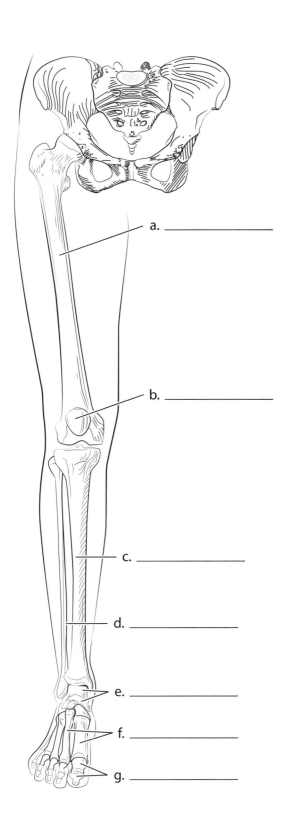

a. _____

b. _____

c. _____

d. _____

e. _____

f. _____

g. _____

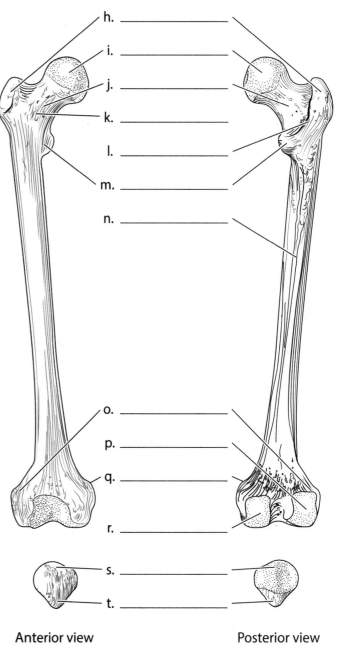

h. _____

i. _____

j. _____

k. _____

l. _____

m. _____

n. _____

o. _____

p. _____

q. _____

r. _____

s. _____

t. _____

Anterior view   Posterior view

TIBIA AND FIBULA

The **tibia** supports the weight of the body and is the bone that articulates with the femur. The **fibula** is more slender and is a bone to which muscles attach. The top of the tibia is expanded into a triangular shape with the **medial tibial condyle** and **lateral tibial condyle** articulating with the condyles of the femur. The quadriceps femoris muscles attach to the **tibial tuberosity** on the anterior surface of the tibia just below the condyles. The **anterior tibial crest** is a large ridge that runs the length of the bone. At the terminal portion of the tibia is the **medial malleolus**. This process, along with the **lateral malleolus** of the fibula, joins with the talus of the foot. The **head** of the fibula is proximal. It is a triangular region with a pointed **apex**. Label the tibia and fibula illustrations.

Color Guide: Color the various regions of the bones, using the same color for the same region seen in both anterior and posterior views on this page.

Answer Key

a. Lateral tibial condyle
b. Medial tibial condyle
c. Tibial tuberosity
d. Apex
e. Head of fibula
f. Anterior tibial crest
g. Shaft of tibia
h. Shaft of fibula
i. Medial malleolus
j. Lateral malleolus

LEARNING HINT

The **fibula** is the smaller of the two bones of the leg (from knee to ankle). Remember this with the phrase "Tell a little fib."

The word **malleolus**, meaning "little hammer," refers to the shape of the expanded distal parts of both the tibia and fibula.

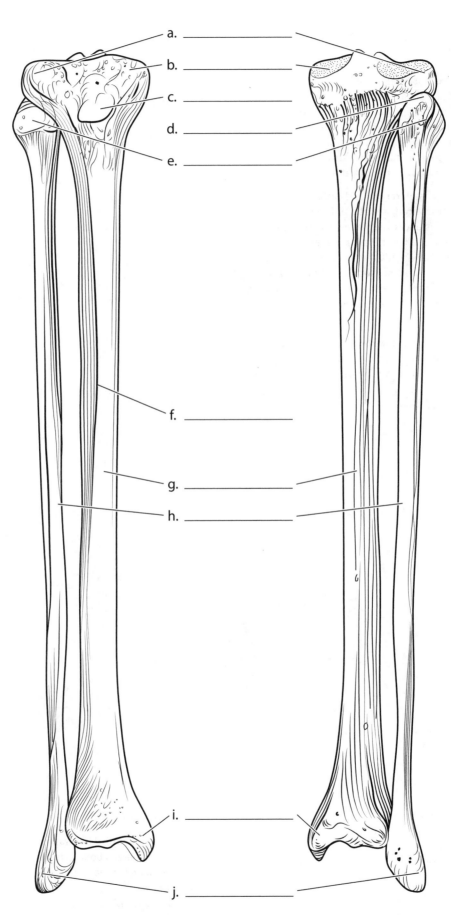

a. _____

b. _____

c. _____

d. _____

e. _____

f. _____

g. _____

h. _____

i. _____

j. _____

Anterior view   Posterior view

LEFT FOOT

The **calcaneus** (heel bone) takes most of the weight of the body when standing. The **talus** connects the foot to the tibia and fibula forming the ankle joint. The first, second, and third **cuneiforms** are so named because they are wedge-shaped bones. They form a natural arch of bone in the foot. The **cuboid** is lateral to the third cuneiform, and the **navicular** is posterior to the cuneiforms.

Note that each of the **metatarsals** and each of the **phalanges** has a distal **head**, a **shaft**, and a proximal **base**. The first metatarsal is under the big toe, and the fifth is under the smallest toe. All of the proximal phalanges are given the same letter in the illustration as are the middle and distal phalanges. Write **proximal**, **middle**, or **distal** in the appropriate space next to the toes. The big toe (hallux) has two phalanges while the other toes have three.

Color Guide: Color in the seven **tarsal** bones of the left foot using a different color for each bone. Color all of the metatarsals one color and the 14 phalanges another color.

Answer Key

1. Phalanges
2. Metatarsals
3. Tarsals
a. Distal phalanges
b. Middle phalanges
c. Proximal phalanges
d. Head
e. Shaft
f. Base
g. First (medial) cuneiform
h. Second (intermediate) cuneiform
i. Navicular
j. Third (lateral) cuneiform
k. Cuboid
l. Talus
m. Calcaneus

LEARNING HINT

Surprisingly, the **third (lateral) cuneiform** bone is not the most lateral bone in that row. But notice: It is the most lateral of the wedge-shaped bones named *cuneiform*.

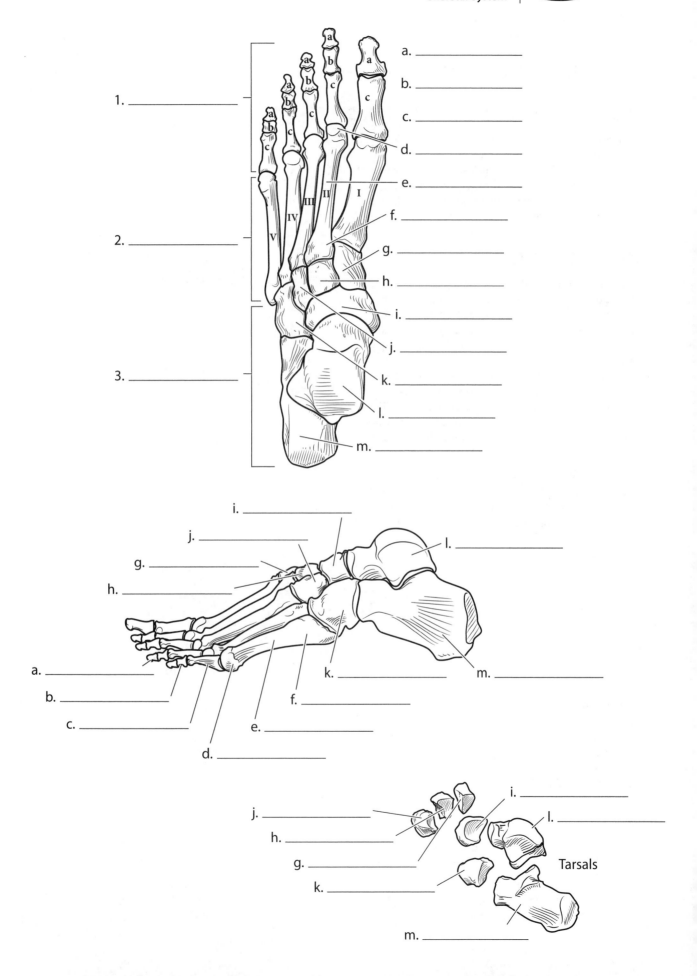

1. _____

2. _____

3. _____

a. _____

b. _____

c. _____

d. _____

e. _____

f. _____

g. _____

h. _____

i. _____

j. _____

k. _____

l. _____

m. _____

i. _____

j. _____

g. _____

h. _____

l. _____

a. _____

b. _____

c. _____

d. _____

e. _____

f. _____

k. _____

m. _____

j. _____

h. _____

g. _____

k. _____

i. _____

l. _____

m. _____

Tarsals

▪ Chapter Four: **Articulations**

CLASSIFICATIONS OF ARTICULATIONS

Articulations are the joints that occur between bones. They can be classified either according to movement or by structure. Joints can be **immovable** (**synarthroses**), **semimovable** (**amphiarthroses**), or **freely movable** (**diarthroses**). The composition of joints can be fibrous, cartilaginous, or synovial.

FIBROUS JOINTS

Fibrous joints are held together by collagenous fibers, the same fibers that make up tendons and ligaments. These joints do not have a joint cavity. A **gomphosis** is a fibrous joint in which a round peg (the tooth) is held into a socket (the aveolar socket with the gingiva). Gomphoses are represented by the teeth held into the maxilla or the mandible. A **syndesmosis** is a fibrous joint like a gomphosis. This joint is found between the distal radius and ulna (or tibia and fibula) and is semimovable. The syndesmoses of the distal tibia and fibula are known as the posterior and transverse **tibiofibular ligaments**.

Color Guide: Color the **periodontal ligaments** in a dark color such as purple. This is the region where the tooth joins to the jaw. Color the **sagittal suture** in the skull and the close-up of the suture in purple as well. Color the **interosseous membrane** in a light blue and the tibiofibular ligaments in purple.

Answer Key

a. Gomphosis (peg suture)
b. Tooth
c. Alveolar socket
d. Gingiva
e. Alveolar ridge
f. Periodontal ligaments
g. Suture
h. Sagittal suture
i. Syndesmosis
j. Tibia
k. Fibula
l. Interosseous membrane
m. Posterior tibiofibular ligament
n. Transverse tibiofibular ligament

a. _____

b. _____

c. _____

d. _____

e. _____

f. _____

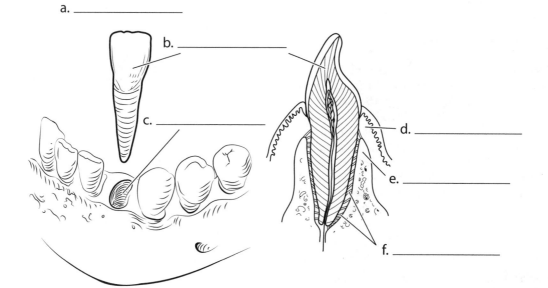

g. _____

h. _____

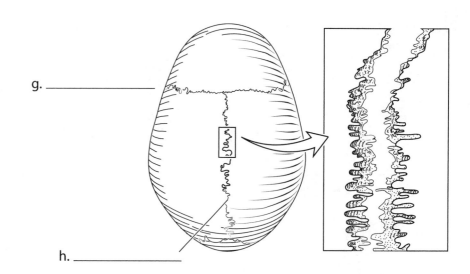

i. _____

j. _____

k. _____

l. _____

m. _____

n. _____

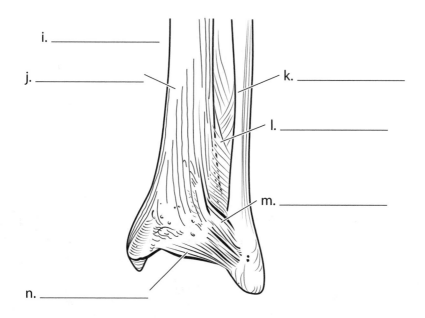

CARTILAGINOUS JOINTS

Cartilaginous joints are bones held together by cartilage and do not have a joint cavity. If the joint is held together by hyaline cartilage, it is known as a **synchondrosis**. If the cartilage is short, then the joint is immovable. An example of this kind of joint is an **epiphyseal plate** of the distal femur. If the cartilage is a little longer, then the joint is a semimovable joint. This is represented by the costal cartilage at the sternal-rib junction. A cartilaginous joint that is composed of fibrocartilage is known as a **symphysis** (symphyses plural). These are semimovable joints. Examples of symphyses are the pubic symphysis and **intervertebral discs**.

Color Guide: Color the cartilaginous joints using pink for the hyaline cartilage and yellow for the fibrocartilage.

Answer Key

a. Synchondrosis
b. First rib
c. Costal cartilage
d. Sternum
e. Femur
f. Epiphyseal plate
g. Symphysis
h. Intervertebral disc
i. Lumbar vertebra
j. Sacrum

LEARNING HINT

Epiphyseal plates are commonly known as "growth plates." They are found in most, if not all, of the long bones.

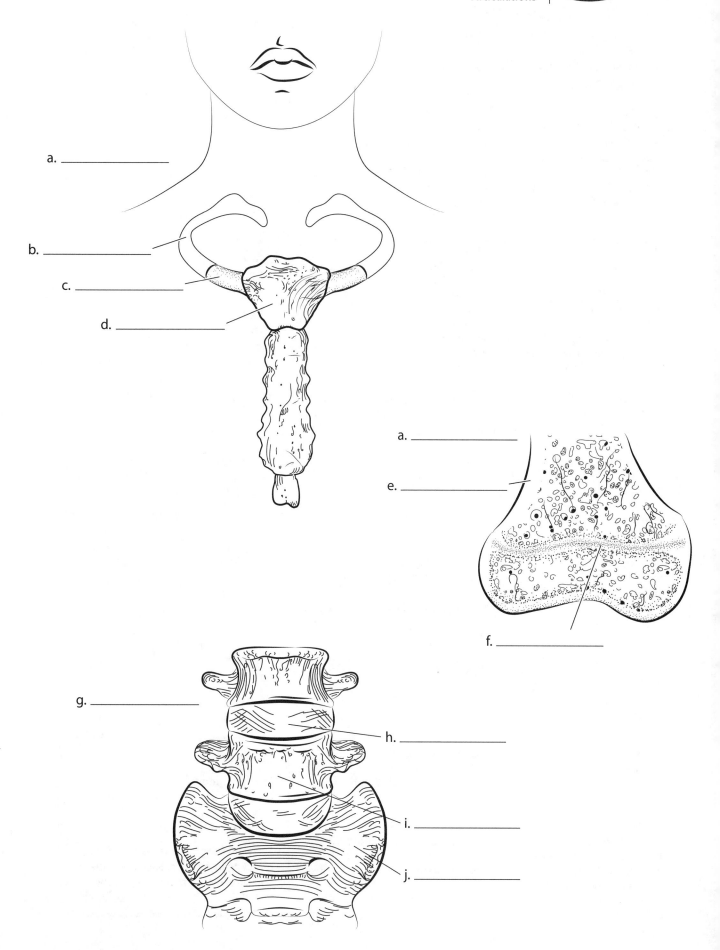

a. _____

b. _____

c. _____

d. _____

a. _____

e. _____

f. _____

g. _____

h. _____

i. _____

j. _____

SYNOVIAL JOINT, TENDON SHEATH, AND BURSA

Synovial joints are complex joints that are all freely movable. There are variations among the joints, but all synovial joints consist of two bones enclosed by a **joint capsule**, **articular cartilages**, and **synovial membranes** that secrete synovial fluid in the **synovial cavity**. Some synovial joints have fibrocartilage pads in the cavity called menisci (**meniscus** singular) within the sinovial cavity.

MODIFIED SYNOVIAL STRUCTURES— BURSAE AND TENDON SHEATHS

There are structures in the body that consist of synovial membranes and fibrous capsules. These are not synovial joints but are associated with joints. A **bursa** is one such structure. It is a fluid-filled sac with an internal synovial membrane that cushions tendons as they pass over bones. The bursa occurs between the tendon and the bone. Another structure is a **tendon sheath**. It also is composed of a synovial membrane and **fibrous sheath**, and it encloses tendons. The sheaths can provide lubrication to the tendon so it does not become irritated as it passes over bones or next to other tendons. In the fingers and toes, there are **annular** fibrous sheaths forming a ring (*annulus* from Latin for "ring") and **cruciate** fibrous sheaths (*cruciate* from Latin for "cross").

Color Guide: Color the articular cartilages of the synovial joint in pink and the synovial cavity in pale blue. Select other colors for the other parts of the synovial joint. Use pale yellow for the bones on this page and brown for the various parts of the tendon sheaths (digital sheaths in the illustration). Color the outside of the bursa green and the inside pale blue.

Answer Key

a. Bone
b. Joint capsule
c. Synovial cavity
d. Meniscus
e. Articular cartilage
f. Synovial membrane
g. Distal phalanx
h. Tendon insertion flexor digitorum profundus
i. Tendon flexor digitorum profundus muscle
j. Middle phalanx
k. Fibrous digital sheath cruciate part
l. Fibrous digital sheath annular part
m. Proximal phalanx
n. Synovial sheath
o. Tendon flexor digitorum superficialis
p. Achilles tendon
q. Bursa
r. Calcaneus

LEARNING HINT

The term **synovial** comes from the Greek words *syn* ("with") and *ovum* ("egg"), as the fluid resembles the texture of raw egg white.

The word **bursa** means "bag" or "purse," reflecting its function: Bursae are little purse-like sacs between tendons and bones.

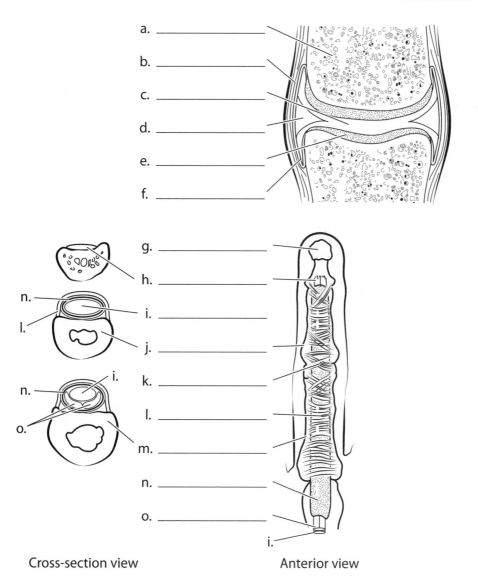

a. _____

b. _____

c. _____

d. _____

e. _____

f. _____

g. _____

h. _____

n. _____

l. _____

i. _____

j. _____

i. _____

k. _____

n. _____

l. _____

o. _____

m. _____

n. _____

o. _____

i. _____

Cross-section view   Anterior view

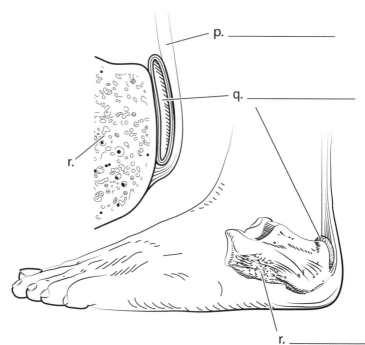

p. _____

q. _____

r. _____

r. _____

SPECIFIC SYNOVIAL JOINTS

Synovial joints are classified by what kind of motion they have. **Gliding joints** move in one plane like two sheets of glass sliding across one another. **Hinge joints** have angular movement like a door hinge. **Rotating (pivot) joints** move like a wheel of a car around an axle. **Condyloid (ellipsoidal) joints** move like hinges in two directions. In these joints, there is a convex surface and a concave surface. **Saddle joints** have two concave surfaces. They allow for greater movement than condyloid joints. **Ball-and-socket joints** allow for the greatest range of movement and are found in the shoulder and hip.

Color Guide: On the next two pages, color the bones in light yellow and the mechanical models in a darker yellow. Use purple to color where the bones meet to indicate the joints.

Answer Key

a. Superior articular process
b. Vertebrae
c. Inferior articular process
d. Gliding (plane)
e. Humerus
f. Ulna
g. Hinge
h. Radius
i. Rotating

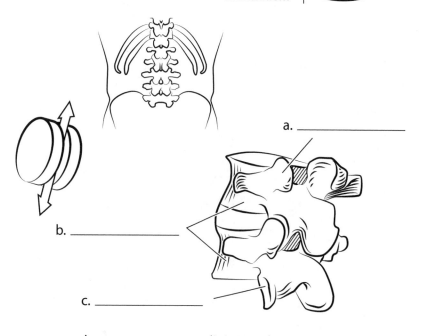

a. _____

b. _____

c. _____

d. _____ (joint type)

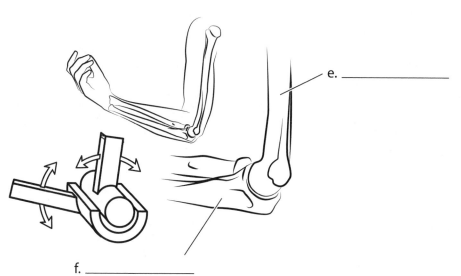

e. _____

f. _____

g. _____ (joint type)

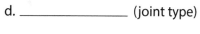

f. _____

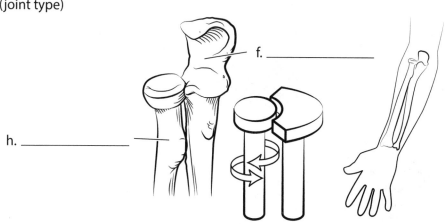

h. _____

i. _____ (joint type)

SPECIFIC SYNOVIAL JOINTS *(continued)*

Answer Key

a. Femur
b. Ball-and-socket
c. Radius
d. Carpals
e. Condyloid
f. Trapezium
g. First metacarpal
h. Saddle

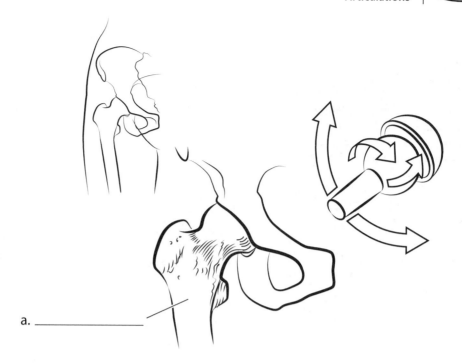

a. _____

b. _____ (joint type)

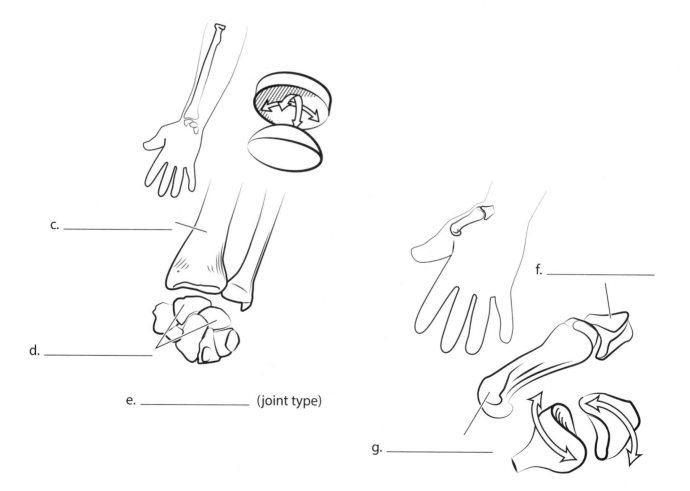

c. _____

d. _____

e. _____ (joint type)

f. _____

g. _____

h. _____ (joint type)

SPECIFIC JOINTS—
TEMPOROMANDIBULAR JOINT

Some joints of the body warrant special attention.
The **temporomandibular joint** or **jaw joint** is both a
gliding joint (moving side to side) and a **hinge joint**. The
condyle of the **mandible** articulates with the **mandibular
fossa** of the temporal bone. An **articular disc** is found in
the joint that decreases the stress on the joint. **Ligaments**
(dense connective tissue that joins bone to bone)
connect the mandible to the temporal bone.

Color Guide: Color the bones (temporal bone, mandible,
coronoid process, and **condylar process**) in light yellow.
Use blue for the capsule and pink for the articular disc.

Answer Key

a. Temporal bone
b. Coronoid process
c. Condylar process (cut)
d. Angle of mandible
e. Mandible
f. Articular disc
g. Capsule
h. Hinge
i. Hinge and glide

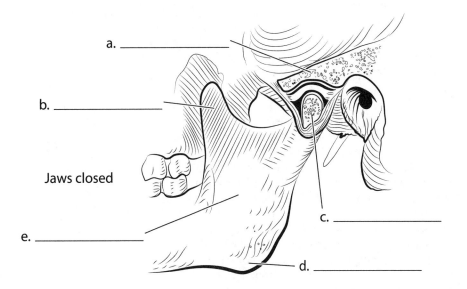

a. _____

b. _____

Jaws closed

e. _____

c. _____

d. _____

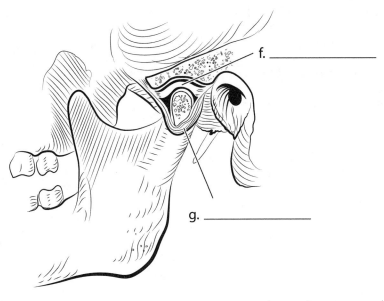

f. _____

Jaws opened slightly
Action:

h. _____

g. _____

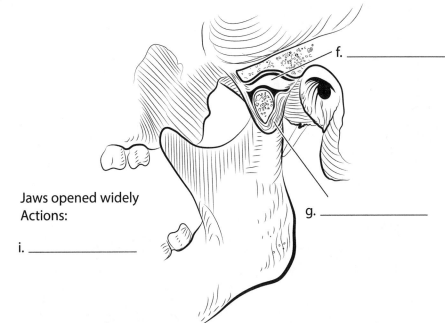

f. _____

Jaws opened widely
Actions:

i. _____

g. _____

SPECIFIC JOINTS—
HUMEROSCAPULAR AND
ACETABULOFEMORAL JOINTS

The **humeroscapular joint** or shoulder joint is a ball-and-socket joint that connects the **humerus** to the **glenoid cavity (fossa)** of the **scapula**. This joint has the greatest range of motion in the body and is covered by an **articular capsule**. Notice how the **biceps brachii tendon** attaches inside the articular capsule and is covered by a synovial sheath. The joint is deepened by the **glenoid labrum**, which is a **fibrocartilage** ring. This ring deepens the glenoid cavity while allowing the humerus greater range of motion than if the ring were made entirely of bone. There are numerous ligaments that connect the scapula to the humerus.

Another ball-and-socket joint is the **acetabulofemoral joint**. It is more stable than the humeroscapular joint because the socket is deeper, but it also has less range of motion. The acetabulofemoral joint also has an **acetabular labrum**, which deepens the hip socket, and numerous ligaments that join the **femur** to the hip. The articular capsule encloses the joint, and the **zona orbicularis** is a circular cluster of fibers that encircle the neck of the femur and help keep the femur in the socket.

Color Guide: Color the bones in light yellow. Use pink for the **articular cartilage** and blue for the articular capsule. For the glenoid labrum and acetabular labrum, use red. Use your choice of colors for the rest of the illustrations.

Answer Key

a.   Articular cartilage
b.   Tendon biceps brachii muscle
c.   Articular capsule
d.   Glenoid cavity (fossa)
e.   Synovial sheath
f.   Humerus
g.   Glenoid labrum
h.   Scapula
i.   Shoulder joint
j.   Zona orbicularis
k.   Acetabular labrum
l.   Femur
m.   Hip joint

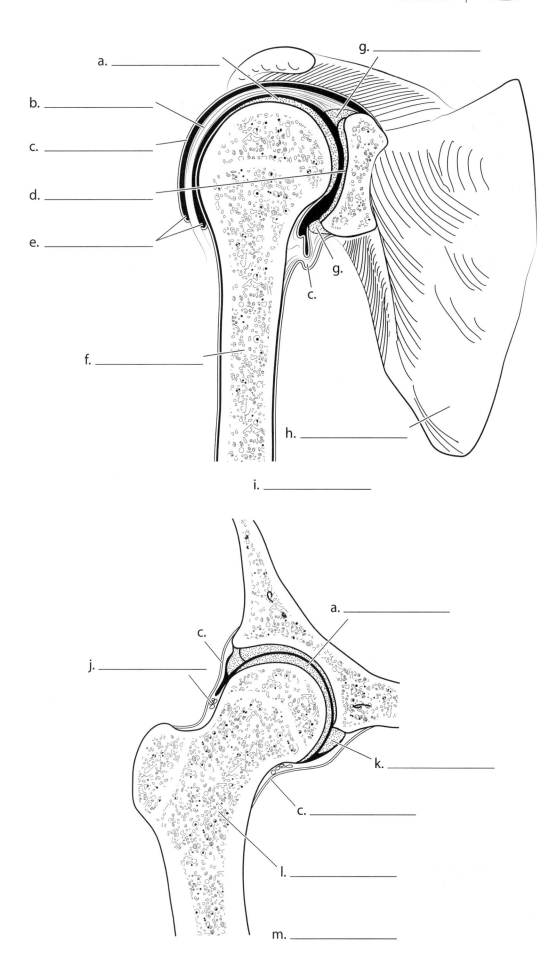

a. _____

g. _____

b. _____

c. _____

d. _____

e. _____

g. _____

c. _____

f. _____

h. _____

i. _____

a. _____

c. _____

j. _____

k. _____

c. _____

l. _____

m. _____

SPECIFIC JOINTS—
TIBIOFEMORAL JOINT

The **tibiofemoral joint** is the largest joint in the body and is particularly vulnerable to injury. The upper illustration is a superficial view of the anterior left knee, and the lower illustration is a deep view of the same knee. The joint is stabilized by the **patellar tendon**, the **medial (tibial)** and **(fibular) lateral collateral ligaments**, the **anterior** and **posterior cruciate ligaments**, and the **medial** and **lateral menisci**. (*Cruciate* means "cross," and it refers to the shape that the ligaments form.) Label the structures in the anterior view, with the **patella** in place in the upper illustration and with it reflected as seen in the lower illustration.

Color Guide: Color the bones a light yellow as in previous illustrations. Color the menisci in pink, and use a selection of colors for the various ligaments.

Answer Key

a. Femur
b. Patella
c. Fibular collateral ligament
d. Patellar tendon
e. Tibial collateral ligament
f. Fibula
g. Tibia
h. Posterior cruciate ligament
i. Anterior cruciate ligament
j. Lateral meniscus
k. Medial meniscus

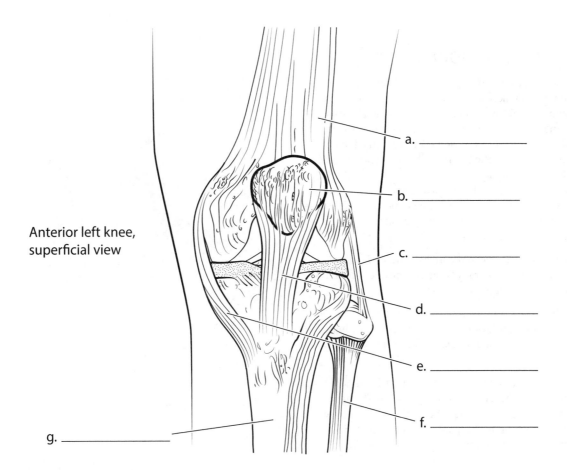

Anterior left knee,
superficial view

a. _____

b. _____

c. _____

d. _____

e. _____

f. _____

g. _____

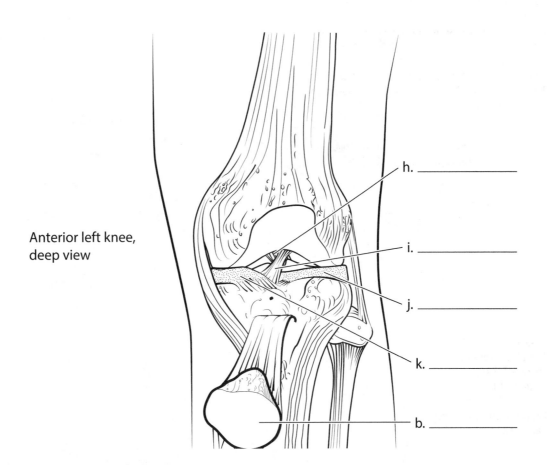

Anterior left knee,
deep view

h. _____

i. _____

j. _____

k. _____

b. _____

MOVEMENT AT JOINTS

A broad range of motion occurs at joints. These motions should be referenced with the body in anatomical position. **Flexion** of a joint is a decrease in the joint angle from the body in anatomic position. When the elbow is bent, the forearm is flexed. Most flexion takes place in a forward direction. The exception to this is the leg, where flexion results in the bending of the knee. **Extension** of the joint is when the joint is returned to anatomic position. **Hyperextension** is a condition where the joint is extended beyond anatomic position. Looking up at the ceiling is hyperextension of the head.

Abduction occurs when the limbs or head are moved in the coronal plane, laterally from the body. **Adduction** is the return of the limbs to the body.

Rotation is the movement of part of the body in a circular pattern. **Lateral rotation** is the movement of the body in a lateral direction, and **medial rotation** is in the opposite direction.

Specific terms describe the rotation of the hands and feet. **Supination** of the hand is lateral rotation of the hand as if to "hold a bowl of soup." **Pronation** is the reverse, or medial rotation of the hand. Starting in anatomical position, if you medially rotate your hands so the palms are facing posteriorly, you are pronating your hands. The same terms are used for lateral movement of the feet, but the feet behave a little differently. If you stand with your feet a bit apart from one another and touch your knees together, the medial part of the foot is bearing most of the weight. Meanwhile, the lateral side of the foot is somewhat lifted; this is pronation of the foot. If you move the foot so that the lateral side (outside) bears most of the weight, this is supination of the foot.

Color Guide: Select a preferred color for the figures, and use any color for the various movements at joints.

Answer Key

a. Hyperextension of the head
b. Flexion of the forearm
c. Extension of the forearm
d. Abduction of the arm
e. Adduction of the arm
f. Medial rotation of the thigh
g. Lateral rotation of the thigh

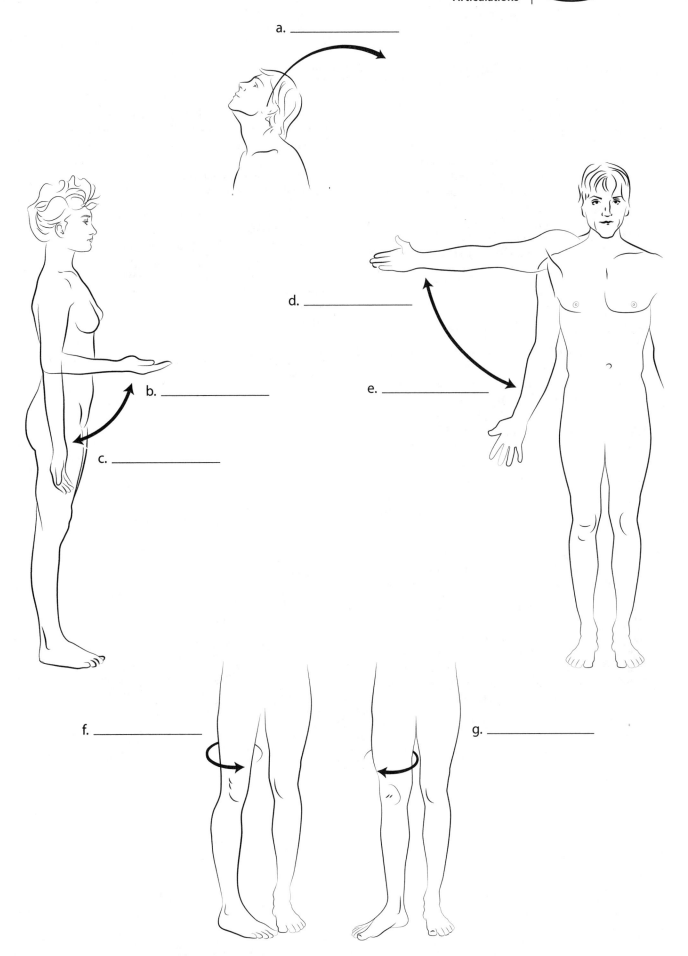

a. _____

b. _____

c. _____

d. _____

e. _____

f. _____

g. _____

▪ Chapter Five: **Muscular System**

OVERVIEW OF THE MUSCULAR SYSTEM

The skeletal muscles make up the largest organ system of the body by weight, comprising a little less than 40 percent of the body mass in lean individuals. There are approximately 640 muscles in the human body, most occurring in pairs. The next few pages are an overview of the superficial muscles of the body, followed by a special flashcard section of 96 muscles illustrated on heavy card stock. You can color these cards and tear them out of the book for study on the go.

ANTERIOR MUSCLES OF THE BODY

The **sternocleidomastoid** muscles originate from the sternum and insert on the mastoid process of the temporal bone. If you place the fingers of both your hands gently on each side of your neck, you can feel how this muscle contracts as you turn your head. The left sternocleidomastoid contracts when your head turns right, and the right sternocleidomastoid contracts when your head turns left.

The **deltoid** muscle, which drapes over the shoulder, is a major abductor of the arm. Because it has a broad origin (both anterior and posterior), it can both flex and extend the arm.

The **pectoralis major** is a muscle that originates in the medial region of the body and inserts on the humerus. The insertion on the humerus is covered by the deltoid.

The term **biceps brachii** translates from the Latin as "the two-headed muscle of the arm." It is the major muscle mass seen over the arm from the anterior view; nonetheless, it neither originates nor inserts on the humerus. The origin is on the scapula, and the insertion is on the radius. Because it crosses the shoulder joint, however, the biceps brachii does flex the arm.

The abdominal region of the body includes two readily observable superficial muscles. The **rectus abdominis** is the muscle that is visible as the "six-pack," and the **external oblique** is a broad abdominal muscle that not only contributes to lateral rotation of the trunk but also compresses the abdomen.

In the lower limb, the **sartorius** is a long, thin strip of muscle that runs from the lateral hip to the medial leg. The main muscles of the anterior thigh are the **quadriceps femoris**, which are four separate muscles that powerfully extend the leg, as in kicking a ball. The **tibialis anterior** muscle can be felt just lateral to the tibia. It dorsiflexes the foot, an action that decreases the angle between the shin and the top of the foot.

Color Guide: Select a different color for each muscle, and color along the length of each muscle.

Answer Key

a. Sternocleidomastoid
b. Pectoralis major
c. Deltoid
d. Biceps brachii
e. Rectus abdominis
f. External oblique
g. Sartorius
h. Quadriceps femoris
i. Tibialis anterior

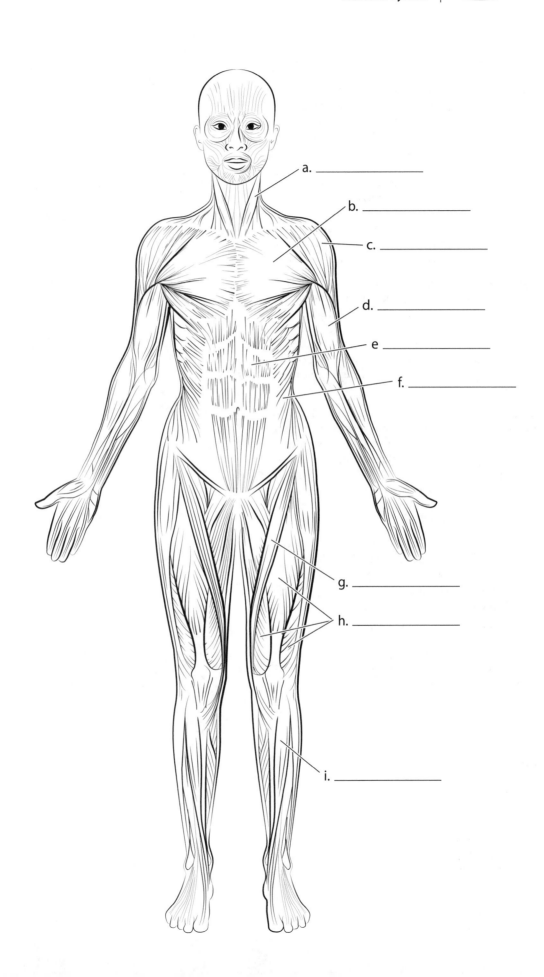

a. _____

b. _____

c. _____

d. _____

e. _____

f. _____

g. _____

h. _____

i. _____

POSTERIOR MUSCLES OF THE BODY

On the posterior side of the body are several muscles that are familiar to many people. Much of the superior back is covered by a pair of muscles forming a diamond shape: the **trapezius** muscles. The trapezius undertakes a few actions, among which are pulling the scapula, or shoulder blade, toward the midline and extending the head, as when looking up at the ceiling. The extensive **latissimus dorsi** muscle, which lies inferior to the trapezius, is another broad muscle. This a powerful extensor of the arm is known as the "swimmer's muscle" because it drives the stroke used in swimming freestyle. The **deltoid**, discussed with the anterior muscles, can also be seen from the back.

The major muscle on the posterior arm is the **triceps brachii**. It originates on the scapula and the humerus, and it inserts on the point of the elbow known as the olecranon process. Another posterior muscle of the upper limb is the **extensor digitorum**, whose name describes what it does—extend the digits. The tendons of this muscle are apparent on the back of the hand as they radiate out to the fingers.

The large **gluteus maximus** is one of the three pairs of gluteal muscles. The gluteus maximus is a strong extensor of the thigh, but its function is not so much for walking as for extending the thigh when climbing stairs or rising from a chair. The long muscles of the thigh seen in this figure are the **adductor magnus**, which adducts the thigh, and the **biceps femoris** and **semitendinosus**, both of which extend the thigh and flex the leg.

The **gastrocnemius** (GAS-trok-NEE-me-uz) is a muscle of the calf that flexes the leg and plantarflexes the foot when a person stands on tiptoes. The gastrocnemius and two other muscles insert on the calcaneus by way of the calcaneal tendon, also known as the Achilles tendon.

Many more muscles are in the Special Flashcard Section.

Color Guide: Select a different color for each muscle, and color along the length of each muscle.

Answer Key

a. Trapezius
b. Deltoid
c. Triceps brachii
d. Latissimus dorsi
e. Extensor digitorum
f. Gluteus maximus
g. Adductor magnus
h. Biceps femoris
i. Semitendinosus
j. Gastrocnemius

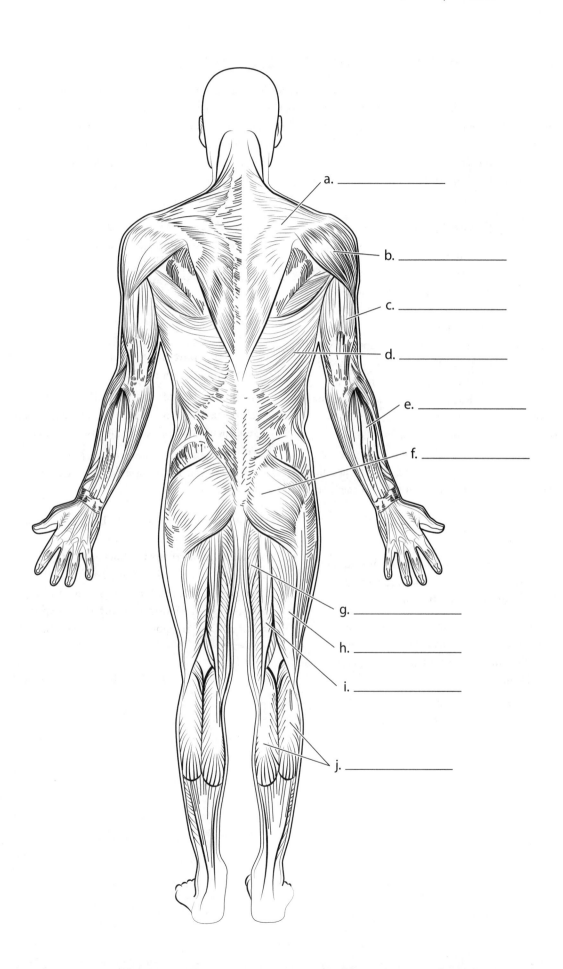

a. _____

b. _____

c. _____

d. _____

e. _____

f. _____

g. _____

h. _____

i. _____

j. _____

SPECIAL FLASHCARD SECTION—MUSCLES OF THE HUMAN BODY

The muscles of the body are numerous, and flashcards are a great tool to learn them. Following is a set of 96 muscles illustrated on heavy card stock, perforated for ease of use. You can color these cards and tear them out of the book for study on the go. The front of each card presents an illustration of the muscle, and the back gives the name of the muscle followed by its origin (abbreviated as "O"), insertion ("I"), and action ("A"). Skeletal muscles are controlled by nerves; this innervation is abbreviated ("N") on the back of the flashcards.

ORIGIN, INSERTION, ACTION

The **origin** of the muscle is the stable part of the muscle. The majority of muscles have origins that are superior, proximal, or medial to the insertion. There are only a few exceptions to this rule. The **insertion** of the muscle is the part of the muscle that has the greatest motion when the muscle contracts. In some cases, a muscle can move either the origin or the insertion, and you should learn the origins and insertions as presented. The **action** of a muscle is what the muscle does. Some muscles are flexors and decrease joint angles. Some are extensors, adductors, abductors, rotators, etc. The action of the muscle is every movement the muscle does.

MUSCLE NAMES

The muscles are named by different criteria, and understanding how they are named can help you to remember the muscle.

• Muscles can be named for their shape. The **trapezius** is a trapezoid-like muscle. The **rhomboideus** muscles are shaped like a rhombus.

• Muscles can be named by the number of heads they have. The **triceps** brachii has three heads.

• Muscles can be named by location. The **rectus abdominis** literally means "the straight muscle of the abdomen." The **tibialis anterior** is the front muscle on the tibia.

• Muscles can be named according to size. The teres **major** is the large muscle and the teres **minor** is the small muscle. (**Teres** means "round.")

• Some muscles are superficial while others are deep. The flexor digitorum **superficialis** is superficial to the flexor digitorum **profundus**.

• Muscles can also be named for their action. There are the **adductors**, **flexors**, **extensor** muscles, etc.

Muscles that cross joints of the body move those joints. The main muscle that causes the joint to move is called the **prime mover** or **agonist**. A muscle that helps the prime mover is called a **synergist**. A muscle that opposes the prime mover is called an **antagonist**. If both the prime mover and the antagonist contract, then the joint is **fixed**.

(continued on p. 109 after flashcards)

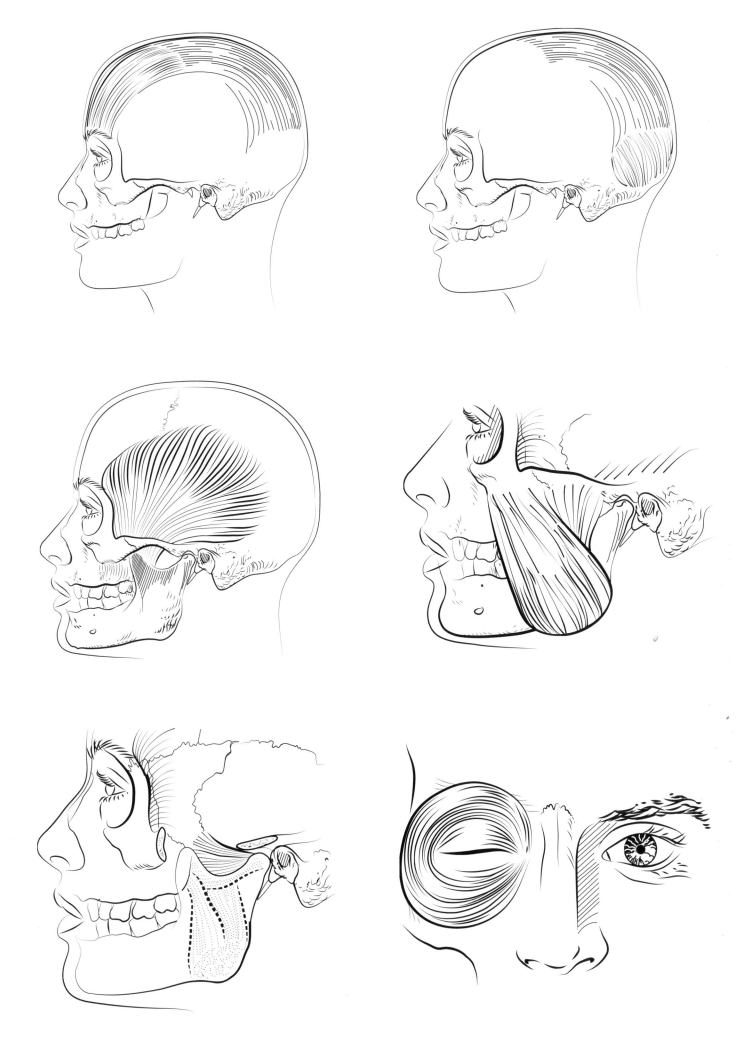

OCCIPITALIS

O: Occipital bone and temporal bone

I: Galea aponeurotica

A: Pulls scalp posteriorly

N: Facial nerve

FRONTALIS

O: Galea aponeurotica

I: Skin near eyebrows

A: Raises eyebrows, pulls scalp anteriorly

N: Facial nerve

MASSETER

O: Zygomatic arch

I: Ramus of mandible

A: Closes mandible

N: Trigeminal nerve, mandibular branch

TEMPORALIS

O: Temporal fossa

I: Coronoid process and ramus of the mandible

A: Closes mandible

N: Trigeminal nerve, mandibular branch

ORBICULARIS OCULI

O: Frontal bone and maxilla on medial orbit

I: Eyelid

A: Closes eye

N: Facial nerve

MEDIAL AND LATERAL PTERYGOIDS

O: Pterygoid processes of sphenoid bone

I: Ramus and condylar process of mandible on medial side

A: Lateral movement of mandible

N: Trigeminal nerve, mandibular branch

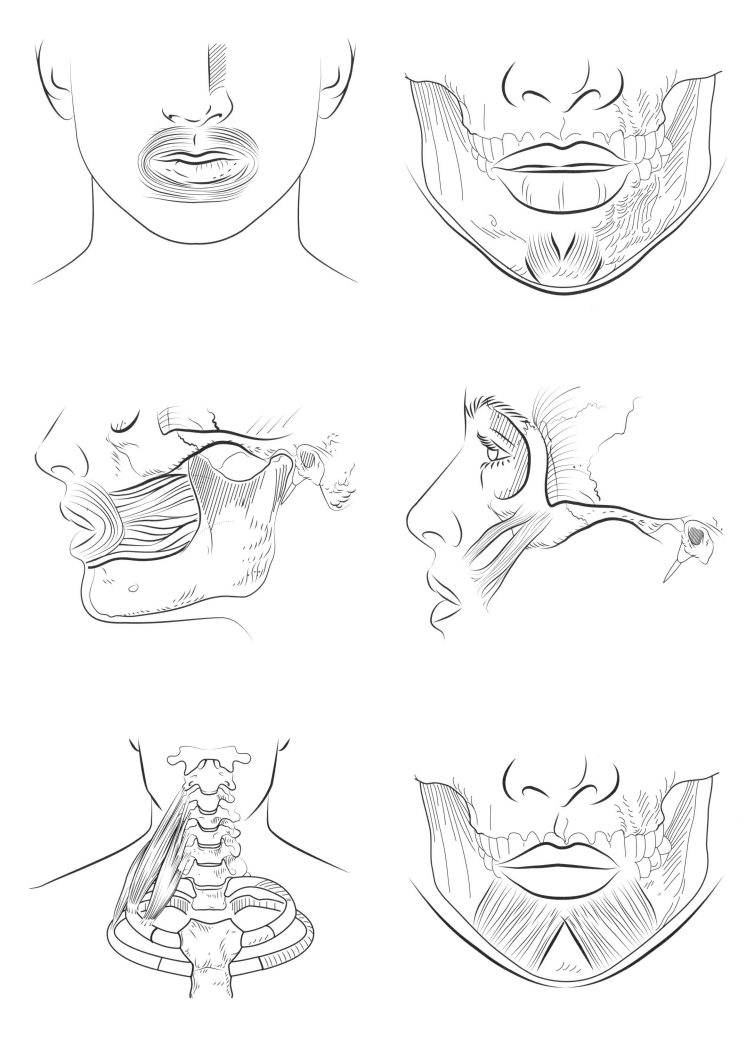

MENTALIS

O: Anterior, medial mandible

I: Skin of chin

A: Elevates lower lip

N: Facial nerve

ORBICULARIS ORIS

O: Muscles encircling mouth

I: Skin of lips

A: Closes mouth

N: Facial nerve

ZYGOMATICUS

O: Zygomatic bone

I: Angle of mouth

A: Elevates corners of mouth
   (in a smile or laugh)

N: Facial nerve

BUCCINATOR

O: Mandible and maxilla

I: Orbicularis oris

A: Tightens cheek

N: Facial nerve

DEPRESSOR LABII INFERIORIS

O: Inferior border of mandible

I: Skin of inferior lip and orbicularis
   oris muscle

A: Depresses lower lip

N: Facial nerve

SCALENUS

O: Transverse process of C2–C6

I: Ribs 1 and 2

A: Flexes and rotates neck, elevates first and
   second ribs

N: Spinal nerves C4–C8

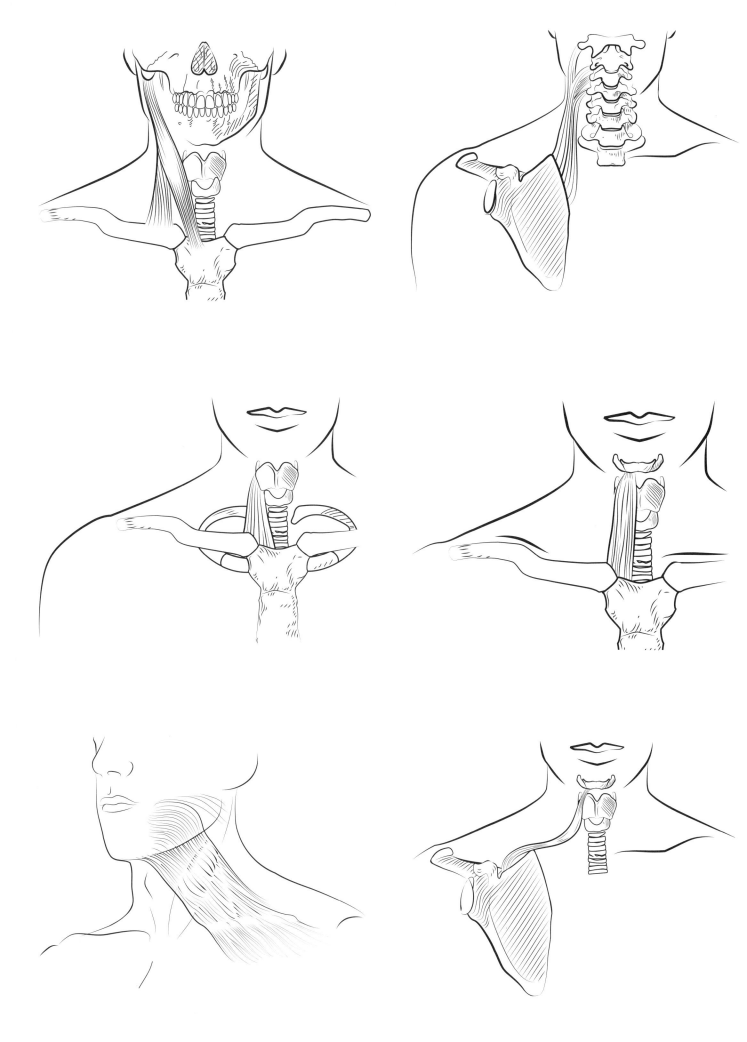

LEVATOR SCAPULAE

O: Transverse processes of C1–C4

I: Superior angle of scapula

A: Elevates scapula, rotates and abducts neck

N: Dorsal scapular nerve and spinal nerves C3–C5

STERNOCLEIDOMASTOID

O: Sternum and clavicle

I: Mastoid process

A: One: rotates and extends head,
   both: flexes neck

N: Accessory nerve

STERNOHYOID

O: Manubrium of sternum

I: Hyoid bone

A: Depresses hyoid bone

N: Spinal nerves C1–C3

STERNOTHYROID

O: Manubrium of sternum

I: Thyroid cartilage of larynx

A: Depresses thyroid cartilage

N: Spinal nerves C1–C3

OMOHYOID

O: Superior border of scapula

I: Hyoid bone

A: Depresses hyoid

N: Spinal nerves C1–C3

PLATYSMA

O: Fascia over pectoralis major and
   deltoid muscles

I: Mandible and skin inferior to lower lip

A: Depresses lower lip

N: Facial nerve

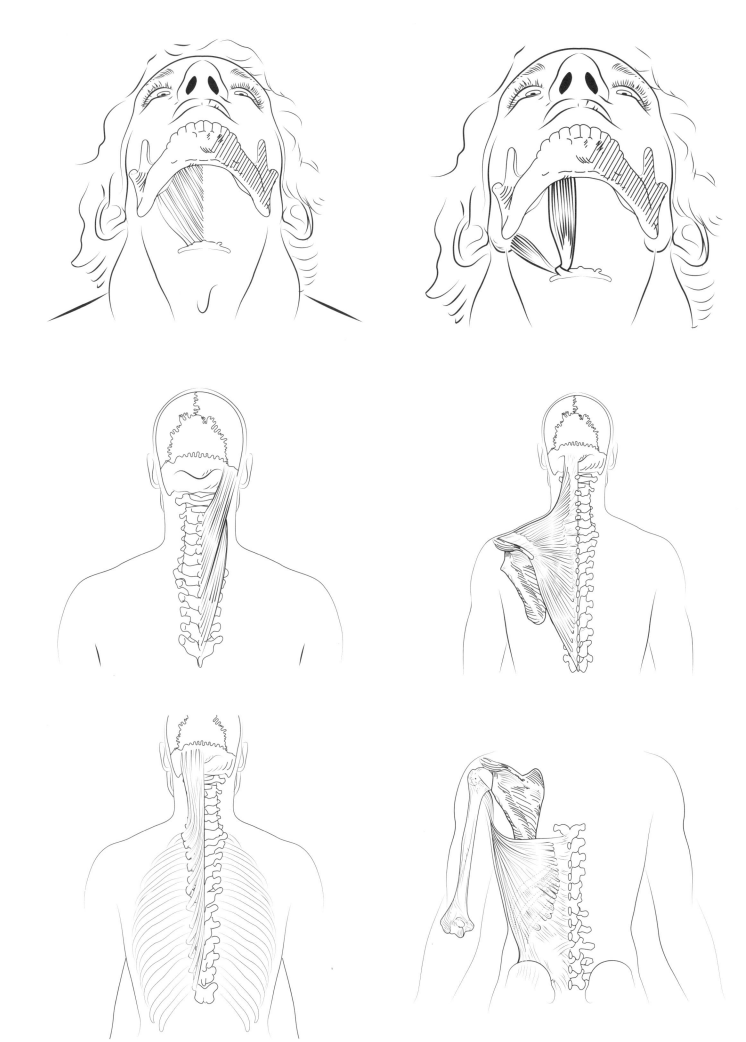

DIGASTRIC

O: Anterior, inferior mandible,
   mastoid notch of temporal bone

I: Hyoid bone

A: Protracts, retracts, and elevates hyoid,
   opens mandible

N: Trigeminal and facial nerves

MYLOHYOID

O: Inner margin of mandible

I: Hyoid bone

A: Elevates floor of oral cavity

N: Trigeminal nerve, mandibular branch

TRAPEZIUS

O: Occipital protuberance, ligamentum nuchae,
   C7–T12

I: Clavicle, acromion, and spine of scapula

A: Abducts and extends head, rotates and
   adducts scapula

N: Accessory nerve

SPLENIUS

O: Ligamentum nuchae, C7–T6

I: C2–C4, occipital bone, temporal bone

A: Extends and rotates head

N: Cervical nerves 2–6

LATISSIMUS DORSI

O: T7–T12, L1–L5, sacrum, iliac crest,
   ribs 10–12

I: Intertubercular groove of humerus

A: Adducts, extends, and medially rotates arm,
   pulls shoulder inferiorly

N: Thoracodorsal nerve

SEMISPINALIS

O: C4–T12

I: Occipital bone, T1–T4

A: Extends head, rotates vertebral column

N: Cervical and thoracic nerves

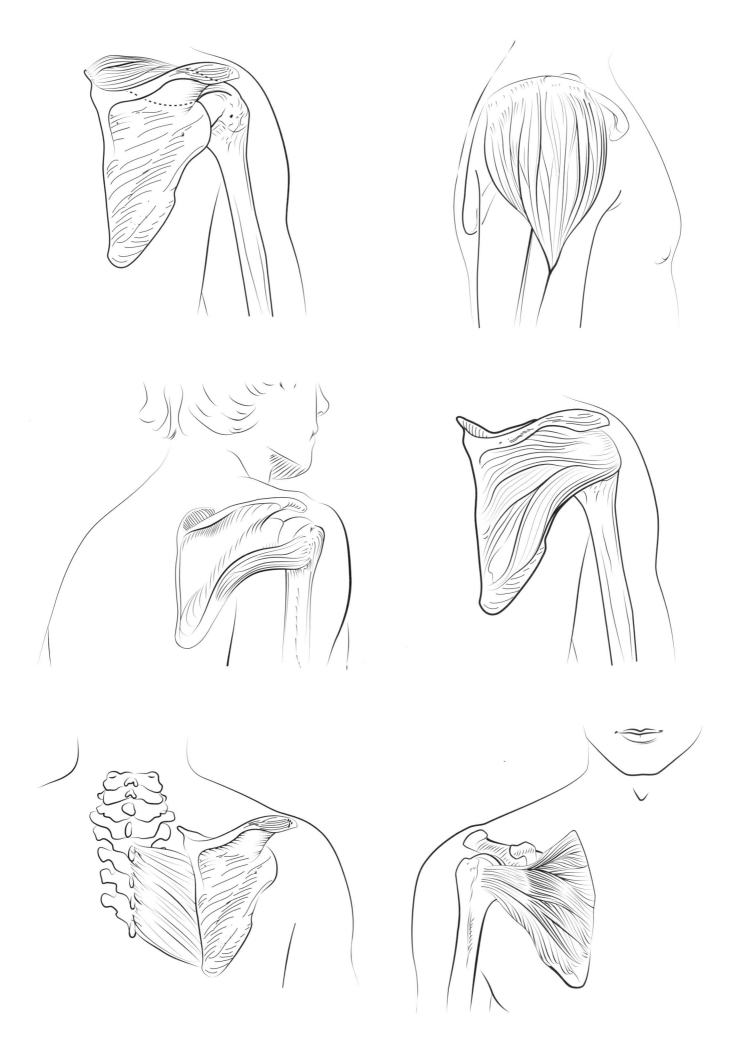

DELTOID

O: Clavicle, acromion, and spine of scapula

I: Deltoid tuberosity

A: Abducts, flexes, extends medially, and laterally rotates arm

N: Axillary nerve

SUPRASPINATUS

O: Supraspinous fossa

I: Greater tubercle of humerus

A: Abducts arm, stabilizes shoulder

N: Suprascapular nerve

INFRASPINATUS

O: Infraspinous fossa

I: Greater tubercle of humerus

A: Extends, laterally rotates arm, stabilizes shoulder

N: Suprascapular nerve

TERES MINOR

O: Axillary border of scapula

I: Greater tubercle of humerus

A: Extends, laterally rotates, adducts arm, stabilizes shoulder

N: Axillary nerve

SUBSCAPULARIS

O: Subscapular fossa

I: Lesser tubercle of humerus

A: Extends, medially rotates arm, stabilizes shoulder

N: Subscapular nerve

RHOMBOIDEUS MAJOR

O: T2–T5

I: Inferior, medial border of scapula

A: Adducts scapula

N: Dorsal scapular nerve

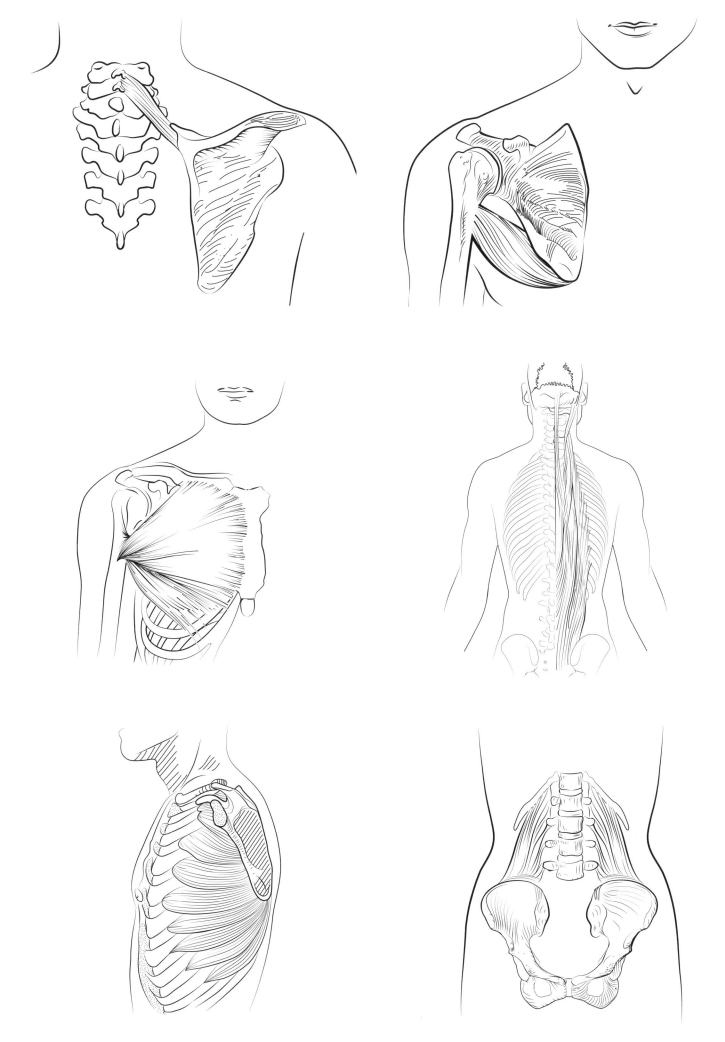

TERES MAJOR

O: Axillary border of scapula

I: Crest of lesser tubercle of humerus

A: Extends, adducts, medially rotates arm

N: Subscapular nerve

RHOMBOIDEUS MINOR

O: Ligamentum nuchae, C6–C7

I: Superior, medial border of scapula

A: Adducts scapula

N: Dorsal scapular nerve

ERECTOR SPINAE (SPINALIS, LONGISSIMUS, ILIOCOSTALIS) AND MULTIFIDUS

O: Vertebral column, ilium, sacrum, ribs

I: Ribs, vertebral column, occipital bone, temporal bone

A: Rotates and extends vertebral column and head

N: Cervical, thoracic, and lumbar nerves

PECTORALIS MAJOR

O: Clavicle, sternum, and ribs 1–7

I: Crest of greater tubercle of humerus

A: Adducts, flexes, and rotates arm medially

N: Pectoral nerve

QUADRATUS LUMBORUM

O: Iliac crest, lower lumbar vertebrae

I: T12, L1–L4, rib 12

A: Abducts vertebral column, depresses rib 12

N: T12, L1–L4

SERRATUS ANTERIOR

O: Ribs 1–8 or 9

I: Vertebral border of scapula

A: Abducts scapula

N: Long thoracic nerve

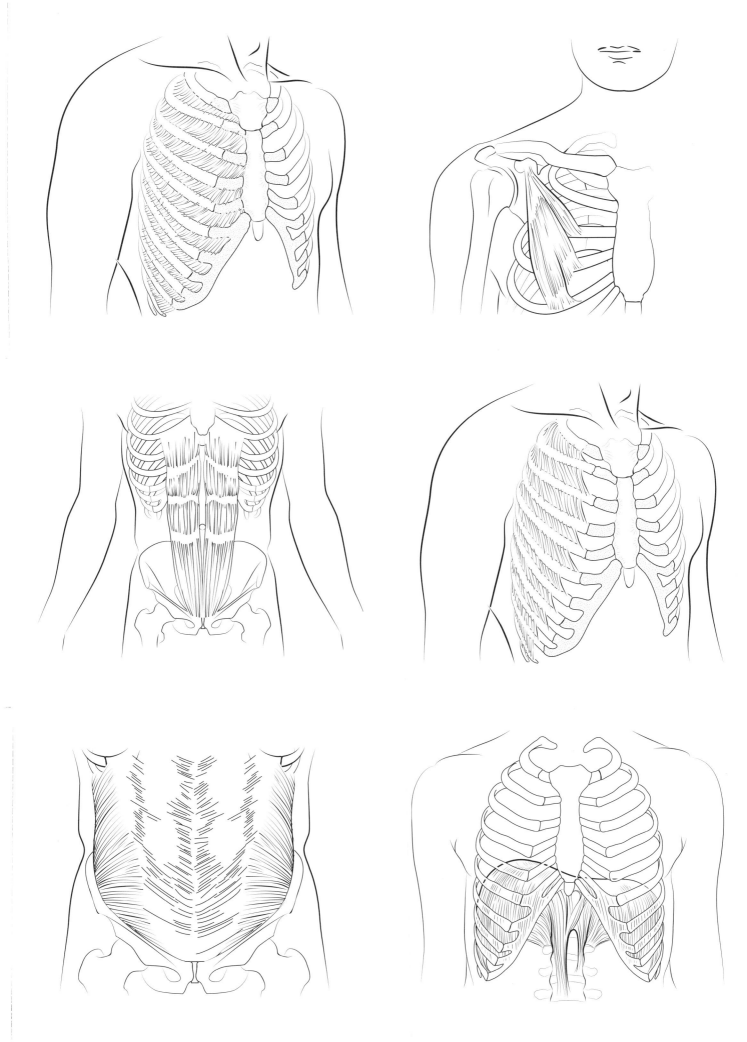

PECTORALIS MINOR

O: Ribs 3–5

I: Coracoid process of scapula

A: Depresses scapula, elevates ribs 3–5

N: Pectoral nerve

INTERNAL INTERCOSTALIS

O: Inferior margin of ribs 1–11

I: Superior margin of ribs 2–12

A: Depresses ribs (decreases thoracic volume)

N: Intercostal nerves

EXTERNAL INTERCOSTALIS

O: Inferior margin of ribs 1–11

I: Superior margin of ribs 2–12

A: Elevates ribs (increases thoracic volume)

N: Intercostal nerves

RECTUS ABDOMINIS

O: Symphysis pubis and pubic crest

I: Cartilages of ribs 5–7 and xiphoid process

A: Flexes lumbar vertebrae, compresses abdomen

N: Intercostal nerves

DIAPHRAGM

O: Xiphoid process, ribs 10–12, lumbar vertebrae

I: Central tendon

A: Inspiration

N: Phrenic nerve

INTERNAL OBLIQUE

O: Inguinal ligament, iliac crest

I: Linea alba, inferior 4 ribs

A: Compresses abdomen, laterally rotates trunk

N: Intercostal nerves, L1

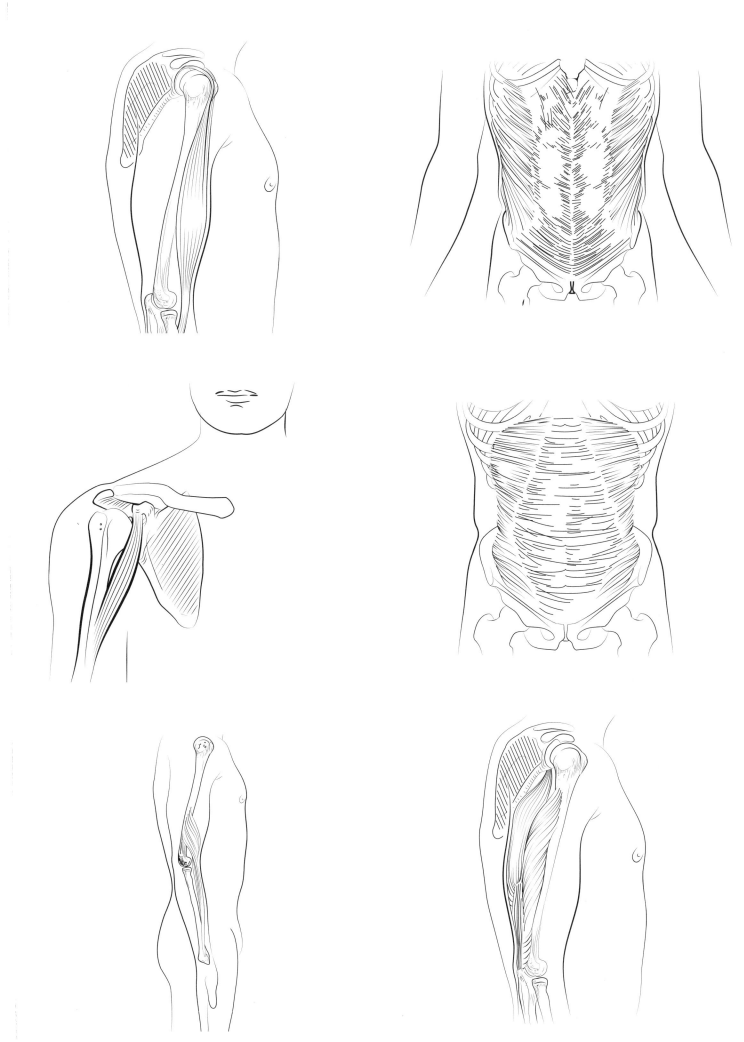

EXTERNAL OBLIQUE

O: Ribs 5–12

I: Iliac crest, inguinal ligament, linea alba

A: Compresses abdomen, laterally rotates trunk

N: Intercostal nerves, L1

BICEPS BRACHII

O: Supraglenoid tubercle, coracoid process

I: Radial tuberosity

A: Flexes arm, flexes and laterally rotates forearm (supinates hand)

N: Musculocutaneous nerve

TRANSVERSUS ABDOMINIS

O: Iliac crest, inguinal ligament, ribs 7–12

I: Linea alba, pubis

A: Compresses abdomen, laterally rotates trunk

N: Intercostal nerves, L1

CORACOBRACHIALIS

O: Coracoid process

I: Medial shaft of humerus

A: Adducts and flexes arm

N: Musculocutaneous nerve

TRICEPS BRACHII

O: Infraglenoid tuberosity of scapula, posterior surface of humerus

I: Olecranon process

A: Adducts arm, extends arm and forearm

N: Radial nerve

BRACHIORADIALIS

O: Lateral supracondylar ridge of humerus

I: Styloid process of radius

A: Flexes forearm

N: Radial nerve

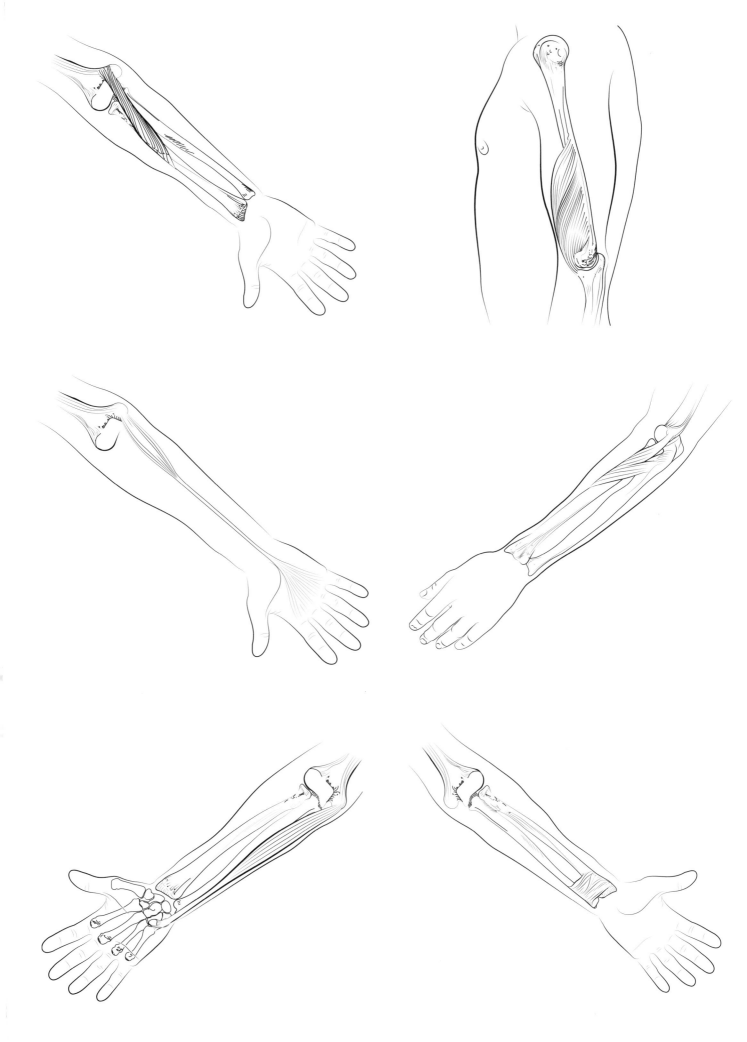

BRACHIALIS

O: Anterior, distal humerus

I: Coronoid process of ulna

A: Flexes forearm

N: Radial and musculocutaneous nerve

PRONATOR TERES

O: Medial epicondyle of humerus, coronoid process of ulna

I: Lateral radius

A: Flexes and medially rotates forearm (pronates hand)

N: Median nerve

SUPINATOR

O: Lateral epicondyle of humerus, proximal ulna

I: Proximal shaft of radius

A: Supinates hand

N: Radial nerve

PALMARIS LONGUS

O: Medial epicondyle of humerus

I: Palmar aponeurosis

A: Flexes hand

N: Median nerve

PRONATOR QUADRATUS

O: Anterior, distal ulna

I: Anterior, distal radius

A: Medially rotates forearm (pronates hand)

N: Median nerve

FLEXOR CARPI ULNARIS

O: Medial epicondyle of humerus olecranon and proximal ulna

I: Pisiform, hamate, metacarpal 5

A: Flexes and adducts hand

N: Ulnar nerve

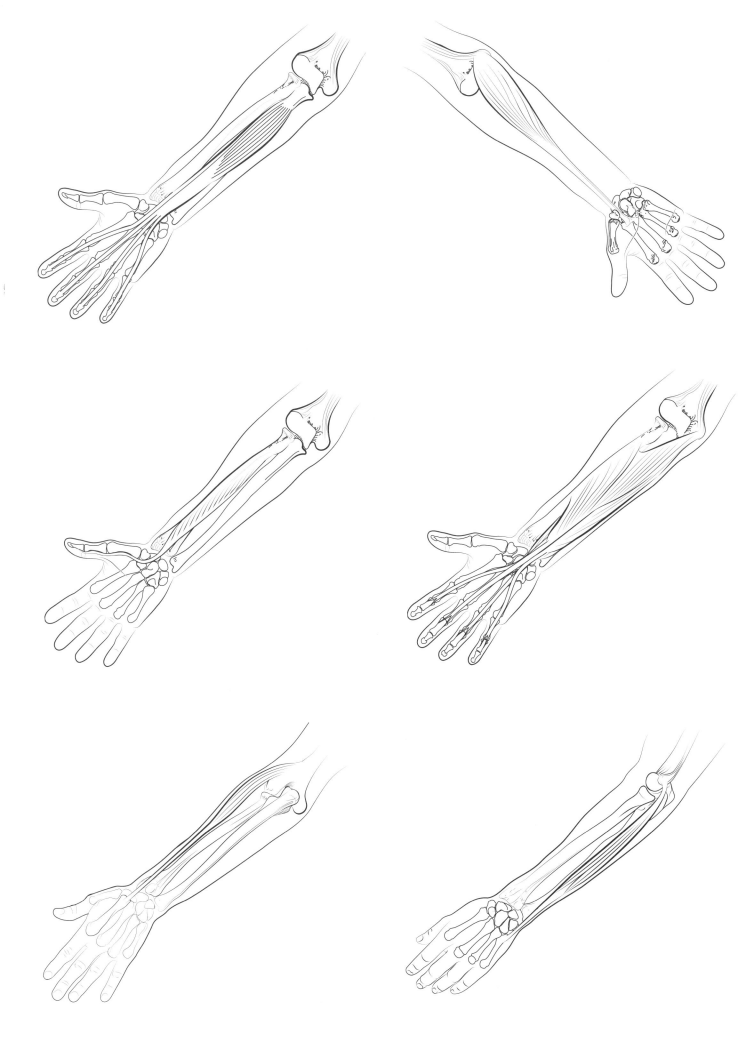

FLEXOR CARPI RADIALIS

O: Medial epicondyle of humerus

I: Metacarpals 2 and 3

A: Flexes and abducts hand

N: Median nerve

FLEXOR DIGITORUM PROFUNDUS

O: Proximal ulna, interosseous membrane

I: Anterior distal phalanges of digits 2–5

A: Flexes phalanges 2–5, flexes hand

N: Median and ulnar nerves

FLEXOR DIGITORUM SUPERFICIALIS

O: Medial epicondyle of humerus, coronoid process of ulna, proximal shaft of radius

I: Middle phalanges of digits 2–5

A: Flexes proximal and middle phalanges of digits 2–5, flexes hand

N: Median nerve

FLEXOR POLLICIS LONGUS

O: Anterior aspect of radius and interosseous membrane

I: Distal phalanx of thumb (pollex)

A: Flexes thumb

N: Median nerve

EXTENSOR CARPI ULNARIS

O: Lateral epicondyle of humerus, posterior ulna

I: Metacarpal 5

A: Extends and adducts hand

N: Radial nerve

EXTENSOR CARPI RADIALIS LONGUS

O: Lateral supracondylar ridge of humerus

I: Metacarpal 2

A: Extends and abducts hand

N: Radial nerve

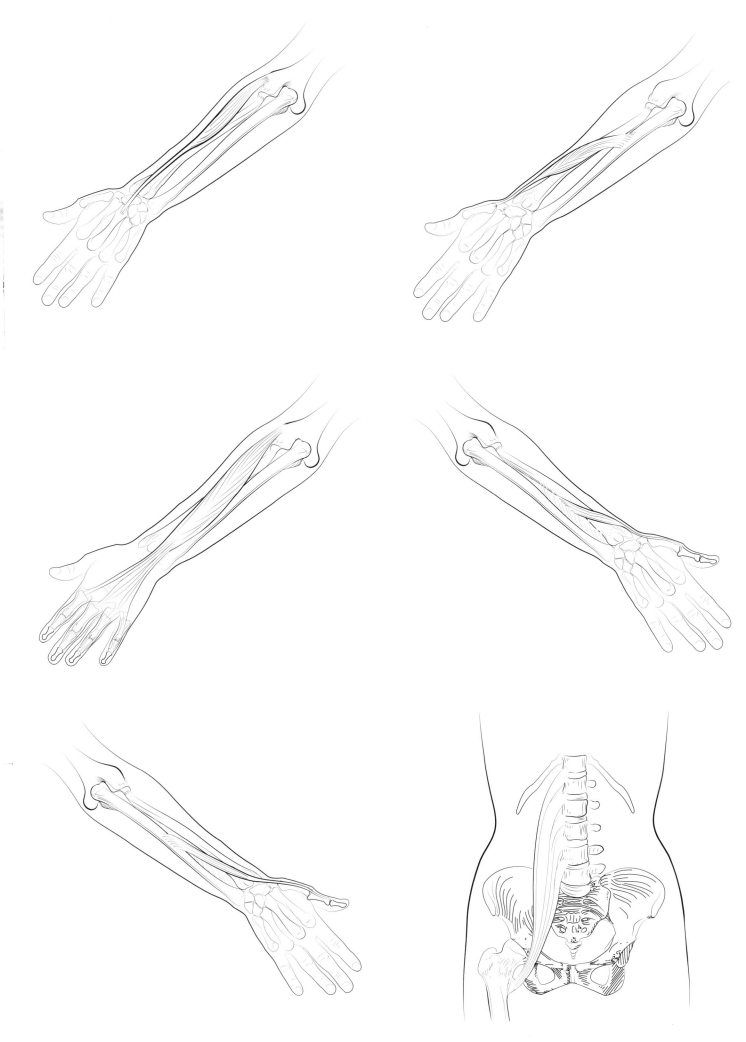

ABDUCTOR POLLICIS LONGUS

O: Posterior radial and ulnar surface, interosseous membrane

I: Metacarpal 1

A: Abducts and extends thumb

N: Radial nerve

EXTENSOR CARPI RADIALIS BREVIS

O: Lateral epicondyle of humerus

I: Metacarpal 3

A: Extends and abducts hand

N: Radial nerve

EXTENSOR POLLICIS BREVIS

O: Posterior radius, interosseous membrane

I: Proximal phalanx of thumb (pollex)

A: Extends thumb

N: Radial nerve

EXTENSOR DIGITORUM

O: Lateral epicondyle of humerus

I: Middle and distal phalanges of digits 2–5

A: Extends all phalanges of digits 2–5, extends hand

N: Radial nerve

PSOAS MAJOR

O: T12, L1–L5

I: Lesser trochanter of femur

A: Flexes thigh and lumbar vertebrae

N: Spinal nerves L1–L4

EXTENSOR POLLICIS LONGUS

O: Posterior ulna, interosseous membrane

I: Distal phalanx of thumb (pollex)

A: Extends thumb

N: Radial nerve

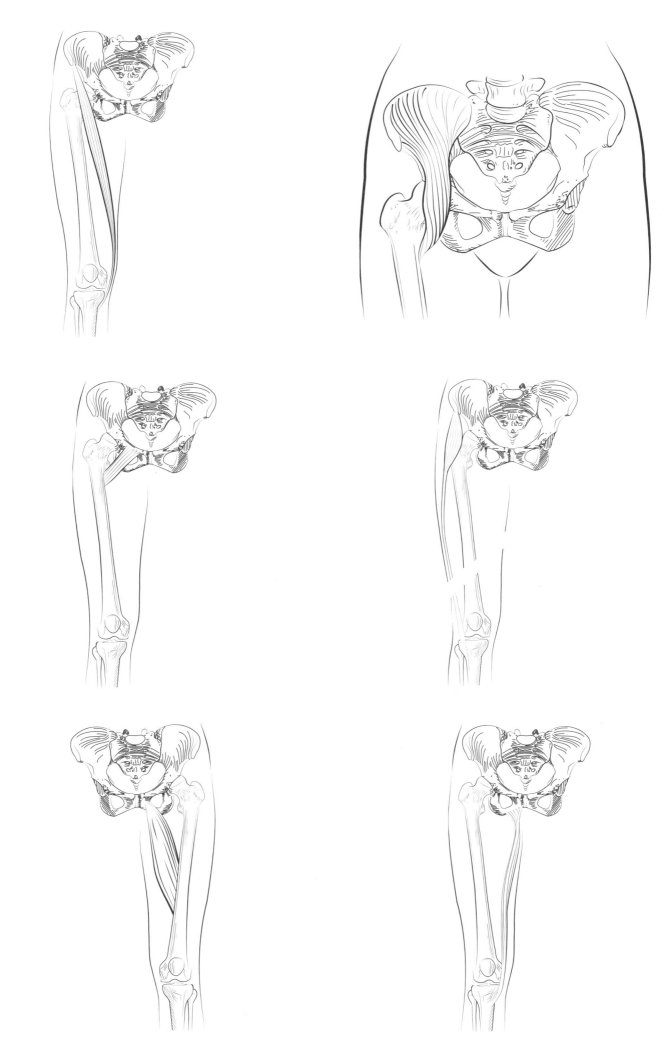

ILIACUS

O: Iliac fossa, sacrum

I: Lesser trochanter of femur

A: Flexes thigh

N: Spinal nerves L2–L3, femoral nerve

SARTORIUS

O: Anterior superior iliac spine

I: Medial side of tibial tuberosity

A: Flexes and laterally rotates thigh, flexes leg

N: Femoral nerve

TENSOR FASCIAE LATAE

O: Anterior superior iliac spine

I: Lateral condyle of tibia by the iliotibial band

A: Flexes, medially rotates, and abducts thigh

N: Gluteal nerve

PECTINEUS

O: Pubis

I: Proximal, posterior femur

A: Adducts and laterally rotates thigh

N: Femoral and obturator nerve

GRACILIS

O: Pubis

I: Proximal portion of medial tibia

A: Adducts thigh, flexes leg

N: Obturator nerve

ADDUCTOR LONGUS

O: Pubis

I: Middle linea aspera of femur

A: Adducts and laterally rotates thigh

N: Obturator nerve

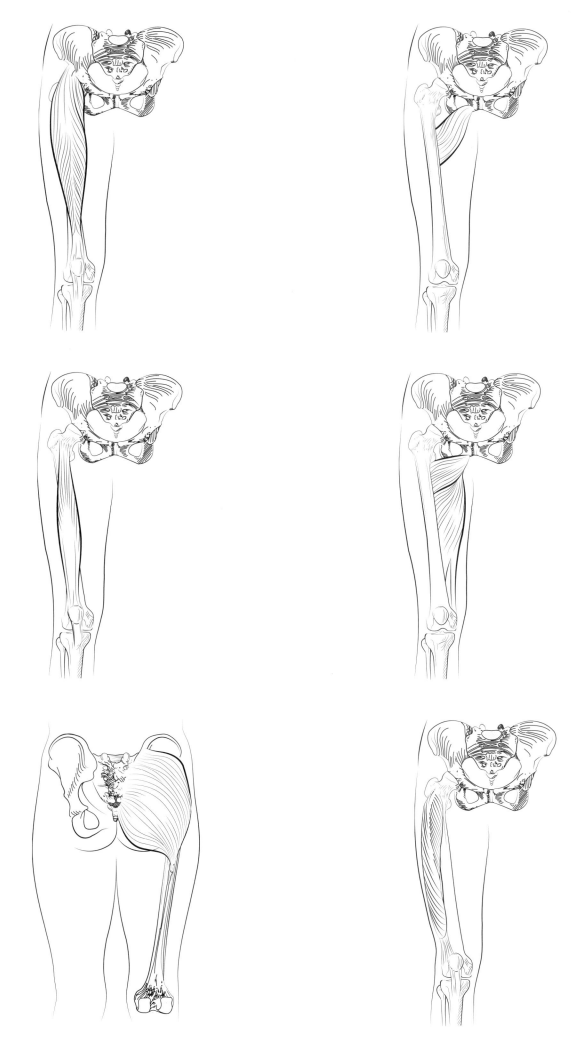

ADDUCTOR BREVIS

O: Pubis

I: Proximal linea aspera of femur

A: Adducts and laterally rotates thigh

N: Obturator nerve

RECTUS FEMORIS

O: Anterior inferior iliac spine

I: Tibial tuberosity

A: Flexes thigh, extends leg

N: Femoral nerve

ADDUCTOR MAGNUS

O: Ischium and pubis

I: Linea aspera and adductor tubercle of femur

A: Adducts, flexes, extends, and laterally
   rotates thigh

N: Obturator and tibial nerve

VASTUS INTERMEDIUS

O: Anterior and lateral part of femur

I: Tibial tuberosity

A: Extends leg

N: Femoral nerve

VASTUS LATERALIS

O: Greater trochanter and linea aspera of femur

I: Tibial tuberosity

A: Extends leg

N: Femoral nerve

GLUTEUS MAXIMUS

O: Lateral surface of ilium, sacrum, coccyx

I: Lateral condyle of tibia by lateral fascia,
   gluteal tuberosity of femur

A: Extends, abducts, and laterally rotates thigh

N: Gluteal nerve

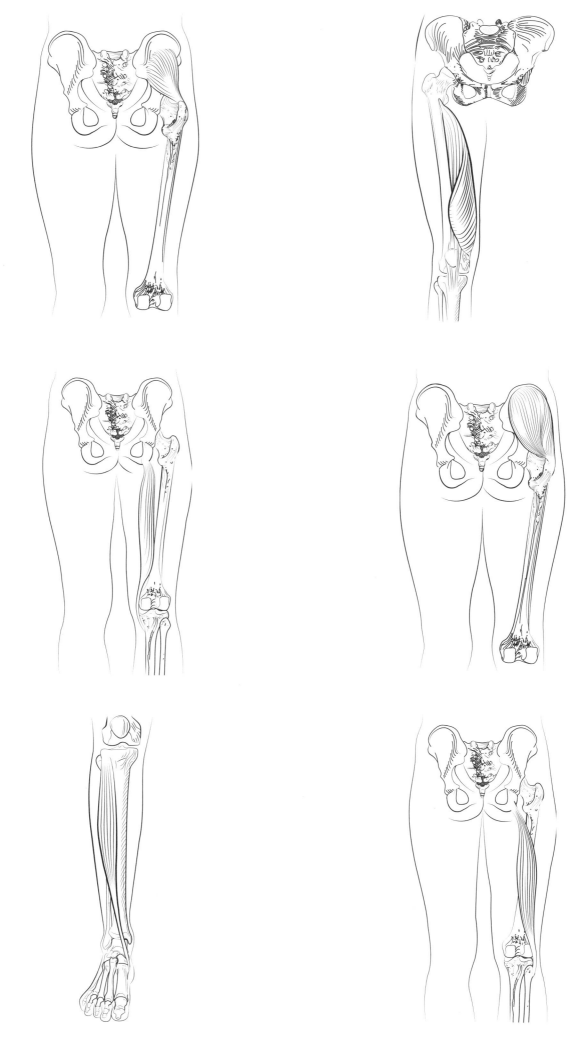

VASTUS MEDIALIS

O: Linea aspera of femur

I: Tibial tuberosity

A: Extends leg

N: Femoral nerve

GLUTEUS MINIMUS

O: Outer ilium

I: Greater trochanter of femur

A: Medially rotates and abducts thigh

N: Gluteal nerve

GLUTEUS MEDIUS

O: Outer ilium

I: Greater trochanter of femur

A: Medially rotates and abducts thigh

N: Gluteal nerve

SEMITENDINOSUS

O: Ischial tuberosity

I: Medial tibia near tibial tuberosity

A: Extends thigh, flexes and medially rotates leg

N: Tibial nerve

BICEPS FEMORIS

O: Ischial tuberosity, distal linea aspera of femur

I: Head of fibula, lateral tibia

A: Extends thigh, flexes and laterally rotates leg

N: Tibial and fibular nerve

TIBIALIS ANTERIOR

O: Lateral tibia

I: First metatarsal and medial cuneiform

A: Dorsiflexes and inverts foot

N: Fibular nerve

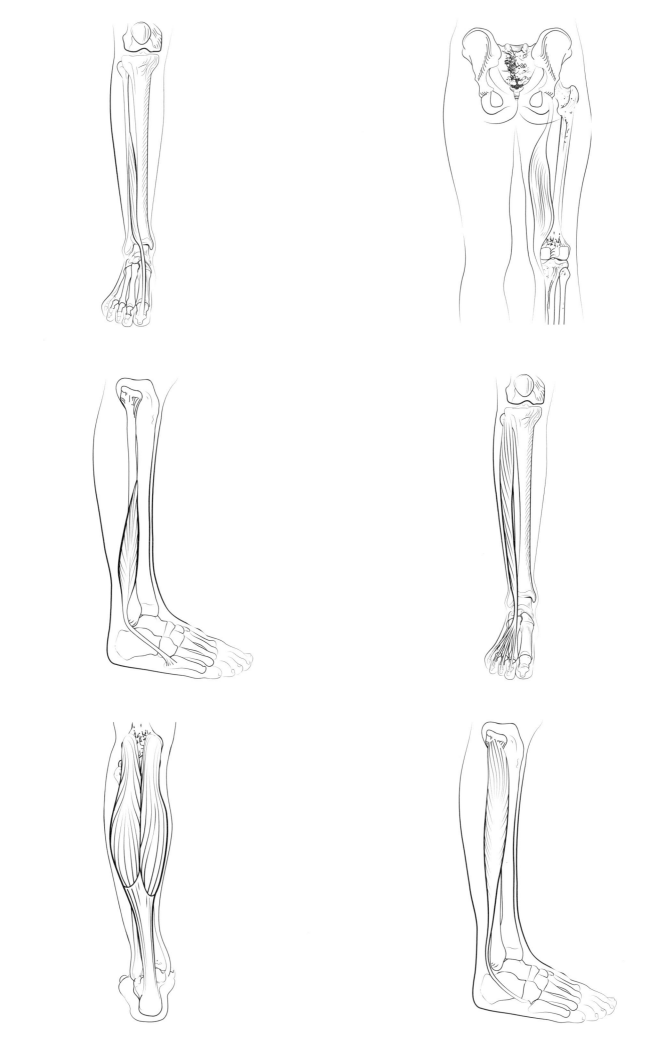

SEMIMEMBRANOSUS

O: Ischial tuberosity

I: Medial tibial condyle

A: Extends thigh, flexes and medially rotates leg

N: Tibial nerve

EXTENSOR HALLUCIS LONGUS

O: Medial shaft of fibula, interosseous membrane

I: Distal phalanx of hallux (first digit)

A: Extends hallux, dorsiflexes and inverts foot

N: Fibular nerve

EXTENSOR DIGITORUM LONGUS

O: Lateral tibial condyle, shaft of fibula

I: Middle and distal phalanges of digits 2–5

A: Extends digits 2–5, dorsiflexes and everts foot

N: Fibular nerve

FIBULARIS BREVIS

O: Fibula

I: Metatarsal 5

A: Plantar flexes and everts foot

N: Fibular nerve

FIBULARIS LONGUS

O: Proximal fibula, lateral condyle of tibia

I: First metatarsal, medial cuneiform

A: Plantar flexes and everts foot

N: Fibular nerve

GASTROCNEMIUS

O: Lateral and medial condyles of femur

I: Calcaneus

A: Flexes leg, plantar flexes foot

N: Tibial nerve

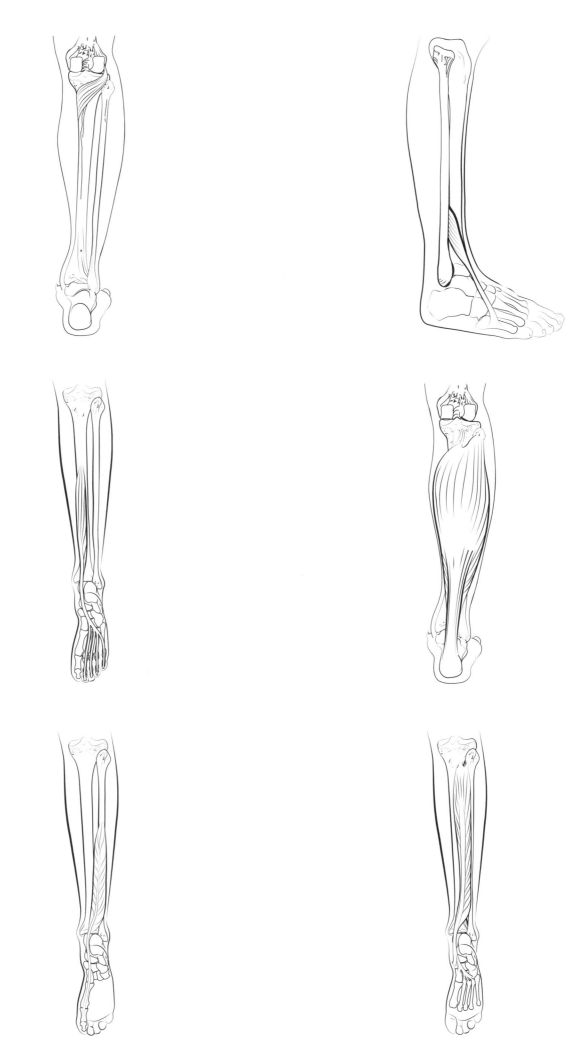

FIBULARIS TERTIUS

O: Distal fibula, interosseous membrane

I: Superior aspect of metatarsal 5

A: Dorsiflexes and everts foot

N: Fibular nerve

POPLITEUS

O: Lateral condyle of femur

I: Proximal tibia

A: Flexes and medially rotates leg

N: Tibial nerve

SOLEUS

O: Posterior tibia and fibula

I: Calcaneus

A: Plantar flexes foot

N: Tibial nerve

FLEXOR DIGITORUM LONGUS

O: Posterior tibia

I: Distal phalanges of digits 2–5

A: Flexes toes, plantar flexes and inverts foot

N: Tibial nerve

TIBIALIS POSTERIOR

O: Posterior tibia and fibula

I: Metatarsals 2–4, navicular, cuneiforms, and cuboid

A: Plantar flexes and inverts foot

N: Tibial nerve

FLEXOR HALLUCIS LONGUS

O: Middle fibula

I: Distal phalanx of hallux

A: Flexes hallux, plantar flexes and inverts foot

N: Tibial nerve

MUSCLE GROUPS

Certain muscles function together, as a group. For example, the **rotator cuff** (**musculotendinous cuff**) muscles stabilize the shoulder joint. These are the supraspinatus, the infraspinatus, the teres minor, and the subscapularis. The **abdominal muscles** are the rectus abdominis, the external oblique, the internal oblique, and the transversus abdominis. The **quadriceps femoris** group is the muscles of the anterior thigh. These are the rectus femoris, the vastus lateralis, the vastus medialis, and the vastus intermedius. The **hamstrings** are muscles on the posterior thigh, and they consist of the biceps femoris, the semitendinosus, and the semimembranosus. These are just a few of the major muscle groups. There are many more functional groups of muscles.

TIPS FOR USING THE FLASHCARDS

Tear out the cards along the perforations, a few at a time. Color each muscle on the front side of the card, and label the origin of the muscle (with a small *O*) and the insertion of the muscle (with a small *I*). Each muscle illustrated is isolated from other muscles so that the origin and the insertion are plainly visible.

When you study muscles, it helps to take two or three at a time and learn just the origins of the muscles. When you know those, then study the insertions and, finally, the actions. After you know that set well, take another group of muscles and add them to the list.

Why study muscles in small groups? Because trying to learn 20 muscles at a time is frustrating. Muscles can be grouped into anatomical regions such as muscles of the head, arm, or torso. Muscles can also be functionally related; for example, muscles that act on the thigh or muscles that flex the hand. Choose ways of grouping the muscles that will help you learn.

▪ Chapter Six: **Nervous System**

OVERVIEW OF THE NERVOUS SYSTEM

The body must react to both the internal and external environments and communicate information between regions of the body. This job is primarily the task of the nervous system. Proper response to the external environment is critical for thermal regulation, response to threats, taking advantage of opportunities such as food availability, and response to many other stimuli. Response to the internal environment is important for sensing muscle tension, digestive processes, maintenance of blood pressure, and other functions. Communication is important for coordination of activities such as walking, digestion, and maintenance of blood pressure. The nervous system also integrates information from the environment, relates past information to the present, and interprets new experiences. The **brain** and the **spinal cord** make up the **central nervous system** (**CNS**). The nerves of the body make up the **peripheral nervous system** (**PNS**). The peripheral nervous system is divided into the **somatic nervous system**, which consists of **spinal nerves** and **peripheral nerves** that innervate the outer regions of the body, and the **autonomic nervous system** (**ANS**). Label and color the parts of the nervous system.

Color Guide: Use pink for the brain, dark yellow for the spinal cord, and light yellow for the peripheral nerves.

Answer Key

a. Central nervous system
b. Brain
c. Spinal cord
d. Peripheral nervous system
e. Spinal nerves
f. Peripheral nerves

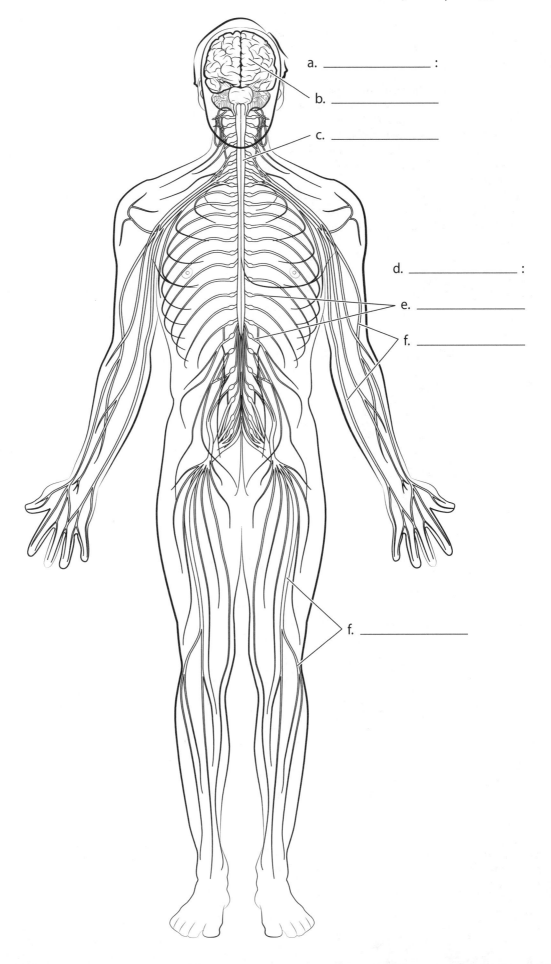

a. _____ :

b. _____

c. _____

d. _____ :

e. _____

f. _____

f. _____

NEURON

The nerve cell or **neuron** is one of the main functional cells in the nervous system. Most electrical conduction in the body is due to the transmission of impulses by the neuron. The neuron consists of branched structures called **dendrites**. The main portion of the nerve cell is called the **soma** or **nerve cell body**, and the elongated part of the neuron is the **axon**. Two neurons are connected by gaps called **synapses**. The nerve cell body is the metabolic center of the cell consisting of a nucleus, an endoplasmic reticulum called the **Nissl bodies**, and a region where the axon attaches called the **axon hillock**.

Color Guide: Color the soma purple, the dendrites blue, and the axon yellow.

Answer Key

a. Dendrites
b. Nerve cell body (soma)
c. Nissl bodies
d. Axon hillock
e. Axon
f. Synapses

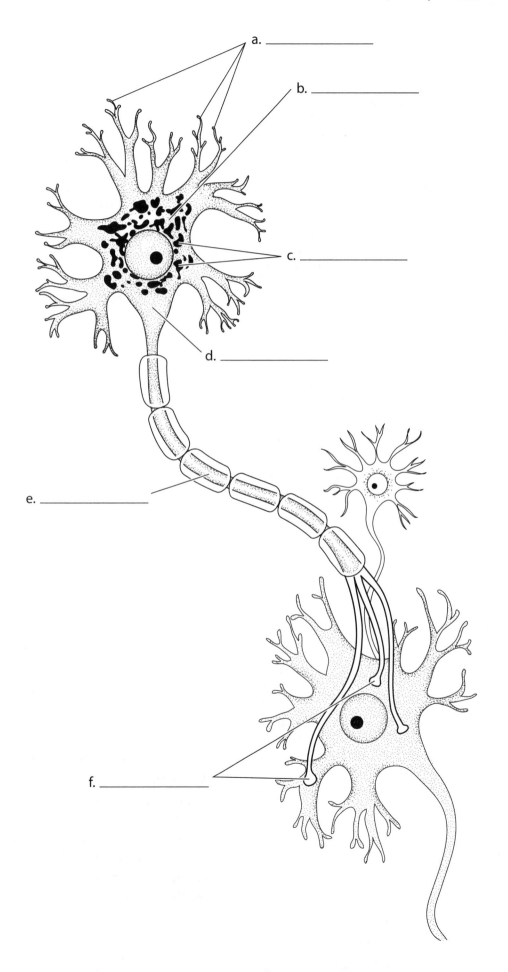

a. _____

b. _____

c. _____

d. _____

e. _____

f. _____

NEUROGLIA

Neuroglia or **glial cells** have many specialized functions in the nervous system. The **neurolemmocyte** or **Schwann cell** is found in the peripheral nervous system. These cells make up the **myelin sheath** that wraps around **axons**.

The other neuroglia are located in the central nervous system. **Astrocytes** are glial cells that, along with the brain capillaries, form the blood-brain barrier. They also have a role in transferring nutrients from the capillaries to the deeper regions of the brain. Another glial cell that functions as a barrier is the **ependymal** cell. These cells are located between the CNS and cavities filled with cerebrospinal fluid. **Microglia** are also found in the CNS, and their function is one of protection. Microglia respond to invasions of the nervous system and destroy microbes.

Oligodendrocytes are neuroglia that produce myelination in the CNS. Myelinated nerve fibers comprise white matter. Myelinated fibers conduct impulses faster than unmyelinated fibers. White matter is mostly associated with transmission of neural impulses from one area to another.

Color Guide: Color each glial cell a different color, and write the name of each cell in the space provided.

Answer Key

a. Astrocyte
b. Ependymal cell
c. Microglial cell
d. Oligodendrocyte
e. Neurolemmocytes (Schwann cells)
f. Myelin sheath
g. Axon

LEARNING HINT

Astrocytes have extensions that make them look like stars.

Ependymal (from the Greek) means "to put a cover on." Ependymal cells cover the inside of CNS cavities.

Oligodendrocytes are small (*oligo-*) dendrocytes, or "cells that look like trees."

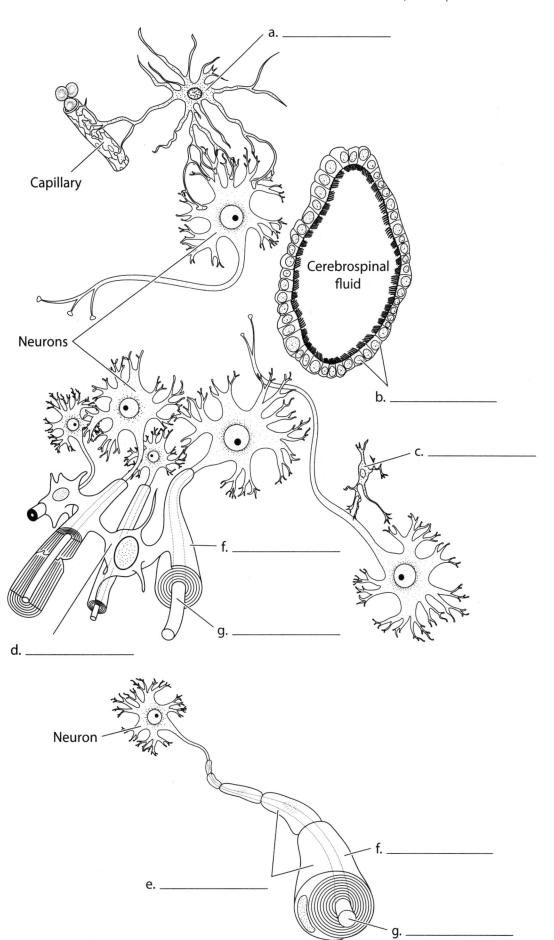

a. _____

Capillary

Cerebrospinal fluid

Neurons

b. _____

c. _____

f. _____

g. _____

d. _____

Neuron

e. _____

f. _____

g. _____

NEURON SHAPES AND SYNAPSES

Neurons come in a few basic shapes. The most common neuron in the CNS is the **multipolar neuron**. It consists of many dendrites and a single axon. **Bipolar neurons** are not very common. They are found in the eye, in the nose, and in the ear and consist of a singular dendrite and an axon. **Pseudounipolar neurons** (unipolar neurons) make up the sensory nerves of the body. They consist of a cluster of dendrites at one end, a long axon leading to the nerve cell body, and another axon leaving the nerve cell body at the same area.

Neurons connect to each other by synapses. The neuron first carrying the information is called the **presynaptic neuron**. This neuron has **synaptic vesicles** that release **neurotransmitters**. The **synaptic cleft** is the space between the neurons, and the **postsynaptic neuron** is the receiving neuron. The neural impulse would travel from "g" to "n" in the lower illustration. Label the various neurons and their parts as well as the synapse between the neurons.

Color Guide: Use the same colors (purple for the soma, blue for the dendrites, and yellow for the axons) for each of the neurons in the upper illustration. Color the presynaptic axon in yellow and the postsynaptic neuron in purple. Select any other colors you want for the other parts of the neurons and synaptic cleft.

Answer Key

a. Dendrites
b. Nerve cell bodies
c. Axons
d. Multipolar neuron
e. Bipolar neuron
f. Pseudounipolar (unipolar) neuron
g. Presynaptic axon
h. Terminal bouton (button knob)
i. Fused vesicle releasing neurotransmitter (exocytosis)
j. Docked neurotransmitter
k. Neurotransmitter
l. Neurotransmitter receptors
m. Synaptic cleft
n. Postsynaptic neuron
o. Synaptic vesicles containing neurotransmitters

a. _____

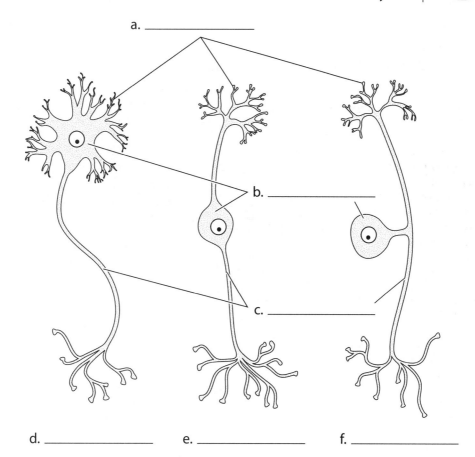

b. _____

c. _____

d. _____   e. _____   f. _____

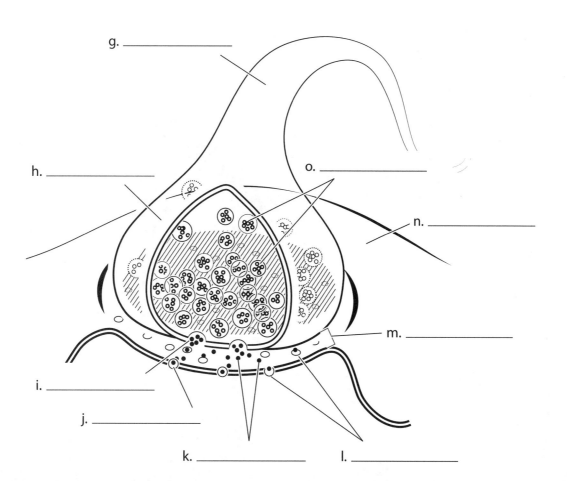

g. _____

h. _____

o. _____

n. _____

m. _____

i. _____

j. _____

k. _____   l. _____

NEURAL DEVELOPMENT

The nervous system develops early as a neural groove. This groove folds in on itself to become a neural tube as early as four weeks after conception. At about six weeks of age, the beginning **cerebral hemispheres** can be seen as lateral enclosures from the neural tube along with the **developing eye** just posterior to the hemispheres. This embryonic brain is divided into three regions, the **prosencephalon** or **forebrain**, the **mesencephalon** or **midbrain**, and the **rhombencephalon** or **hindbrain**. Label the parts of the embryonic brain and the adult derivatives of that brain.

Color Guide: Select different colors for the prosencephalon, mesencephalon, and rhombencephalon. Use these same colors for the derivatives of the embryonic brain: Make the forebrain the same color as the prosencephalon, the midbrain the same color as the mesencephalon, and the hindbrain the same color as the rhombencephalon. You will use these colors for the same structures on subsequent pages.

Answer Key

a. Prosencephalon
b. Mesencephalon
c. Rhombencephalon
d. Spinal cord
e. Cerebral hemisphere
f. Developing eye
g. Forebrain
h. Midbrain
i. Hindbrain

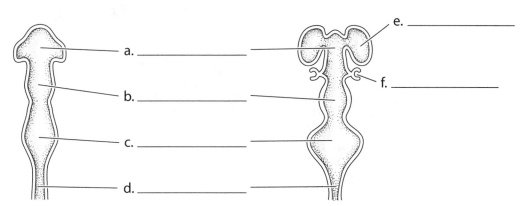

a. _____

b. _____

c. _____

d. _____

e. _____

f. _____

Frontal section
4-week embryo

Frontal section
6-week embryo

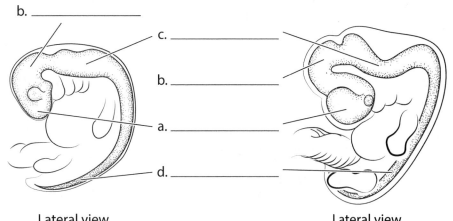

b. _____

c. _____

b. _____

a. _____

d. _____

Lateral view
4-week embryo

Lateral view
6-week embryo

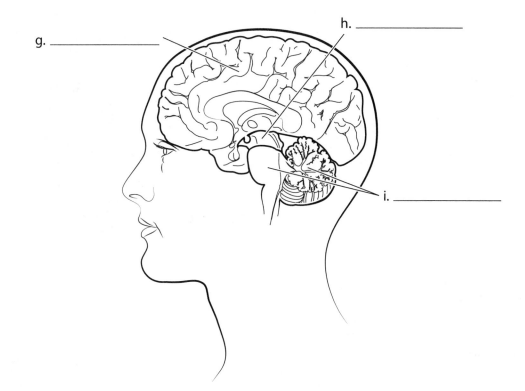

g. _____

h. _____

i. _____

LATERAL ASPECT OF THE BRAIN

The most obvious features of a lateral view of the brain are the lobes of the **cerebrum** and the **cerebellum**. The most anterior lobe is the **frontal lobe**, which is responsible for intellect and abstract reasoning, among other things. The division between the frontal lobe and the **parietal lobe** is the **central sulcus**. Just anterior to the central sulcus is the **precentral gyrus**, an area that sends motor impulses to muscles of the body. Just posterior to the central sulcus is the **postcentral gyrus**. The postcentral gyrus receives sensory information from the body. On the lateral aspect of the brain is the **lateral fissure**, and inferior to this is the **temporal lobe** of the brain. Hearing, taste, smell, and the formation of memories all have centers here. The most posterior part of the cerebrum is the **occipital lobe**, which has visual interpretation areas. The major lobes of the cerebrum are named for the bones of the skull that cover them—hence the names frontal lobe, parietal lobe, temporal lobe, and occipital lobe. Label the regions seen in a lateral view of the brain and the spinal cord.

Color Guide: Use the same colors for the forebrain, midbrain, and hindbrain as you did on the previous page. Color the precentral and postcentral gyri, and then color the lobes of the brain using darker colors or shading for the various parts of the forebrain (letters "a" through "h"). Shade in the cerebellum as well.

Answer Key

a. Temporal lobe
b. Lateral fissure
c. Frontal lobe
d. Precentral gyrus
e. Central sulcus
f. Postcentral gyrus
g. Parietal lobe
h. Occipital lobe
i. Cerebellum

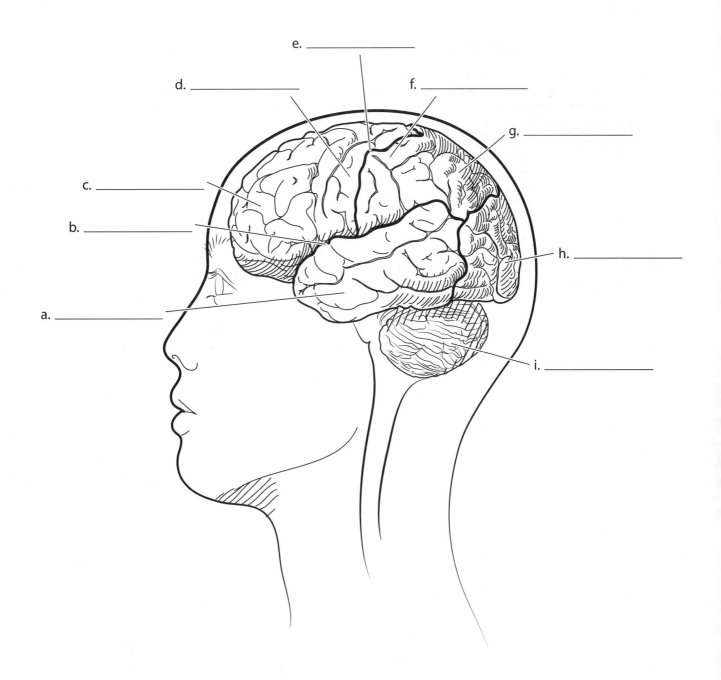

e. _____

d. _____

f. _____

g. _____

c. _____

b. _____

h. _____

a. _____

i. _____

SUPERIOR ASPECT OF THE BRAIN

From the superior aspect, the two **cerebral hemispheres** are divided by the **longitudinal fissure**. (A fissure is a deep cleft or depression.) The **frontal lobes** are separated from the **parietal lobe** by the **central sulcus**. The **precentral gyrus (primary motor cortex)** and the **postcentral gyrus (primary somatosensory cortex)** are on either side of the central sulcus. The **gyri** are the raised areas of the cerebral cortex, and the **sulci** are the shallow depressions of the cerebral cortex. Together, these compose the **convolutions** of the brain.

Color Guide: Label and color the regions of the superior aspect of the brain. Use the same color for the brain as you used for the forebrain (but different shades for each section).

Answer Key

a. Frontal lobe
b. Longitudinal fissure
c. Precentral gyrus
d. Central sulcus
e. Postcentral gyrus
f. Parietal lobe
g. Gyri
h. Occipital lobe
i. Sulci

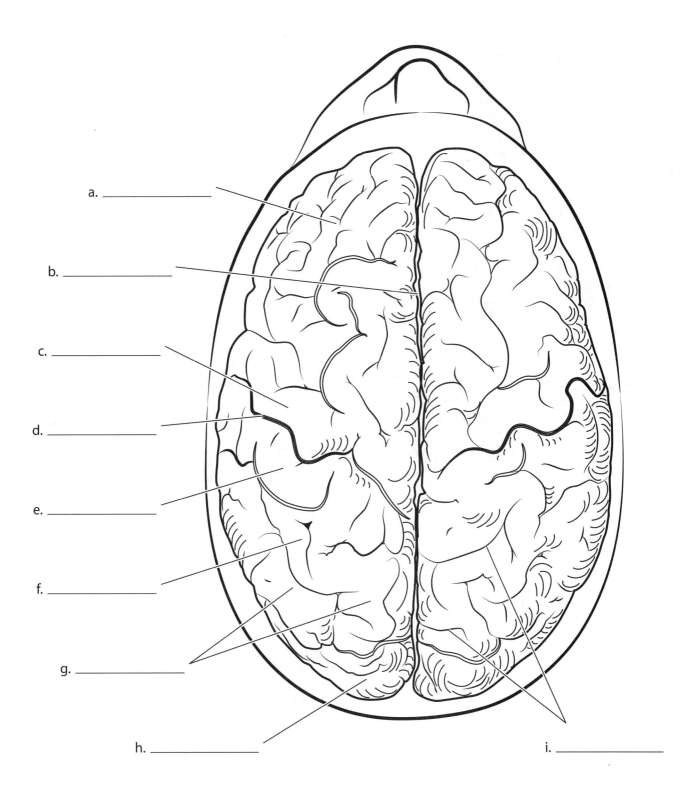

a. _____

b. _____

c. _____

d. _____

e. _____

f. _____

g. _____

h. _____

i. _____

INFERIOR ASPECT OF THE BRAIN

When seen from an inferior view, many different features can be seen on the brain. The **frontal lobe** is anterior, and the **temporal lobe** and **cerebellum** are visible as well. The cerebellum has small folds called folia. The **medulla oblongata** is attached to the spinal cord, and the **pons** is anterior to the medulla oblongata. Anterior to the pons are the **mammillary bodies**, which are responsible for the olfactory (smell) reflex. The **pituitary gland** is next to the mammillary bodies. Anterior to the pituitary is the **optic chiasma**, an x-shaped structure that has the optic nerves anteriorly and the optic tracts posteriorly. The olfactory tracts are seen in this view of the brain as two parallel structures on either side of the longitudinal fissure. The blood vessels of the brain are not visible in this illustration because they obstruct some of the neural structures. They are covered in the cardiovascular section. The cranial nerves will be covered in subsequent pages. Label the structures seen in an inferior view.

Color Guide: Color the lobes of the brain in the same color that you used for the other forebrain drawings. Color the cranial nerves yellow, and use the same color as you did earlier for the hindbrain. Make the pons, medulla oblongata, and cerebellum different shades of the same color. Use different colors for "c," "d," and "f."

Answer Key

a. Frontal lobe
b. Cranial nerves
c. Optic chiasma
d. Pituitary
e. Temporal lobe
f. Mammillary body
g. Pons
h. Medulla oblongata
i. Cerebellum

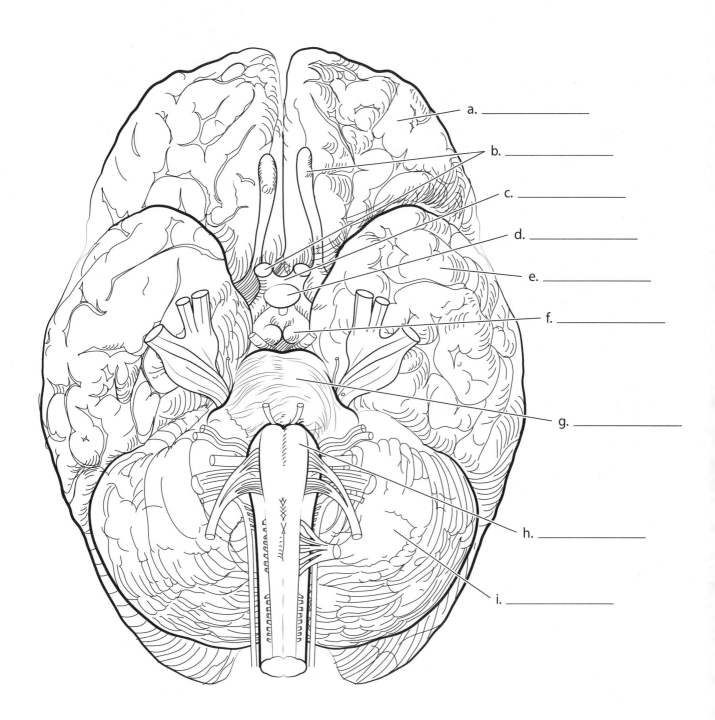

a. _____

b. _____

c. _____

d. _____

e. _____

f. _____

g. _____

h. _____

i. _____

MIDSAGITTAL SECTION OF THE BRAIN

When the brain is sectioned in the midsagittal plane, many internal features are visible. One of the most obvious features is the crescent-shaped **corpus callosum**. Superficial to this is the cerebral hemisphere with the **frontal lobe**, **parietal lobe**, and **occipital lobe**. Locate the **thalamus, hypothalamus,** and **mammillary body** along with the **optic chiasma** and the **pituitary gland**. The **pineal gland** is a small structure at the posterior aspect of the thalamus. These structures are all part of the forebrain. The midbrain is a small section with the **cerebral peduncles** forming the inferior aspect of the midbrain and the **cerebral aqueduct** as a narrow tube between the peduncles and the **corpora quadrigemina**. The corpora consist of the **superior colliculi**, which are responsible for visual reflexes, and the **inferior colliculi**, which are responsible for auditory reflexes. Posterior and inferior to the midbrain is the hindbrain. It consists of the **pons**, the **cerebellum**, and the **medulla oblongata**. The pons is a large oval-shaped structure. The cerebellum is visible with the arbor vitae (white matter of the cerebellum) and a triangular space known as the **fourth ventricle**. The medulla oblongata is the terminal part of the hindbrain. Label the features of the midsagittal section of the brain.

Color Guide: Use different shades of the same color for the different lobes of the brain. Select different colors for the various structures seen in the midsagittal section of the brain.

Answer Key

a. Optic chiasma
b. Mammillary body
c. Hypothalamus
d. Frontal lobe
e. Thalamus
f. Corpus callosum
g. Pineal gland
h. Parietal lobe
i. Superior colliculus
j. Cerebral aqueduct
k. Occipital lobe
l. Inferior colliculus
m. Cerebellum
n. Fourth ventricle
o. Medulla oblongata
p. Pons
q. Cerebral peduncle
r. Pituitary gland

LEARNING HINT

Here are a few translations that might help you remember terms:

callosum = "tough"
thalamus = "den" or "chamber"
colliculi = "little hills"
ventricles = "small cavities"

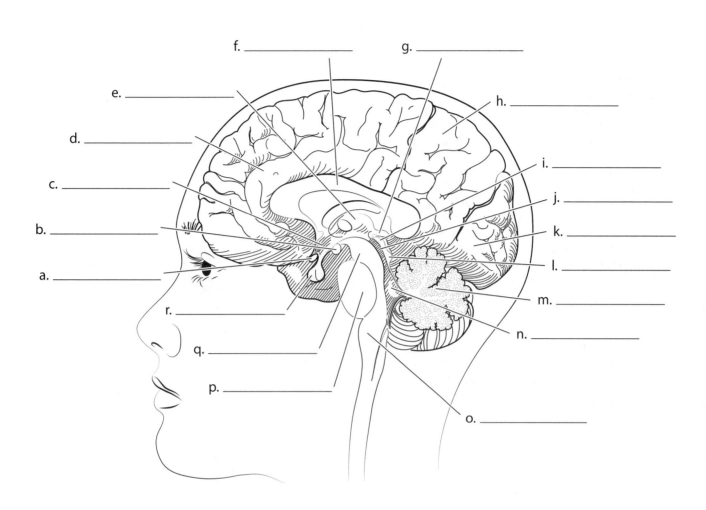

e. _____

d. _____

c. _____

b. _____

a. _____

f. _____

g. _____

h. _____

i. _____

j. _____

k. _____

l. _____

m. _____

n. _____

r. _____

q. _____

p. _____

o. _____

CORONAL SECTION OF THE BRAIN

When the brain is sectioned in the coronal plane, the **convolutions** are obvious. The **gray matter** is on the external aspect of the brain, and the **white matter** is internal. There are deep sections of gray matter in the brain, and these are known as **basal nuclei**. The external gray matter is known as the **cerebral cortex** and is divided into the **gyri** (raised areas) and **sulci** (depressed areas). The **longitudinal fissure** is the deep cleft that separates the **cerebral hemispheres**. The cerebral hemispheres are connected by the **corpus callosum**. Deep in the hemispheres are spaces known as the **lateral ventricles**, and the **third ventricle** is a space in the middle part of the brain. On the sides of the third ventricle is the **thalamus**, and the floor of the third ventricle is the **hypothalamus**. The **pituitary** is suspended from the hypothalamus by the **infundibulum**.

Color Guide: Use dark gray to color in the cerebral cortex. Color the ventricles blue and the basal nuclei a light gray, and leave the white matter in this illustration white.

Answer Key

a. Longitudinal fissure
b. Cerebral cortex (gray matter)
c. Corpus callosum
d. Lateral ventricle
e. White matter
f. Thalamus
g. Third ventricle
h. Basal nuclei

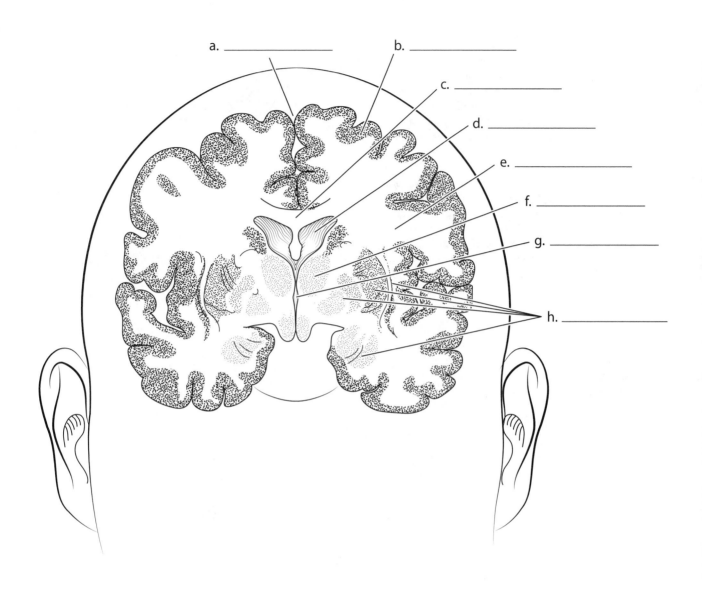

a. _____

b. _____

c. _____

d. _____

e. _____

f. _____

g. _____

h. _____

LIMBIC SYSTEM

The limbic system is deep in the cerebrum and performs numerous functions. The system has an important role in memory and in emotions (both positive and negative). The sense of smell enters the limbic system and has interpretive centers there. The **cingulate gyrus** is a curved part of the system and coordinates sensory input with emotions. The **hippocampus** and **amygdala** are also parts of the limbic system. The amygdala plays a role in both arousal and aversion, and the hippocampus is involved in memory formation. The **hippocampal gyrus** is part of the temporal lobe and takes sensory information to the hippocampus. Memory apparently enters the limbic system, and damage to the limbic system impairs memory formation. The storage of memory occurs in other parts of the brain. The **mammillary body** receives olfactory inputs, and the **fornix** connects the mammillary body to the hippocampus. Label the parts of the limbic system.

Color Guide: Use a different color for each part of the limbic system. Color the cerebrum with the same color that you have used on previous pages.

Answer Key

a. Cingulate gyrus
b. Fornix
c. Thalamus
d. Hippocampal gyrus
e. Hippocampus
f. Amygdala
g. Mammillary body
h. Olfactory bulb
i. Hypothalamus

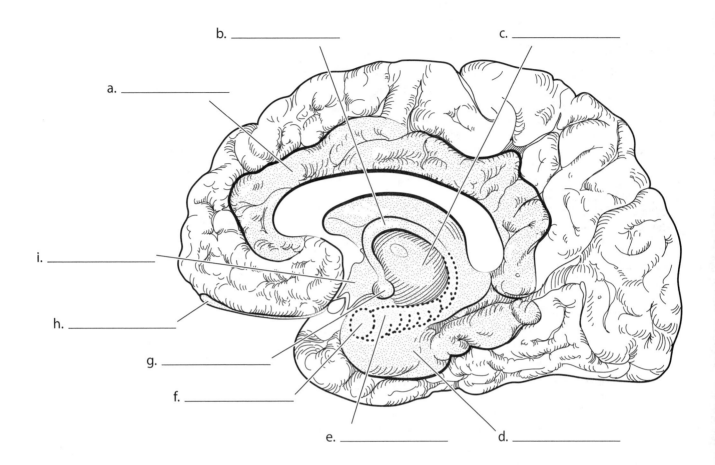

b. _____

c. _____

a. _____

i. _____

h. _____

g. _____

f. _____

e. _____

d. _____

FUNCTIONAL AREAS OF THE CEREBRUM

The cerebrum can be described not only physically but also in terms of the functional areas. The functions of language are many and have different areas of specialization. The **motor speech area (Broca's area)** is typically on the left side of the frontal lobe, and it involves the formation of words. Coordination of the tongue and other parts of the vocal apparatus occur here. **Wernicke's area** is located in the parieto-temporal region and is involved in the syntax of speech. Wernicke's area allows for the formation of sentence structure while Broca's area is involved in the articulation of speech.

The **primary motor cortex** is located in the **precentral gyrus**, and it determines what body muscles to move. The **motor association area** is just anterior to the primary motor cortex. The **primary somatosensory cortex** receives sensory information from the body and has a sensory association area just posterior to it.

The posterior part of the brain includes the **visual area** and the **association area**. If this area is damaged, then sight can be impaired or lost completely. The **angular gyrus** is one of the areas associated with reading. The temporal lobe includes the **primary auditory cortex** and the **auditory association area**. Label these functional areas of the brain.

Color Guide: Color each functional area in a different color. You may want to use different shades of colors for related areas. For example, you may want to color the primary motor cortex with one shade of green and the related motor association area with another shade of green.

Answer Key

a. Premotor (motor association) area
b. Primary motor cortex
c. Primary somatosensory cortex
d. Wernicke's area
e. Angular (reading) gyrus
f. Visual area
g. Visual association area
h. Auditory cortex
i. Motor speech area

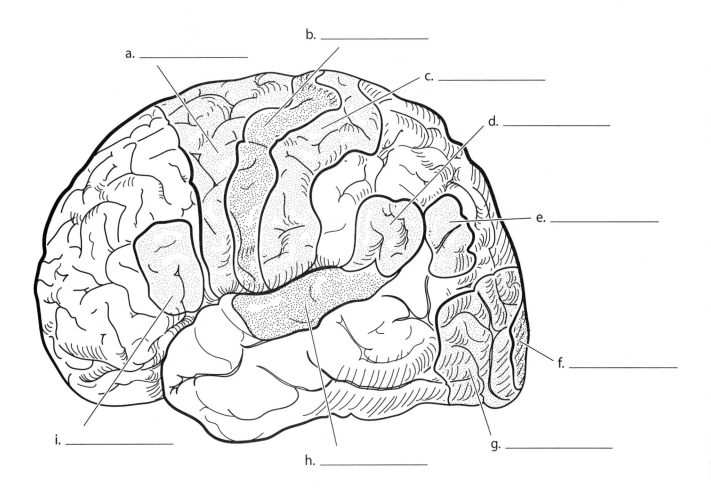

VENTRICLES

The brain has hollow cavities enclosed in nervous tissue
called ventricles. Each cerebral hemisphere has a **lateral
ventricle**, and these lead into a central **third ventricle** via
the **interventricular foramina**. Cerebrospinal fluid (CSF)
is produced from blood capillaries called choroid plexuses
in the ventricles, and this fluid flows slowly through
the ventricles. There are choroid plexuses in all of the
ventricles of the brain. The CSF from the lateral ventricles
flows into the third ventricle. From the third ventricle,
the CSF flows into the **cerebral aqueduct** to the **fourth
ventricle**, which is located anterior to the cerebellum.
From the fourth ventricle, CSF exits to the space between
the brain and the skull. CSF cushions the brain from
mechanical damage and "floats" the brain in a fluid
medium. The CSF is returned to the cardiovascular system
by venous sinuses. Label the ventricles, foramina, and the
cerebral aqueduct.

Color Guide: Color in each ventricle with a different color.

Answer Key

a. Lateral ventricle
b. Third ventricle
c. Cerebral aqueduct
d. Interventricular foramen
e. Fourth ventricle

a. _____

b. _____

c. _____

d. _____

e. _____

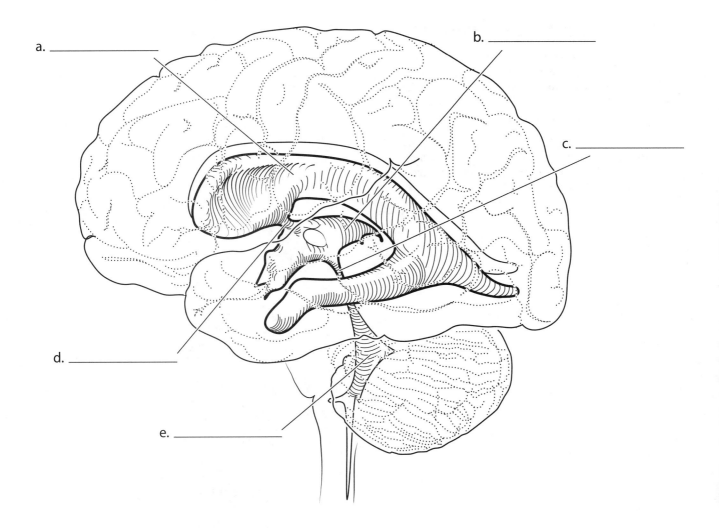

CEREBROSPINAL FLUID PATHWAY

Both the brain and spinal cord have layers that cover
the nervous tissue. These are known as the **meninges**.
The **cerebrospinal fluid** (CSF) is produced in the **choroid
plexus** and then exits to the outside of the brain where it
is absorbed in the **venous sinus**.

Color Guide: Color the structures and trace the flow of
cerebrospinal fluid in the schematic from its source to its
reabsorption in the cardiovascular system.

Answer Key

a. Cerebrospinal fluid
b. Choroid plexus
c. Venous sinus
d. Interventricular foramen
e. Third ventricle
f. Cerebral aqueduct
g. Fourth ventricle

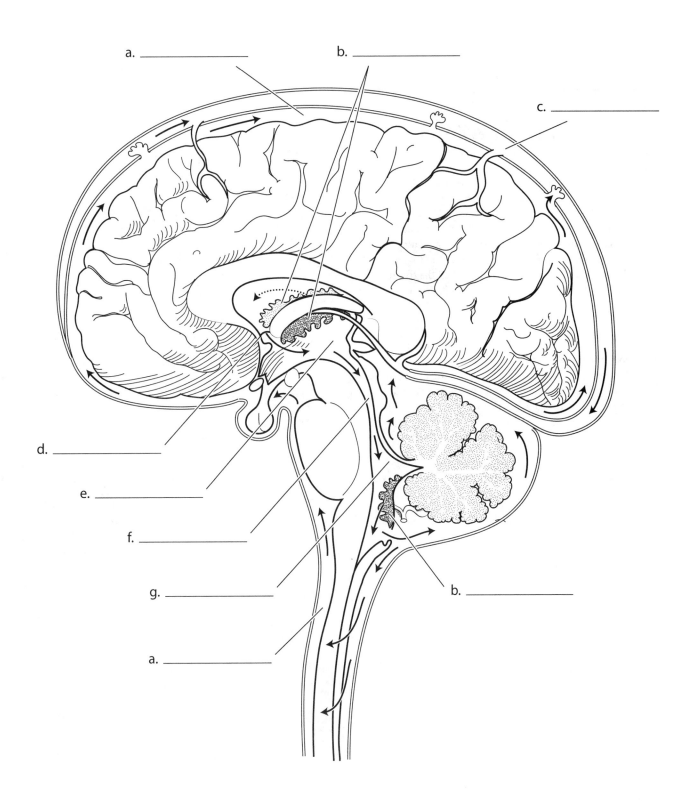

a. _____

b. _____

c. _____

d. _____

e. _____

f. _____

g. _____

b. _____

a. _____

SPINAL CORD

The spinal cord is attached to the brain at the foramen magnum. It expands just below this junction as the **cervical enlargement**. This enlargement is due to the increased neural connections with the upper limbs. Another increase in the diameter of the cord is the **lumbar enlargement**, which is due to the neural connections with the lower limbs. The end of the cord is the **conus medullaris** found at the region of the first or second lumbar vertebra. The spinal cord is shorter than the vertebral canal because it matures early and the vertebral column continues to grow. The neural fibers continue in the vertebral canal as the **cauda equina**, a structure that resembles a horse's tail. The cord is attached to the coccyx by an extension of the pia mater called the **filum terminale**, which becomes enclosed in the **coccygeal ligament**.

Color Guide: Color the cervical enlargement one color, the lumbar enlargement another color, and the conus medullaris yet another color. Use yellow for the main part of the spinal cord and use a different color for the cauda equina. Color the nerves a light yellow.

Answer Key

a. Dura mater
b. Cervical enlargement
c. Spinal nerves
d. Lumbar enlargement
e. Conus medullaris
f. Cauda equina
g. Filum terminale
h. Coccygeal ligament

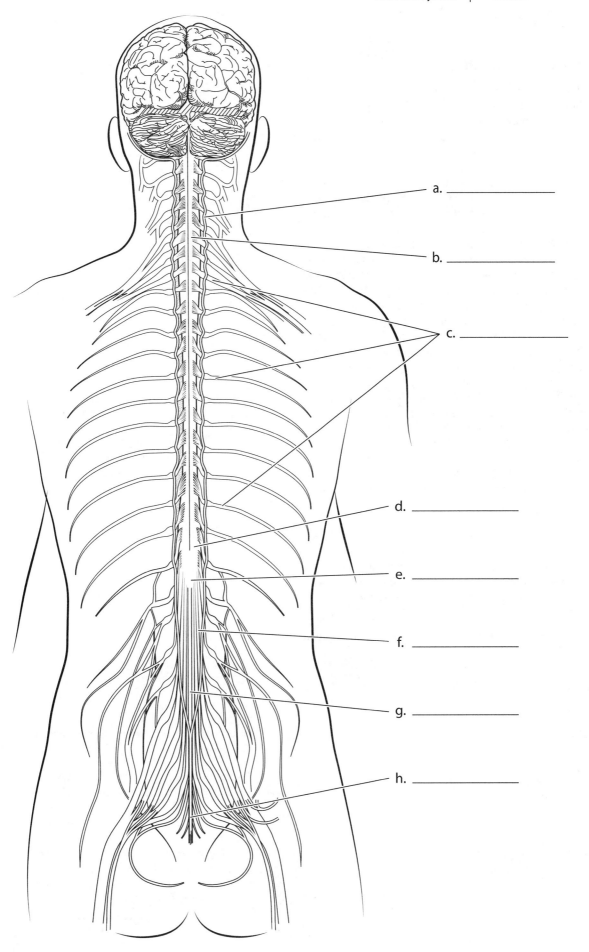

a. _____

b. _____

c. _____

d. _____

e. _____

f. _____

g. _____

h. _____

CRANIAL NERVES

The cranial nerves are those nerves that attach to the brain. They are paired and are numbered (typically by Roman numerals) from anterior to posterior. The **olfactory nerve** is a sensory nerve that receives the sense of smell from the nose and transmits it to the brain. The **optic nerve** takes visual impulses from the eye while the **oculomotor nerve** mostly takes motor impulses to several muscles that move the eye. The **trochlear nerve** takes motor impulses to the superior oblique muscle. The trochlear nerve is so named because it innervates a muscle that passes through a loop called the trochlea. The **trigeminal nerve** is a large nerve located laterally in the pons. It is a mixed nerve (having both sensory and motor functions) that has three branches. The ophthalmic branch innervates the upper head while the maxillary branch innervates the region around the maxilla. The mandibular branch innervates the jaw. The **abducens nerve** is posterior to the trigeminal and is located exiting the brain between the pons and the medulla oblongata. It is a motor nerve to the lateral rectus muscle of the eye. On the anterior portion of the medulla oblongata is the **facial nerve**, which is both a sensory and motor nerve to the face and the tongue. The **vestibulocochlear nerve** is a sensory nerve that receives impulses from the ear. It picks up auditory stimuli as well as information about equilibrium. The **glossopharyngeal nerve** is a nerve that carries both sensory and motor impulses. It innervates the tongue and throat. A large nerve on the side of the medulla oblongata is the **vagus nerve**. It is also a mixed nerve carrying both sensory and motor impulses. The vagus nerve innervates organs in the thoracic and abdominal regions. The **accessory nerve** is inferior to the vagus nerve and is a motor nerve to the neck muscles. The **hypoglossal nerve** is a motor nerve to the tongue.

Color Guide: Label the cranial nerves and color each pair a different color.

Answer Key

a. Olfactory
b. Optic
c. Oculomotor
d. Trochlear
e. Trigeminal
f. Abducens
g. Facial
h. Vestibulocochlear
i. Glossopharyngeal
j. Vagus
k. Accessory
l. Hypoglossal

LEARNING HINT

There are **12 pairs of cranial nerves**, and many memory devices have been used to help remember them in sequence. Here is one such mnemonic: "Often old orcas try to arrange fancy vacations, grabbing Vegas and Hawaii." Each letter represents the initial letter of an organ system: Olfactory, Optic, Oculomotor, Trochlear, Trigeminal, Abducens, Facial, Vestibulocochlear, Glossopharyngeal, Vagus, Accessory, and Hypoglossal.

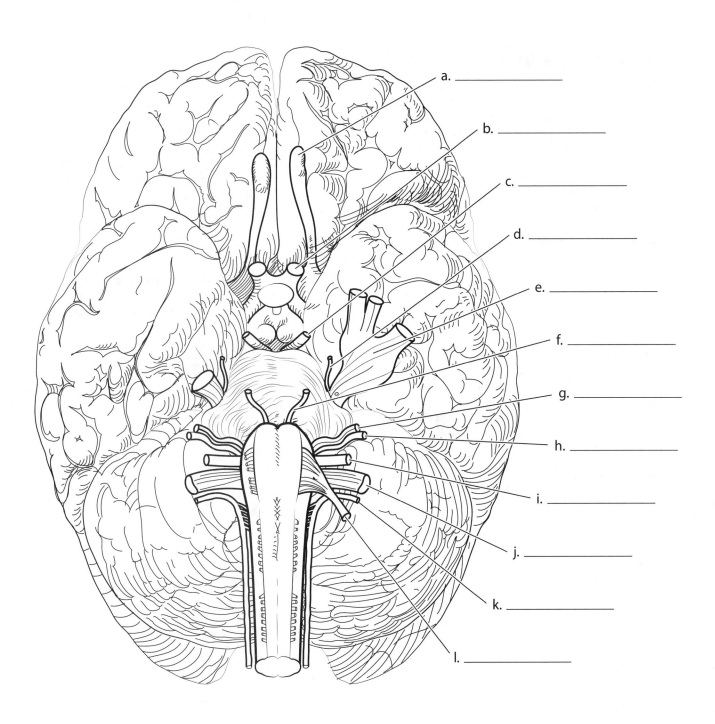

a. _____

b. _____

c. _____

d. _____

e. _____

f. _____

g. _____

h. _____

i. _____

j. _____

k. _____

l. _____

SPINAL CORD AND SPINAL NERVES

When seen in cross section, the spinal cord is composed of an internal arrangement of gray matter resembling a butterfly and an external white matter. The two thin strips of gray matter are the **posterior gray horns**, and the more rounded sections are the **anterior gray horns**. The **lateral gray horns** are found in the thoracic and lumbar regions. The hole in the middle of the spinal cord is the **central canal**, and the gray matter that surrounds the central canal is the **gray commissure**. The spinal cord has two main depressions in it, the **posterior median sulcus** and the **anterior median fissure**. Label the parts of the spinal cord.

Attached to the spinal cord are the **spinal nerves** that take impulses from the spinal cord to the peripheral nerves and impulses to the spinal cord. The spinal nerves are mixed nerves that pass through the intervertebral foramina of the vertebral column. The spinal nerve splits into a **dorsal root** and a **ventral root**. The **dorsal root ganglion** is a swelling of the dorsal root within its intervertebral foramen. The dorsal root ganglion contains the nerve cell bodies of the sensory neurons coming from the body. The ganglion leads to the dorsal root, which branches into the rootlets. These branches carry sensory information to the posterior gray horn of the spinal cord. The ventral root carries motor information from the anterior gray horn and innervates muscles.

Both the brain and spinal cord have layers that cover the nervous tissue. These are known as the **meninges**, and there are three layers. The outermost layer is the **dura mater**, a tough connective tissue layer. Underneath this layer is the **arachnoid mater**, which is so named because it looks like a spider web. Deep to this is the subarachnoid space, which is filled with cerebrospinal fluid. The deepest of the layers is the **pia mater** located on the surface of the nervous tissue. Label the meninges and the structures associated with the spinal cord in both the horizontal view and the vertical view.

Color Guide: Use the same colors for the same meninges in both the upper and lower illustration. Do likewise for the parts of the spinal cord, the ganglia, and the nerves.

Answer Key

a. Pia mater
b. Ventral root
c. Dorsal root
d. Dorsal root ganglion
e. Posterior median sulcus
f. Arachnoid mater
g. Spinal nerve
h. Dura mater
i. Anterior gray horn
j. Lateral gray horn
k. Central canal
l. Anterior median fissure
m. Posterior gray horn

LEARNING HINT

The term **meninges** comes from the Greek word for "membrane." There are three types. The outer, durable one is the **dura mater** ("tough mother"). The **arachnoid mater** is named for its spider-web appearance (*arachnid* is another word for spider), and the **pia mater** ("soft mother") is the one next to the spinal cord.

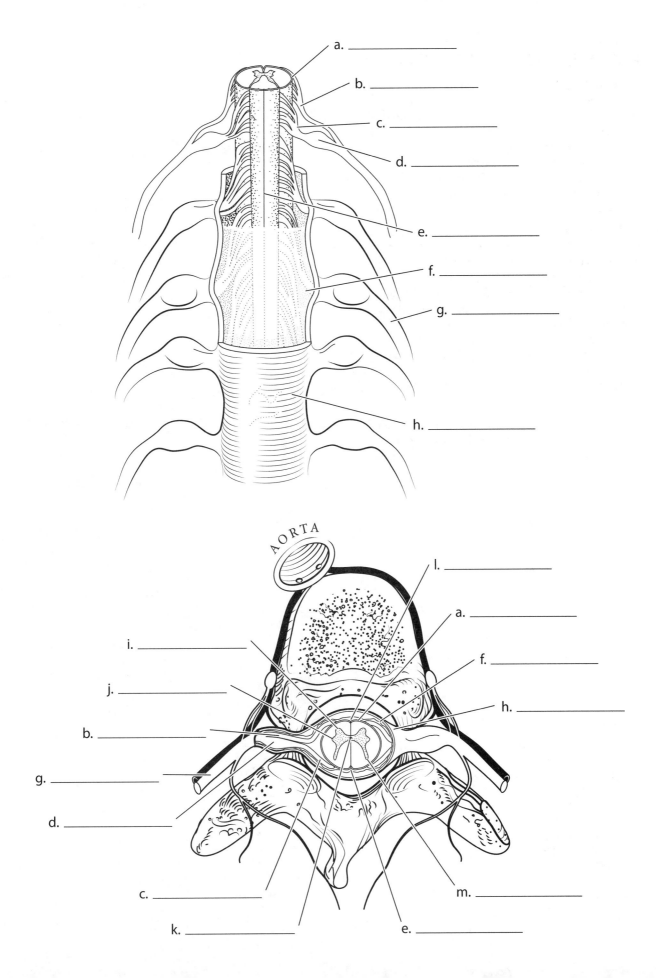

a. _____

b. _____

c. _____

d. _____

e. _____

f. _____

g. _____

h. _____

AORTA

l. _____

a. _____

i. _____

f. _____

j. _____

h. _____

b. _____

g. _____

d. _____

c. _____

m. _____

k. _____

e. _____

PLEXUSES AND THORACIC NERVES

There are 31 pairs of spinal nerves grouped by region of the vertebral column. The **cervical nerves** are the most superior, and there are eight pairs of them. The first cervical nerves arise superior to the first cervical vertebra. The **thoracic nerves** arise as 12 pairs. They lead to nerves that innervate the muscles between the ribs and associated skin. There are five pairs of **lumbar nerves** and five pairs of **sacral nerves**. The last pair of spinal nerves is the **coccygeal nerves**.

A **plexus** is a weblike arrangement of nerves that is near the spinal cord and gives rise to the **terminal nerves**. The most superior plexus is the **cervical plexus**, which arises from the first five cervical spinal nerves. The **brachial plexus** receives input from the fifth through eighth cervical nerves and the first pair of thoracic nerves. The **lumbar plexus** arises from the first four pairs of lumbar nerves, and the **sacral plexus** is associated with the last two pairs of lumbar nerves and the first four pairs of sacral nerves. Sometimes the lumbar and sacral plexuses are grouped together as the **lumbosacral plexus**.

Color Guide: Use one color to color in the short segments of the spinal nerves and label the plexuses. Color each plexus a different color.

Answer Key

a. Cervical plexus
b. Brachial plexus
c. Lumbar plexus
d. Sacral plexus
e. Cervical nerves
f. Thoracic nerves
g. Lumbar nerves
h. Sacral nerves
i. Coccygeal nerves

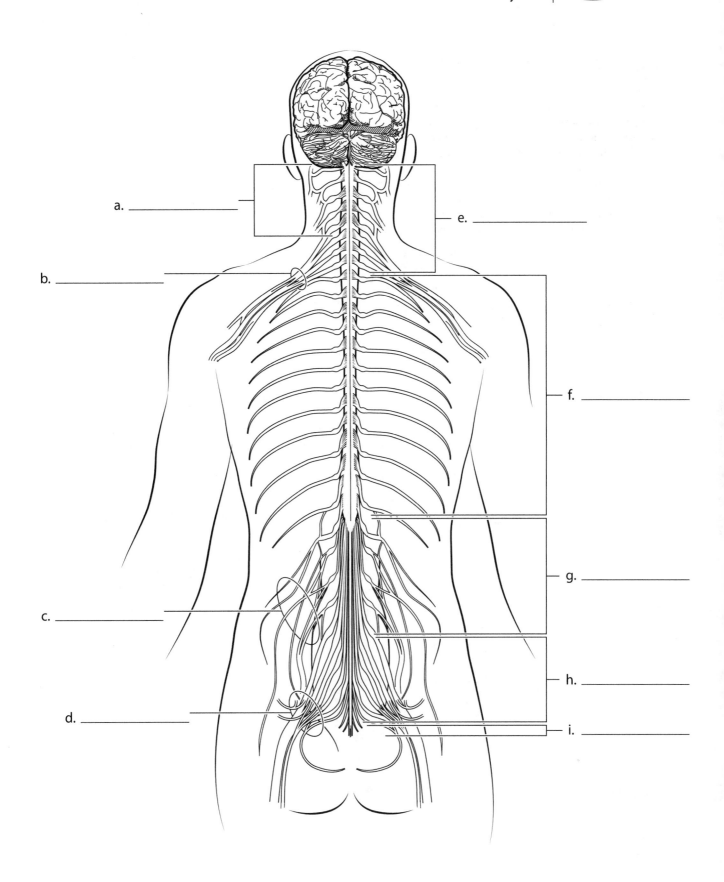

NERVES OF CERVICAL PLEXUS

The **cervical plexus** is a complex interweaving of branches from the first five pairs of cervical nerves. The **hypoglossal nerve** enters this plexus from the head. The **ansa cervicalis** is an arched structure (*ansa* is Latin for "loop") that has many nerves innervating the anterior throat muscles. The major nerves of the cervical plexus are the two **phrenic nerves** that descend to the diaphragm and stimulate the diaphragm to contract. Label the major features of the cervical plexus, and color the hypoglossal nerve, the ansa cervicalis, and the phrenic nerve.

Contributions to the accessory nerve leave the cervical plexus from **C2**, **C3**, and **C4**.

Color Guide: Use a different color for each nerve of the cervical plexus and the associated nerves.

Answer Key

a. C1
b. C2
c. C3
d. C4
e. C5
f. Hypoglossal nerve
g. Ansa cervicalis
h. Phrenic nerve

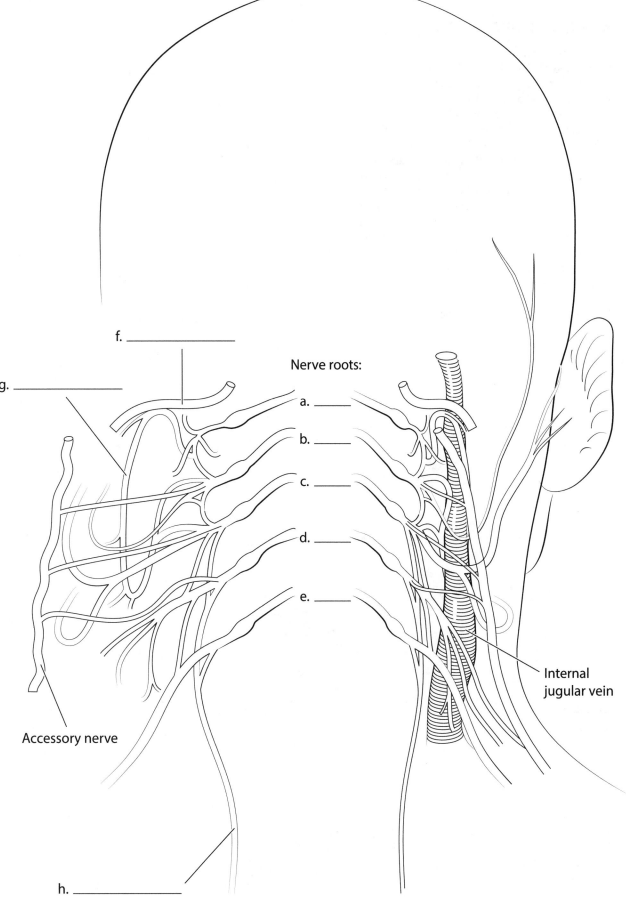

f. _____

g. _____

Nerve roots:

a. _____

b. _____

c. _____

d. _____

e. _____

Internal jugular vein

Accessory nerve

h. _____

NERVES OF BRACHIAL PLEXUS

The brachial plexus is associated with spinal nerves
C4–C8 and **T1**. It leads to major nerves of the shoulder
and arm. The **axillary nerve** arises from the brachial
plexus and innervates the deltoid and the teres minor
muscles. It also receives stimulation from the skin of
the shoulder and lateral upper limb. The **radial nerve**
innervates the triceps brachii muscle and the extensors
of the forearm and hand. The **musculocutaneous nerve**
innervates the anterior muscles of the arm (biceps brachii,
brachialis, and coracobrachialis) and the skin on the
lateral side of the forearm. The median nerve runs the
length of the arm and forearm and innervates the anterior
muscles of the forearm and the muscles associated with
the thumb. The **ulnar nerve** passes along the posterior
side of the medial epicondyle of the humerus and gives
that tingling sensation of the "funny bone" when hit. It
innervates the muscles of the medial side of the anterior
hand. Label these nerves and related structures.

Color Guide: Select a different color for each nerve.

Answer Key
a. C4
b. C5
c. C6
d. C7
e. C8
f. T1
g. Axillary nerve
h. Musculocutaneous nerve
i. Radial nerve
j. Median nerve
k. Ulnar nerve

Nerve roots:

a. _____

b. _____

c. _____

d. _____

e. _____

f. _____

g. _____

h. _____

i. _____

k. _____

j. _____

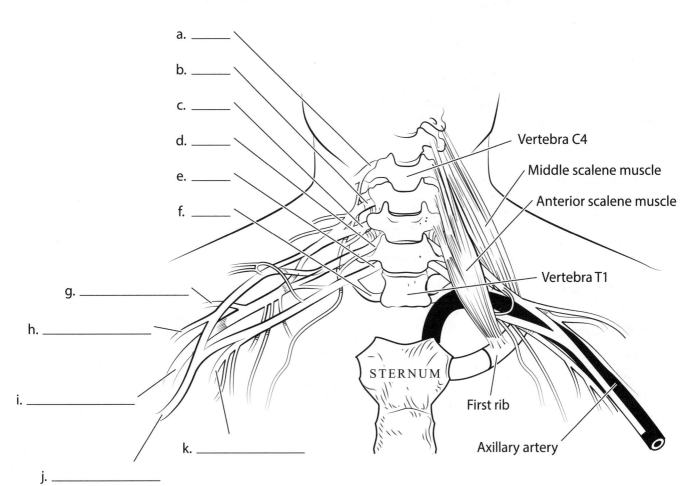

Vertebra C4

Middle scalene muscle

Anterior scalene muscle

Vertebra T1

STERNUM

First rib

Axillary artery

NERVES OF LUMBAR PLEXUS

The lumbar plexus leads to nerves on the anterior
and the medial aspect of the thigh. A large **femoral
nerve** arises from the lumbar plexus and innervates
the four muscles of the quadriceps femoris group on
the anterior thigh. The **obturator nerve** innervates the
adductor muscles of the medial thigh. The **genitofemoral
nerve** takes sensory impulses from the anterior thigh
(both sexes), skin of the anterior scrotum (males), and
mons pubis and labia majora (females), and it carries
motor impulses to the cremaster muscle (males). The
iliohypogastric nerve innervates the muscles of the
abdomen and the skin of the belly. The **ilioinguinal nerve**
innervates the same muscles as does the iliohypogastric
nerve, and it receives sensory information from the base
of the penis and the scrotum in males and from the labia
majora in females. The **lateral femoral cutaneous nerve**
receives sensory information from the skin of the lateral
thigh. Label these nerves in the illustration.

Color Guide: Color in each nerve with a different color.

Answer Key

a. T12
b. L1
c. L2
d. L3
e. L4
f. L5
g. Iliohypogastric nerve
h. Ilioinguinal nerve
i. Lateral femoral cutaneous nerve
j. Femoral nerve
k. Genitofemoral nerve
l. Obturator nerve

Nerve roots:

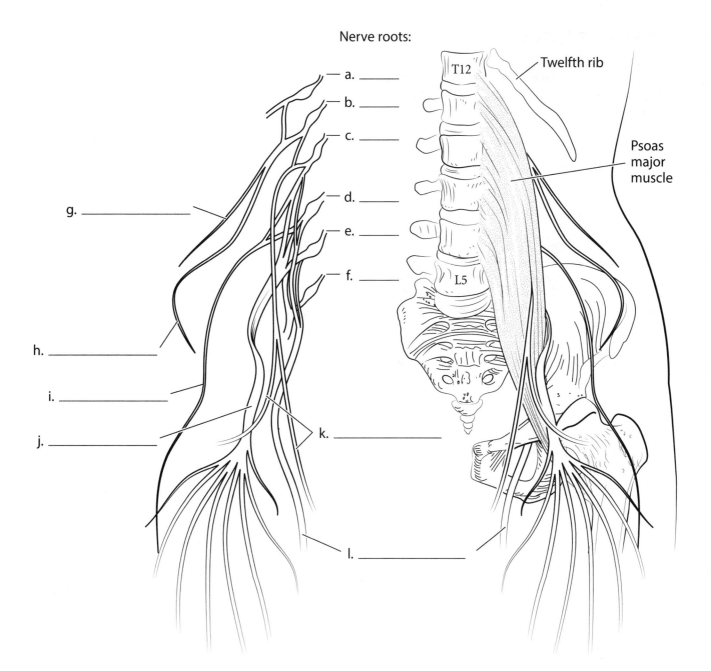

a. _____
b. _____
c. _____
d. _____
e. _____
f. _____
g. _____
h. _____
i. _____
j. _____
k. _____
l. _____

T12
L5
Twelfth rib
Psoas major muscle

NERVES OF SACRAL PLEXUS

The sacral plexus has nerves that provide genital innervation and also has motor nerves to the posterior hip, thigh, and anterior and posterior leg. The **pudendal nerve** innervates the penis and scrotum in males; the clitoris, labia, and distal vagina in females; and the muscles of the pelvic floor in both sexes, so it is both a sensory and motor nerve. The sacral plexus also has the **superior** and **inferior gluteal nerves**, which innervate the gluteal muscles, and the **tibial nerve** and **common fibular nerve**. These last two nerves are grouped together as the **sciatic nerve**, a large nerve of the posterior thigh. The tibial nerve innervates the hamstring muscles, the muscles of the calf, and the muscles originating on the foot. The common fibular nerve innervates the short head of the biceps femoris muscle, the muscles on the lateral side of the leg, and the anterior surface of the leg. **Cutaneous branches** innervate the skin, and **muscular branches** take motor information to the muscles. Label these nerves.

Color Guide: Color each nerve of the sacral plexus with a different color.

Answer Key

a. L4
b. L5
c. S1
d. S2
e. S3
f. S4
g. S5
h. Coccygeal nerve
i. Superior gluteal nerve
j. Inferior gluteal nerve
k. Pudendal nerve
l. Common fibular nerve
m. Tibial nerve
n. Sciatic nerve
o. Cutaneous branches
p. Muscular branches

Nerve roots:

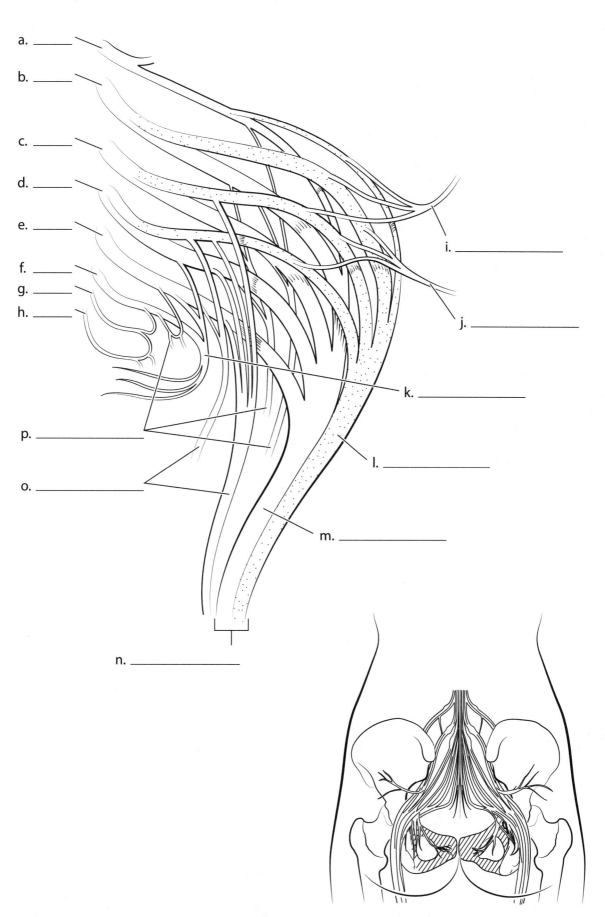

a. _____

b. _____

c. _____

d. _____

e. _____

f. _____

g. _____

h. _____

i. _____

j. _____

k. _____

p. _____

l. _____

o. _____

m. _____

n. _____

DERMATOMES

Dermatomes are regions of the skin innervated by
nerves. The nerves receive sensory inputs from the
skin and take that information back to the spinal cord.
The clinical importance of dermatomes is the role
they play in assessing spinal cord damage. If there is
a significant spinal cord injury, then the regions below
the level of the injury may not transmit sensory signals
to the brain. Lack of sensation in specific areas of the skin
provides a base of understanding of where the trauma
may be located. Label the innervations of the dermatomes.

Color Guide: Color in the regions that are innervated by
the cervical nerves with one color, and choose separate
colors for the thoracic, lumbar, and sacral innervation.

Answer Key

a. C2
b. C5
c. C6
d. C7
e. T1
f. T4
g. T10
h. T12
i. C7
j. S5
k. L1
l. S1
m. L5

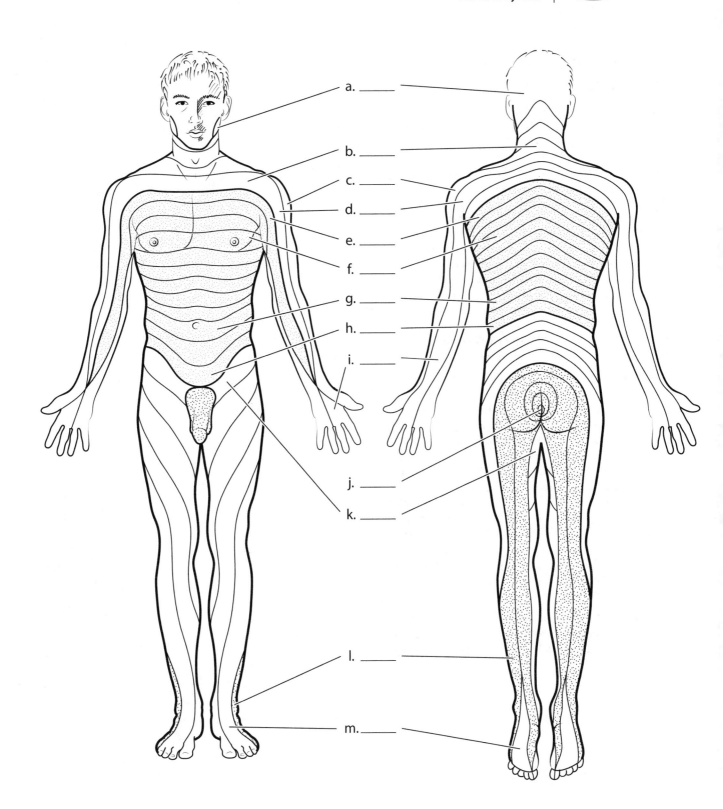

a. _____

b. _____

c. _____

d. _____

e. _____

f. _____

g. _____

h. _____

i. _____

j. _____

k. _____

l. _____

m. _____

AUTONOMIC NERVOUS SYSTEM— SYMPATHETIC DIVISION

The **autonomic nervous system** (**ANS**) regulates automatic functions of the human body. Changes in heart rate, pupil dilation, digestive functions, and blood flow to the kidney are all controlled by the ANS. There is some possibility of conscious regulation of parts of the ANS, but for the most part, it functions without conscious control. There are two divisions of the autonomic nervous system. The resting state of the body is controlled by the **parasympathetic division**. Digestion, kidney filtration, erection of the clitoris, erection of the penis, and pupil constriction are some of the functions of the parasympathetic division. This division is also known as the **craniosacral division** because the nerves exit the central nervous system (CNS) in these locations. The cranial segments go to the eye, salivary glands, heart, lungs, digestive system, and kidneys. The sacral segments go to the lower digestive tract, bladder, and reproductive organs.

The **sympathetic division** controls the "fight or flight" response of the body, shutting down the digestive functions, inhibiting erections, shunting blood away from the kidneys, and dilating the pupils. The sympathetic division increases heart rate; dilates capillaries in the lungs, brain, and muscle tissue; and stimulates the adrenal glands. This division is also known as the **thoracolumbar division** because the nerves exit the CNS in the thoracic and lumbar regions of the spinal cord. Ganglia associated with the sympathetic division are located on either side of the ventral portion of the vertebral column. They are called the **sympathetic chain ganglia**, and the neurons from the thoracolumbar division synapse with nerve cells in these ganglia.

Color Guide: Use bright red and orange colors to color in the regions of the sympathetic division, and trace each arrow to the organ that it innervates with the same bright color.

Answer Key

a. Preganglionic
b. Postganglionic
c. Ganglia
d. Sympathetic trunk
e. T1
f. L2

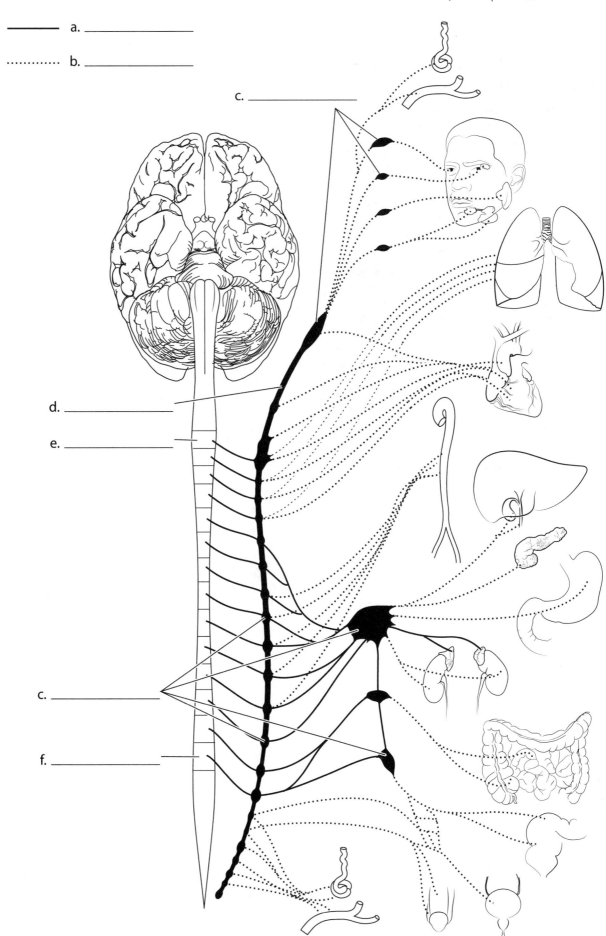

a. _____

b. _____

c. _____

d. _____

e. _____

c. _____

f. _____

AUTONOMIC NERVOUS SYSTEM— PARASYMPATHETIC DIVISION

The parasympathetic and sympathetic divisions are antagonistic to one another, and organs under the influence of the ANS have dual innervation. Typically, one division either inhibits the organ from functioning or causes an increase in activity in the organ. This occurs due to the difference in neurotransmitters secreted by the separate divisions. At the terminal end of the parasympathetic division, the neurotransmitter is acetylcholine. At the terminal end of the sympathetic division, the neurotransmitter is mostly norepinephrine.

The neurons leaving the CNS are called **preganglionic neurons**. In the case of the parasympathetic division, the preganglionic neurons secrete acetylcholine as neurotransmitters. The **ganglia** of the parasympathetic division are next to, or in, the organ they innervate. The **postganglionic neurons** secrete acetylcholine as well. In the sympathetic division, the preganglionic neurons secrete acetylcholine in the sympathetic chain ganglia. The postganglionic neurons mostly secrete norepinephrine to stimulate or inhibit the organs they innervate.

Color Guide: Use blue/green (calming) colors for this illustration to highlight the parasympathetic nervous system.

Answer Key

a. Preganglionic
b. Postganglionic
c. Ganglia
d. Oculomotor (III)
e. Facial (VII)
f. Glossopharyngeal (IX)
g. Vagus (X)
h. S2
i. S4

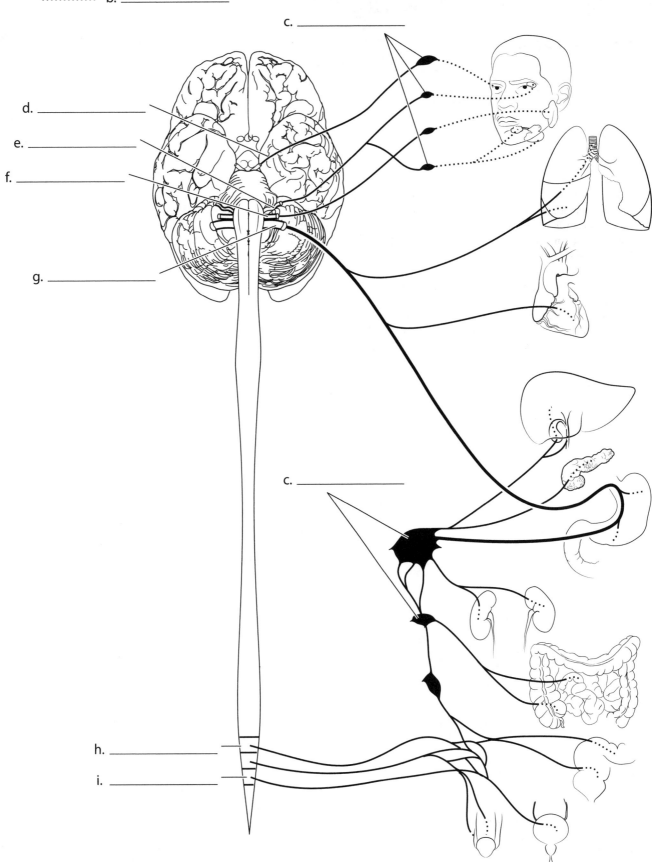

a. _____

b. _____

c. _____

d. _____

e. _____

f. _____

g. _____

c. _____

h. _____

i. _____

Chapter Seven: **Sense Organs**

SKIN RECEPTORS

There are several sense receptors in the skin. Some
are receptive to mechanical vibration, some to
temperature, and some to pain. The receptors for
mechanical vibration pick up light touch or are
involved in perception of pressure. There are **hair
receptors** that wrap around the hair follicles, and
as the hair moves, it stimulates the neurons. Light
touch is perceived by both **Meissner's corpuscles
(tactile corpuscles)** and **Merkel's disks**. These
receptors are found in the superficial layers of the
skin (**epidermis** and upper **dermis**). In the deeper
layers, **Pacinian corpuscles (lamellar corpuscles)**
pick up pressure. **Pain receptors** are naked nerve
endings located throughout the skin that pick up
variable stimuli including extreme temperatures,
acids, strong mechanical vibration, etc. Other
receptors in the skin are **thermoreceptors** that are
receptive to smaller changes in temperature. Label
these structures on the figure.

Color Guide: Use dark colors for the sensory
receptors in the skin and light colors for the
epidermis and dermis.

Answer Key
a. Meissner's (tactile) corpuscle
b. Merkel's disks
c. Pain receptor
d. Hair receptors
e. Pacinian (lamellar) corpuscle
f. Epidermis
g. Dermis

a. _____   b. _____

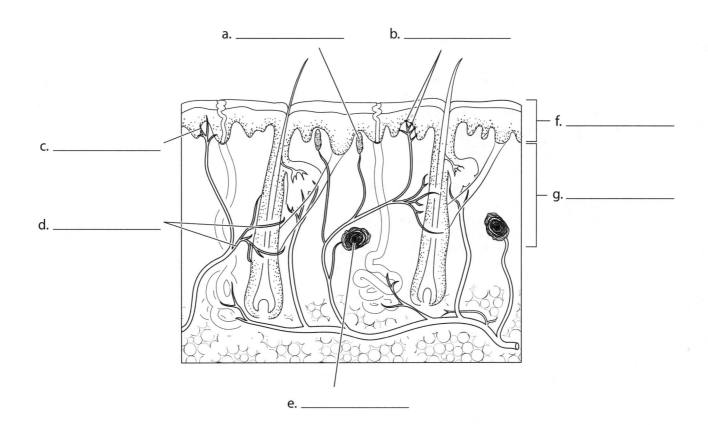

c. _____

d. _____

f. _____

g. _____

e. _____

TONGUE

The tongue is the region where taste is perceived. The tongue has regions that are sensitive to different tastes, and these vary from person to person. Not only do people taste material in different places on the tongue, but the sensitivity to specific tastes is different among individuals. Taste buds are located on the sides of papillae of the tongue. The **lingual tonsils** are found on the posterior tongue, and the **palatine tonsils** are on the sides of the oral cavity. Posterior and inferior to the tongue is the **epiglottis**. The papillae of the tongue come in a few shapes. **Vallate papillae** are shaped like mesas. They have a flat top. **Filiform papillae** are line-shaped while **fungiform papillae** are shaped like mushrooms. Label the papillae.

The **taste buds** consist of epithelial cells and nerve cells. Taste is sensed if the material to be tasted is in solution and comes into contact with the **taste pore**. The taste buds have taste hairs that extend into the taste pore and connect with taste cells, which in turn synapse with **sensory nerve fibers** that take the sense of taste to the brain. Label the various structures in the illustration.

Color Guide: Use separate colors for each group of papillae in the upper illustration, and use the same colors for these papillae in the lower figures. Color the taste bud with another color, and use light colors for the nearby structures, including the epiglottis and tonsils.

Answer Key

a. Epiglottis
b. Palatine tonsil
c. Lingual tonsil
d. Vallate papilla
e. Fungiform papilla
f. Filiform papillae
g. Taste bud
h. Taste pore
i. Sensory nerve fibers

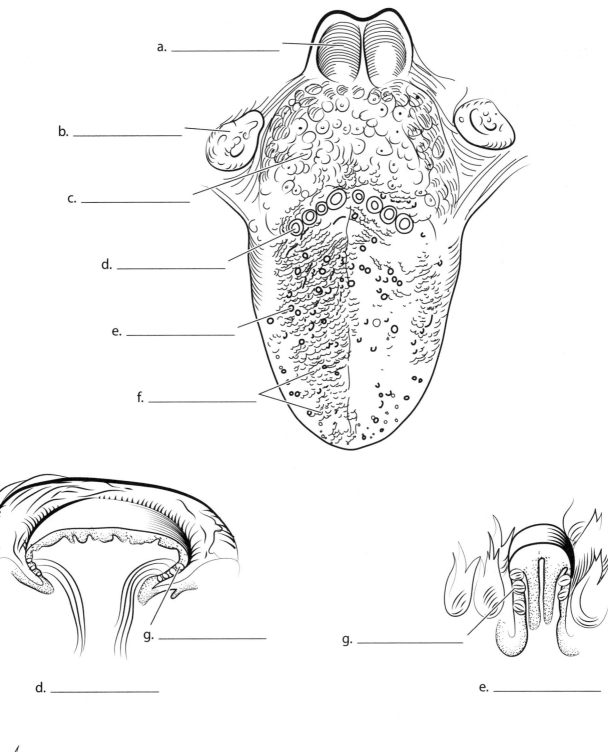

a. _____

b. _____

c. _____

d. _____

e. _____

f. _____

g. _____

d. _____

g. _____

e. _____

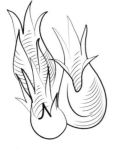

i. _____

h. _____

f. _____

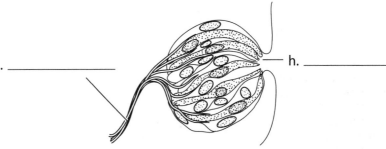

g. _____

NOSE

The sense of smell is more complex than the sense of
taste. There are only five primary tastes but many different
kinds of smells. The region that is sensitive to smell is
the **olfactory epithelium**, which is located in the superior
portion of the **nasal cavity**. The olfactory epithelium
consists of elongated epithelial cells that are **supporting
cells** with neurons called **olfactory cells**. These olfactory
cells have **olfactory hairs** on their surface. Chemicals
that are inhaled come into contact with a mucous sheet
and are picked up by the olfactory cells. The sensation of
smell is transmitted by the **olfactory nerves** through the
cribriform plate of the ethmoid bone, and they synapse
in the **olfactory bulb** at the base of the frontal lobe of
the brain.

Color Guide: Select specific colors for structures "a"
through "c," and use these colors in both the upper and
lower figures. Select light colors for the rest of the figures.

Answer Key

a. Olfactory bulb
b. Olfactory axon bundle (filaments)
c. Olfactory epithelium
d. Nasal cavity
e. Olfactory cells
f. Supporting cells
g. Cribriform plate
h. Olfactory hairs

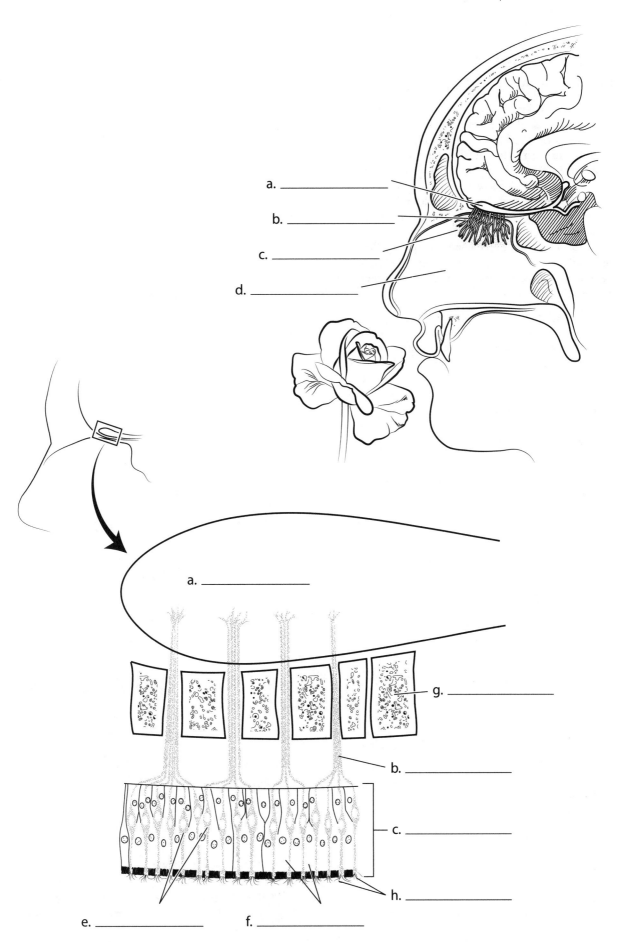

a. _____

b. _____

c. _____

d. _____

a. _____

g. _____

b. _____

c. _____

h. _____

e. _____

f. _____

ANTERIOR SURFACE OF THE EYE AND LACRIMAL APPARATUS

The eye is located in the orbit of the skull and has several external features. Above the eye is the **eyebrow**. The corners of the eye have either a **lateral commissure** or a **medial commissure**. Next to the medial commissure is the **caruncle**, a small thickened tissue in the medial corner of the eye. The outer surface of the eye is protected by the **upper** and **lower eyelids**. The blink reflex rapidly closes the eyelids to keep dust from hitting the outer surface of the eye. Label the **sclera** (the white of the eye), **iris** (the colored part of the eye), **pupil** (the opening that lets light into the back of the eye), and the **eyelids**. There is a transparent extension of the sclera called the **cornea**, and it covers the iris and pupil.

The eyes are kept moist and are subject to potential bacterial infection. Tears have antimicrobial properties and are formed by the **lacrimal gland**. They contain digestive enzymes and wash microbes from the surface of the eye. Tears drain from the eye into the **lacrimal canaliculi**. These canaliculi lead into the **nasolacrimal duct** and then into the **nasal cavity**.

Color Guide: Leave the sclera white. Color the rest of the structures of the eye with your choice of colors.

Answer Key

a. Lacrimal gland
b. Upper eyelid
c. Sclera
d. Lacrimal canaliculus
e. Medial commissure
f. Nasal cavity
g. Lateral commissure
h. Pupil
i. Iris
j. Lower eyelid
k. Caruncle
l. Nasolacrimal duct

LEARNING HINT

A **commissure** is a structure that joins together. The eyelids are joined together on each end by commissures.

The structures involved in the production and drainage of tears are called the **lacrimal glands**. The related English word *lachrymose* means "tearful."

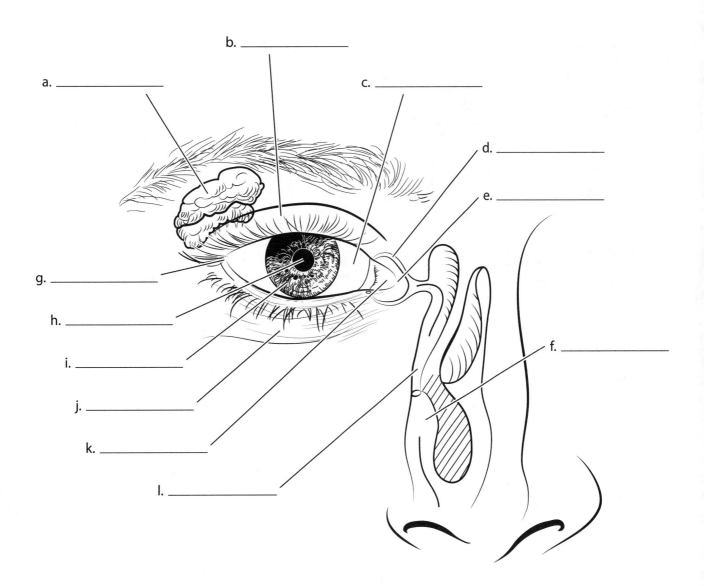

a. _____

b. _____

c. _____

d. _____

e. _____

f. _____

g. _____

h. _____

i. _____

j. _____

k. _____

l. _____

MUSCLES OF THE EYE

The lateral and superior views of the eye show the major muscles controlling the eye. The **lateral rectus** is the muscle that turns the eye to the side. The **medial rectus** turns the eye toward the midline. The **superior rectus** makes you look up while the **inferior rectus** makes you look down. The **superior oblique** turns the eye inferiorly and laterally while the **inferior oblique** makes the eye turn superiorly and laterally. The **levator palpebrae superioris** elevates the eyelid. Label the muscles of the eye and the **optic nerve** where it exits the tendinous ring.

Color Guide: Use different shades of red for the eye muscles. Leave the eyeball white, and select your preferred color for the skin. Color the optic nerve yellow.

Answer Key

a. Lateral rectus
b. Superior rectus
c. Levator palpebrae superioris
d. Superior oblique
e. Inferior oblique
f. Inferior rectus
g. Optic nerve
h. Medial rectus

d. _____

c. _____

b. _____

a. _____

g. _____

f. _____

e. _____

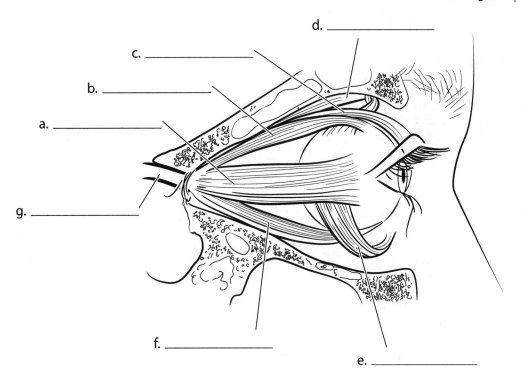

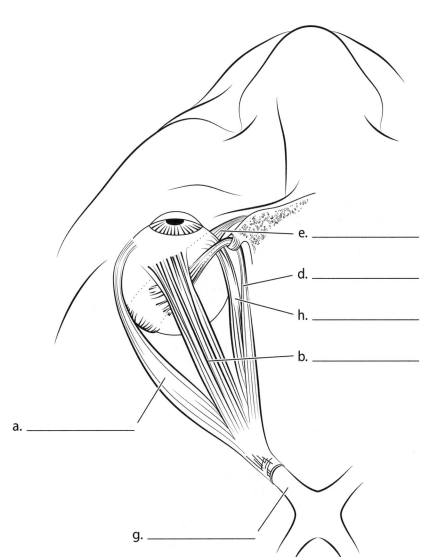

e. _____

d. _____

h. _____

b. _____

a. _____

g. _____

MEDIAN SECTION OF THE EYE

The **cornea** is the outermost part of the eye, and it is responsible for most of the light refraction in the eye (the bending of light rays). On the periphery of the cornea is the **sclera**, which helps maintain eye shape. The space behind the cornea is the **anterior cavity**, which is found in front of the **lens**. It is composed of two smaller chambers, the **anterior chamber** and the **posterior chamber**. The anterior chamber is between the cornea and the **iris**, the part that determines eye color. The posterior chamber is between the iris and the **lens**. The lens is made of protein and is held to the wall of the eye by the **suspensory ligaments**. These ligaments are pulled by the **ciliary muscle** on the wall of the eye. When the ligaments tighten, the lens flattens and the eye focuses on distant objects. The fluid in the anterior cavity is known as **aqueous humor**, and it is released by the ciliary body and reabsorbed in the **scleral venous sinus**.

Behind the lens is the **posterior cavity**. This cavity is filled with a jellylike material called **vitreous humor**. Light travels through this medium to the back of the eye where it strikes the **retina**. The retina is the region of the eye where light waves are converted to nerve impulses. The **fovea** is a small area of the retina where there is a high concentration of cones (cells that determine color and visual acuity). Behind the retina is the **choroid**, a darkened layer that absorbs light, making vision sharp during the daytime. Behind this layer is the sclera, the white of the eye, where muscles attach. At the posterior of the eye, you can see the **optic disk**. This is where the **optic nerve** takes visual impulses from the eye to the brain.

Color Guide: Leave the sclera, "h," white. Use the same color for the anterior cavity, "o," as for the posterior chamber, "i," and the anterior chamber, "j." Use different colors for each layer or specific structure of the eye.

Answer Key

a. Scleral venous sinus
b. Ciliary muscle
c. Retina
d. Choroid
e. Fovea
f. Optic nerve
g. Optic disk
h. Sclera
i. Posterior chamber
j. Anterior chamber
k. Cornea
l. Lens
m. Iris
n. Suspensory ligament
o. Anterior cavity
p. Posterior cavity
q. Vitreous humor

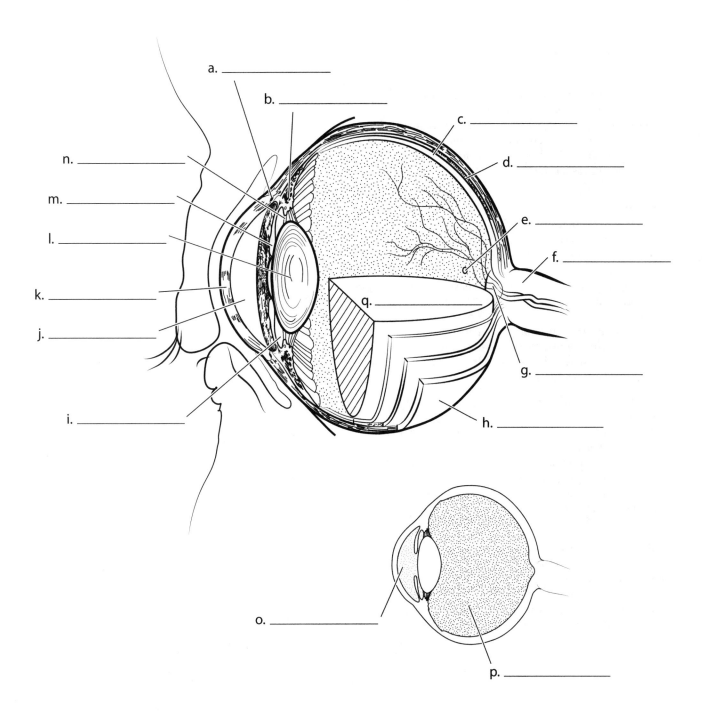

a. _____

b. _____

c. _____

n. _____

m. _____

d. _____

l. _____

e. _____

f. _____

k. _____

q. _____

j. _____

g. _____

i. _____

h. _____

o. _____

p. _____

POSTERIOR VIEW OF THE EYE

In the posterior view of the eye, you can see the **blood vessels** in the choroid that bring nutrients to the back of the eye. Color these vessels. They enter the eye at a region known as the **optic disk**, which is the same place where the **optic nerve** exits the eye. This is the blind spot of the eye. You should also label and color the **fovea centralis** of the eye and the **macula lutea**.

Retina

The retina is the tunic or layer of the eye that converts light energy into nerve impulses. There are two main types of photosensitive cells in the retina. **Rods** are more numerous and determine motion and night vision. There are many rods in the eye, but they are not very sensitive in determining visual detail. This is because many rods connect to one neuron fiber. The other photosensitive cells are **cones**. There are fewer cones per neuron so they produce a sharper visual image. There are three types of cones that have sensitivities to different wavelengths of light. Label and color the rods and cones in the retina.

The retina consists of three layers. The **photoreceptor layer** contains the rods and cones. This is at the posterior layer of the retina. In front of this is the **bipolar layer** that has neurons that synapse with the rods and cones. The layer closest to the posterior cavity is the **ganglionic layer**. The axons of the ganglion cells conduct impulses from the ganglionic layer along the span of the eye and form the **optic nerve**. Label these layers.

Color Guide: The word *lutea* means yellow, so color the macula lutea, "a," in yellow. Use red for the light blood vessels, "c," and select other colors for the other features of the eye. In the lower illustration, use different colors for rods and cones, and shade in each of the layers ("f," "g," and "h") with light colors.

Answer Key

a. Macula lutea
b. Fovea centralis
c. Blood vessels
d. Optic disk
e. Optic nerve
f. Ganglionic layer
g. Bipolar layer
h. Photoreceptor layer
i. Cone
j. Rod

LEARNING HINT

The term **macula lutea** means "yellow spot," and the **fovea centralis** at its center contains a great number of photosensitive cells.

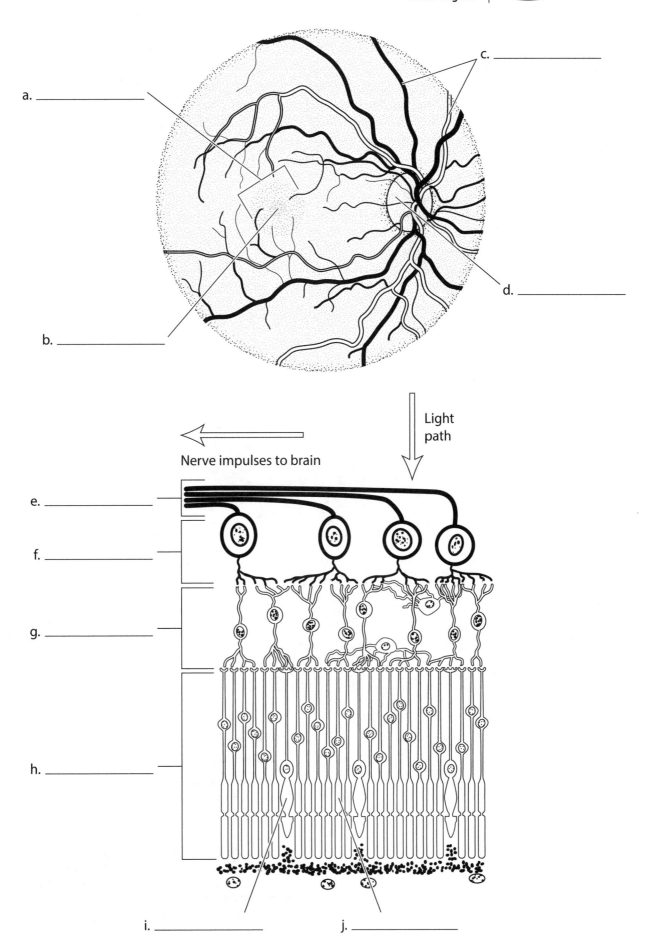

a. _____

c. _____

b. _____

d. _____

Light path

Nerve impulses to brain

e. _____

f. _____

g. _____

h. _____

i. _____

j. _____

OVERVIEW OF THE EAR

The ear consists of three major regions, the **outer ear**, the **middle ear**, and the **inner ear**. The outer ear consists mainly of two parts, the **auricle** (**pinna**), including the **ear lobe** and the **external auditory canal**. The middle ear begins at the **tympanic membrane** (eardrum). Inside the tympanic membrane is the tympanic cavity, another part of the middle ear. Here you should label the ear **ossicles** and the **auditory tube** (Eustachian tube). The inner ear consists of three major regions, the cochlea, the vestibule, and the semicircular ducts.

Color Guide: Use your choice of flesh colors for the skin ("a" and "e"). Use a different color for each major region of the ear.

Answer Key

a. Auricle (pinna)
b. External auditory canal
c. Ossicles
d. Inner ear
e. Ear lobe
f. Tympanic membrane
g. Auditory tube
h. Outer ear
i. Middle ear

LEARNING HINT

The word **cochlea** means "snail" in Latin. Like a snail shell, the cochlea is a spiral structure.

The **external auditory canal** and the **auditory tube** have similar functions and similar-sounding names. But the auditory canal comes first both in the alphabet (*C* before *T*) and in function: Sound first strikes the external auditory canal, and then enters the (internal) auditory tube.

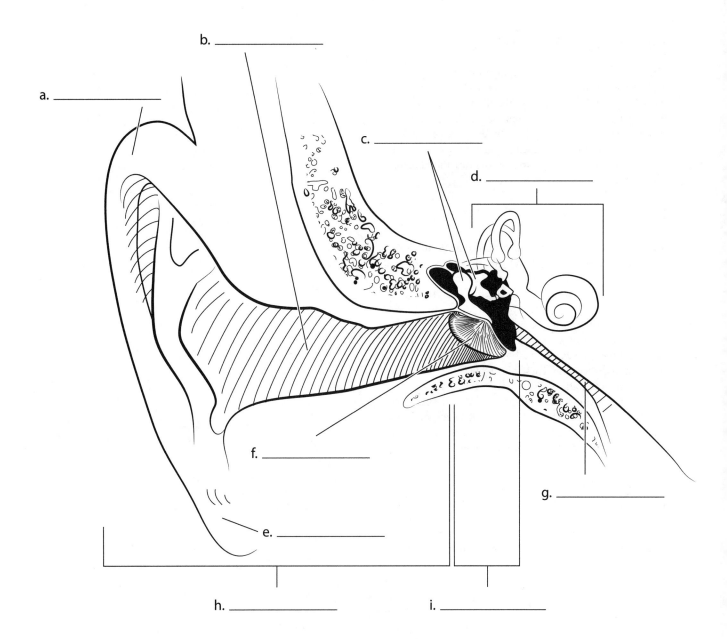

a. _____

b. _____

c. _____

d. _____

e. _____

f. _____

g. _____

h. _____

i. _____

MIDDLE EAR

The middle ear consists of the **tympanic cavity** and structures in that cavity. It is connected to the nasopharynx by the **auditory tube**. This tube allows for equalization of pressure from the middle ear and the external environment. The three ear ossicles transfer sound from the tympanic membrane to the **oval window** of the inner ear. Label the three ear ossicles, the **malleus**, **incus**, and **stapes**.

INNER EAR

The inner ear consists of the **cochlea**, the **vestibule**, and the **semicircular ducts**. In Latin, the name *cochlea* means "snail shell," and this structure spirals like a snail. Its function is to translate the mechanical vibrations of sound into nerve impulses. The cochlea has an oval window that attaches to the stapes and a **round window** that allows for changes in pressure to occur in the inner ear. Label the cochlea. The vestibule has two parts, the **utricle** and the **saccule**. These are involved in equilibrium. They determine static equilibrium whereby a person can determine the position of the body at rest. They also register acceleration. The semicircular ducts respond to angular acceleration. There are three semicircular ducts, the **posterior**, the **anterior**, and the **lateral ducts**.

Color Guide: In the upper illustration, color the oval window where the stapes connects, and use lighter colors for the auditory tube and tympanic cavity. In the lower illustration, color the utricle and saccule of the vestibule a different color. Color each of the semicircular ducts a different color.

Answer Key

a. Malleus
b. Incus
c. Stapes
d. Oval window
e. Tympanic membrane
f. Tympanic cavity
g. Auditory (Eustachian) tube
h. Semicircular ducts
i. Anterior duct
j. Posterior duct
k. Lateral duct
l. Vestibule
m. Utricle
n. Saccule
o. Round window
p. Cochlea

LEARNING HINT

Several structures of the internal ear are named with the Latin word for their shapes, such as the **malleus** (meaning "hammer"—think of *mallet*), **incus** ("anvil"), and **stapes** ("stirrup"). Both **utricle** and **saccule** mean "small bag" or "small sack."

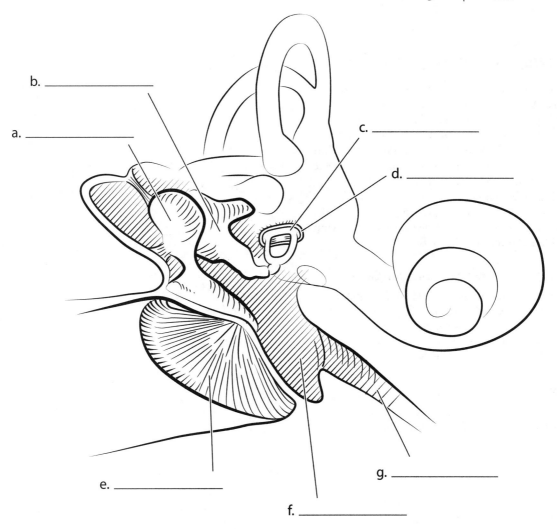

b. _____

a. _____

c. _____

d. _____

e. _____

f. _____

g. _____

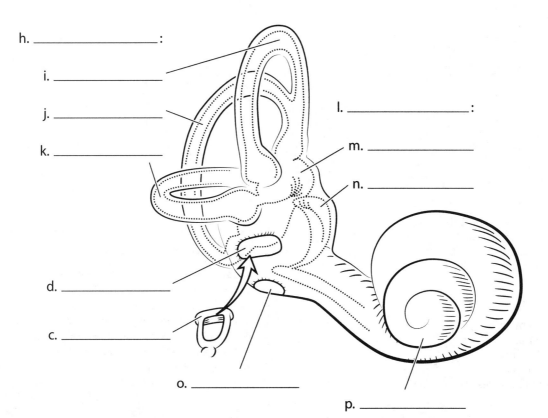

h. _____ :

i. _____

j. _____

k. _____

l. _____ :

m. _____

n. _____

d. _____

c. _____

o. _____

p. _____

LABYRINTHS OF THE INNER EAR

The outer part of the inner ear consists of the **bony labyrinth**, an encasement of bone. (This is the darker gray, stippled area in the upper illustration.) Inside the bony labyrinth is the **membranous labyrinth**, consisting of delicate tissue. Like the durable outer tire of a bicycle wheel that surrounds a soft inner tube, the outer bony labyrinth encases and protects the more fragile membranous labyrinth. Between these two labyrinths is the fluid called **perilymph**. Deeper, inside the membranous labyrinth, is a fluid called **endolymph**. Label these structures and fluids.

Cross Section of a Semicircular Canal

The outer part of the canal is the bony labyrinth. The fluid lying between the bony labyrinth and the membranous labyrinth is perilymph, and the fluid within the membranous labyrinth is endolymph. Label these structures and fluids.

Color Guide: Use light blue to color the endolymph, pink for the perilymph, and beige for the surrounding bone. Use light yellow for the **vestibulocochlear nerve**.

Answer Key

a. Membranous labyrinth
   b. Semicircular ducts
   c. Utricle
   d. Saccule
   e. Cochlear duct
f. Perilymph
g. Endolymph
h. Bony labyrinth
   i. Semicircular canals
   j. Vestibule
   k. Cochlea
l. Vestibulocochlear nerve

LEARNING HINT

A **labyrinth** (pronounced LAB-ur-inth) is a maze, and the bony and membranous labyrinths form mazelike tubes in the temporal bone. Since *peri*- means "around" and *endo*- means "inside," the words **perilymph** (outside the membranous labyrinth) and **endolymph** (inside the membranous labyrinth) indicate their locations.

a. _____ :

b. _____   c. _____   d. _____   e. _____

f. _____

g. _____

h. _____ :

i. _____

j. _____

k. _____

l. _____

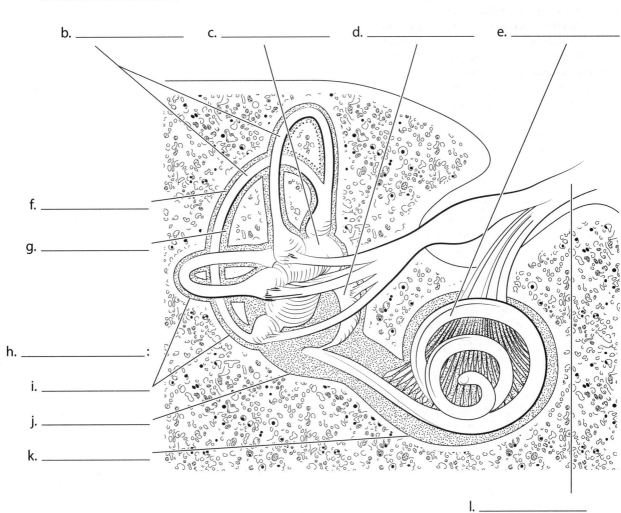

b. _____

f. _____

g. _____

h. _____

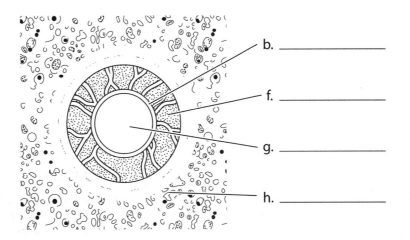

CROSS SECTION OF COCHLEA

Look at the cross section of cochlea. Each coil of the cochlea has three chambers and three membranes. The upper chamber in the illustration is the **scala vestibuli**. It is connected to the oval window. The **vestibular membrane** is the tissue that forms the bottom of the scala vestibuli. Below this is the **scala media** that houses the **spiral organ** (or the **organ of Corti**). The bottom chamber is the **scala tympani**. Between the scala tympani and the scala media is the **basilar membrane**. Label these features.

Spiral Organ

The scala media is the region of the cochlea involved in hearing. It is bounded by the vestibular membrane on top and the basilar membrane on the bottom. Attached to the basilar membrane are the **hair cells**. These cells are attached to the **tectorial membrane**, which vibrates when sound impulses enter the cochlea. The tectorial membrane tugs on the hair cells, converting the sound impulse to a neural impulse, which travels by the **cochlear nerve** to the temporal lobes of the brain, where hearing is interpreted. Label these structures.

Color Guide: In the upper figure, color each space (scala) a different color. In the lower illustration, color in the details of the spiral organ with the colors of your choice.

Answer Key

a. Scala vestibuli
b. Vestibular membrane
c. Scala media
d. Scala tympani
e. Basilar membrane
f. Hair cell
g. Tectorial membrane

LEARNING HINT

Scala means "stairs" or "ladder" in Latin. Thinking of the cochlea as a kind of spiral staircase may help you understand the terminology on the facing page.

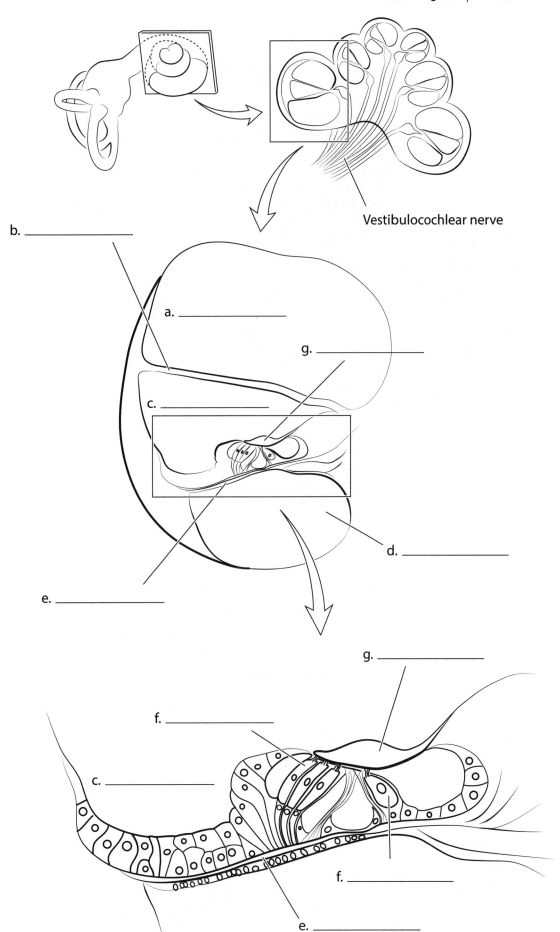

Vestibulocochlear nerve

b. _____

a. _____

g. _____

c. _____

d. _____

e. _____

g. _____

f. _____

c. _____

f. _____

e. _____

■ Chapter Eight: **Endocrine System**

OVERVIEW OF THE ENDOCRINE SYSTEM

The endocrine system is a collection of glands or organs that secrete hormones, which are chemical messengers that control heart rate, development, growth, reproduction, digestion, etc. Hormones are released from endocrine glands and typically travel through blood vessels and reach target areas receptive to them.

Organs in the brain include the **pineal gland**, which secretes **melatonin**, regulating sleep cycles, alertness, and temperature. The **hypothalamus** produces hormones stored in the posterior pituitary and secretes hormones that affect the anterior pituitary. The **pituitary gland** secretes numerous hormones, some of which stimulate other endocrine glands.

The **thyroid gland** is inferior to the larynx and is shield-shaped. Thyroid hormones control metabolic rate and decrease calcium levels in the blood. The **parathyroid glands** are on the posterior surface of the thyroid gland and secrete parathyroid hormone, increasing blood calcium levels. The hormones of the **pancreas**, such as insulin and glucagon, regulate blood sugar levels.

The **adrenal glands** are superior to the kidneys, producing epinephrine (adrenaline) and hormones that control mineral balance, inflammation, and metabolic functions. Testosterone is a hormone primarily of the male **testes**. Estrogen and progesterone, produced in the **ovaries**, regulate the female reproductive system. The reproductive hormones also influence secondary sex characteristics such as beard growth in males and breast development in females.

Color Guide: Start with each of the endocrine glands, and color them in with dark or bright colors. Shade in the rest of the body lightly using your preferred color.

Answer Key

a. Pineal body (gland)
b. Hypothalamus
c. Pituitary gland (hypophysis)
d. Parathyroid glands (posterior view)
e. Thyroid gland
f. Adrenal glands
g. Pancreas
h. Ovary
i. Testis

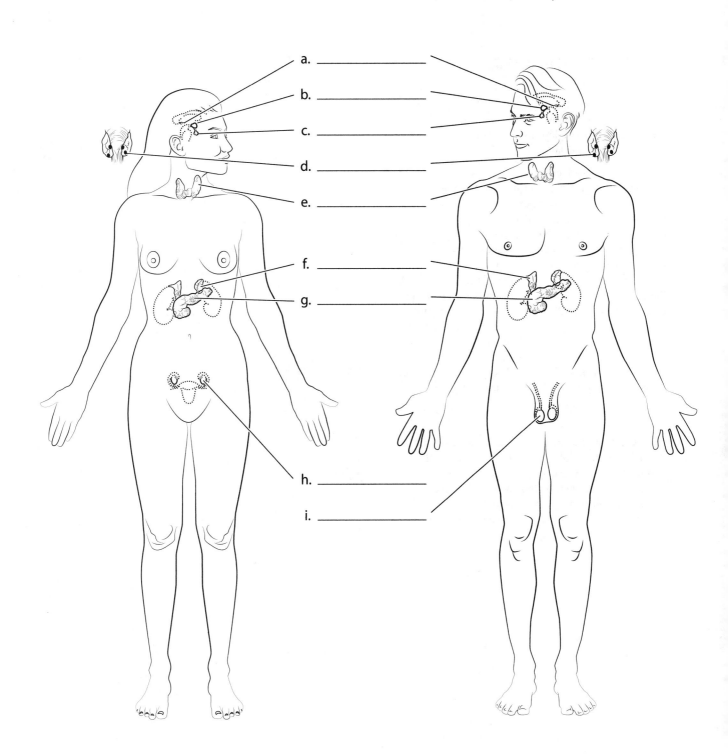

a. _____

b. _____

c. _____

d. _____

e. _____

f. _____

g. _____

h. _____

i. _____

ORGANS OF THE HEAD

The **pineal gland** is a small gland located posterior to the **corpus callosum** in the brain. It has the shape of a pine nut but is a little bit smaller. It secretes the hormone melatonin; melatonin levels increase during the night and decrease during the day.

The **pituitary gland**, or **hypophysis**, is suspended from the brain by a stalk called the **infundibulum**. The pituitary sits in the **hypophyseal fossa**, which is a depression in the **sphenoid bone**. The pituitary is a complicated gland that has numerous functions. The **adenohypophysis** or **anterior pituitary** originates from the oral cavity during development and consists of epithelium. It produces several hormones, which will be discussed later. The anterior pituitary has cells that pick up histological stain differently. These are **acidophilic cells** and **basophilic cells**. The **neurohypophysis** or **posterior pituitary** is derived from the brain during development and does not make its own hormones but stores hormones produced in the hypothalamus. Label the pineal gland, the corpus callosum, and the pituitary gland. Label the parts of the pituitary.

Color Guide: In the upper illustration, color the pineal gland and pituitary gland in different colors. In the middle illustration, use purple for the adenohypophysis and yellow for the neurohypophysis. In "e," color the acidophilic cells red and the lighter-shaded basophilic cells purple or blue. Use yellow to color the lower right illustration of the neurohypophysis.

Answer Key
a. Pituitary gland (hypophysis)
b. Pineal gland
c. Corpus callosum
d. Hypophyseal fossa
e. Adenohypophysis (anterior pituitary)
f. Sphenoid bone
g. Infundibulum
h. Neurohypophysis (posterior pituitary)
i. Basophilic cell
j. Acidophilic cell

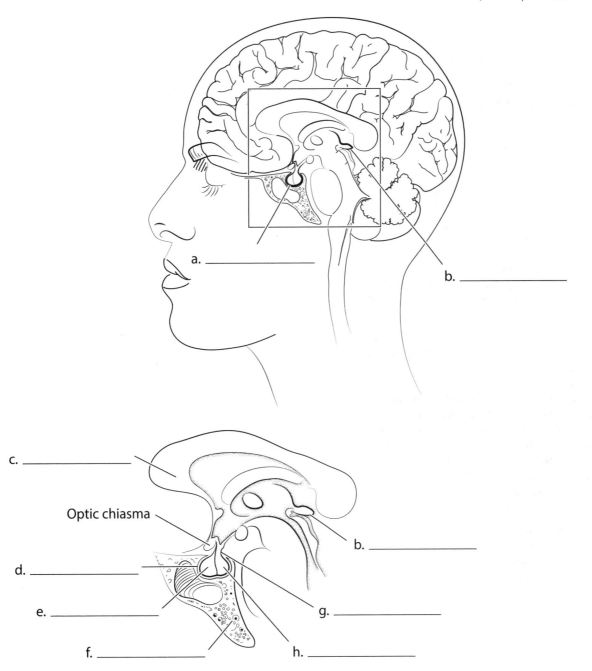

a. _____

b. _____

c. _____

Optic chiasma

b. _____

d. _____

e. _____

f. _____

g. _____

h. _____

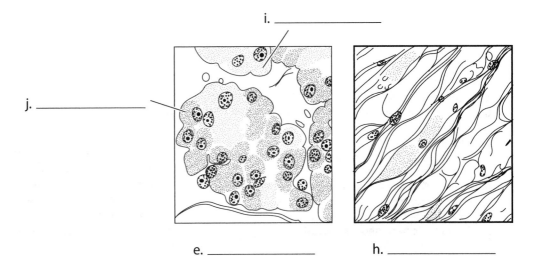

i. _____

j. _____

e. _____

h. _____

HORMONES SECRETED BY THE PITUITARY AND THEIR TARGET ORGANS

The **adenohypophysis** produces and secretes many hormones that have diverse target areas. **Growth hormone (GH)** is released by the pituitary and causes growth and division of cells, such as muscle and bone cells, throughout the body. **Prolactin** is more specific in its function. It initiates milk production in the mammary glands. **Follicle stimulating hormone (FSH)** and **luteinizing hormone (LH)** are gonadotropins that cause the ovaries and testes to release hormones. **Thyroid stimulating hormone (TSH)** causes the thyroid gland to secrete hormones, and **adrenocorticotropic hormone (ACTH)** has an influence on the adrenal cortex.

The posterior pituitary, or **neurohypophysis**, stores and secretes a hormone called **oxytocin**. This hormone has many functions. It causes milk letdown during nursing and has multiple functions as a neurotransmitter in the brain. It is secreted during orgasm in the female and is also released when the infant is nursing. Oxytocin causes uterine contractions and has an effect on kidney water balance. The other hormone stored in the neurohypophysis is **antidiuretic hormone** or **ADH**. It is also known as **vasopressin**. It causes absorption of water from the collecting ducts of the kidney, decreasing the volume of water in urine.

Color Guide: Select one color for the impacts of the adenohypophysis, indicated in the lower illustration as "a" through "g." Select another color for the neurohypophysis and its impacts shown in structures "h" through "j." Use the same color scheme in the upper illustration.

Answer Key

a. Adenohypophysis
b. Thyroid stimulating hormone
c. Prolactin
d. Growth hormone
e. Adrenocorticotropic hormone
f. Luteinizing hormone
g. Follicle stimulating hormone
h. Neurohypophysis
i. Oxytocin
j. Antidiuretic hormone (vasopressin)

LEARNING HINT

To remember the hormones secreted by the pituitary, draw a chart with two main sections: **adenohypophysis** and **neurohypophysis**. Under these heads, list each hormone and its impact on the human body.

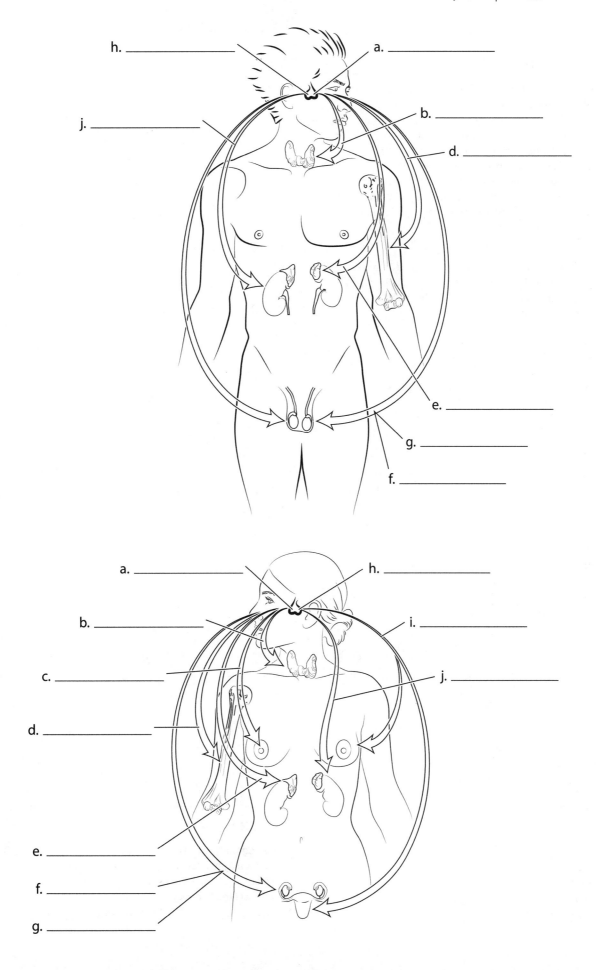

h. _____

a. _____

j. _____

b. _____

d. _____

e. _____

g. _____

f. _____

a. _____

h. _____

b. _____

i. _____

c. _____

j. _____

d. _____

e. _____

f. _____

g. _____

THYROID GLAND

The thyroid gland is just inferior to the thyroid cartilage of the larynx. It has two main **lobes** and a small connection between them called the **isthmus**. The histology of the thyroid is very distinctive. There are cells called **follicular cells** forming a sphere, and these make up the follicle. Inside the follicle is the **colloid** where thyroid hormones are stored. The **parafollicular cells** are between the follicles. Label the main parts of the thyroid gland, the follicular cells, the parafollicular cells, and the colloid.

Color Guide: Color each lobe of the thyroid in brown, and use a lighter shade of brown for the isthmus. Use red for the follicular cells and blue for the colloid. Select another color for the parafollicular cells.

Answer Key

a. Thyroid gland
b. Right lobe
c. Isthmus
d. Left lobe
e. Colloid
f. Follicular cells
g. Parafollicular cells

LEARNING HINT

In geography, an **isthmus** is a strip of land connecting two landmasses. In the endocrine system, the isthmus is a small strip of tissue that connects the two lobes of the thyroid.

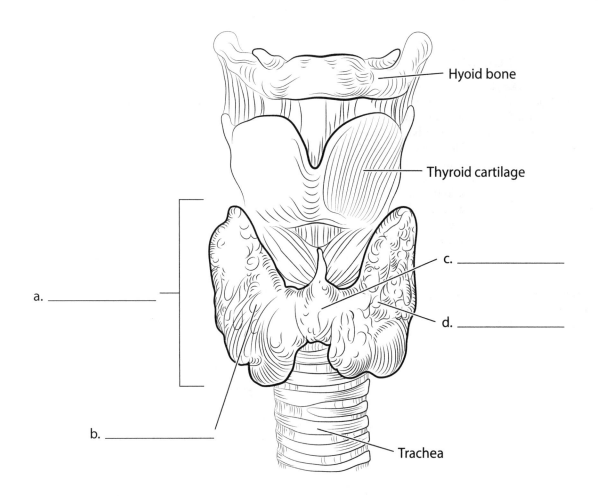

Hyoid bone

Thyroid cartilage

a. _____

b. _____

c. _____

d. _____

Trachea

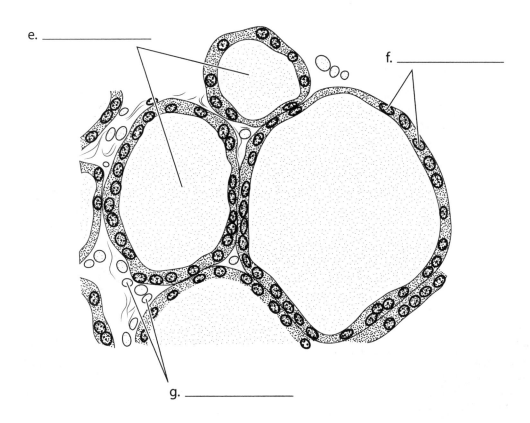

e. _____

f. _____

g. _____

PARATHYROID GLANDS

There are typically four glands on the posterior
of the thyroid gland, and these are known as the
parathyroid glands. They secrete a hormone called
parathormone, which regulates calcium balance in the
blood. Parathormone increases blood calcium levels by
causing more absorption of calcium from the digestive
tract, increased osteoclast activity in the bones, and
reabsorption of calcium from the kidney. The **principal**
or **chief cells** secrete parathyroid hormone. The **oxyphilic
cells** are less common, and their function is poorly
understood. Label the parathyroids on the posterior
thyroid gland.

Color Guide: Use a light color for the parathyroid glands
and brown for the thyroid gland. Color the chief cells pink
and the oxyphilic cells purple or blue.

Answer Key

a. Thyroid gland
b. Parathyroid glands
c. Principal (chief) cells
d. Oxyphilic cells

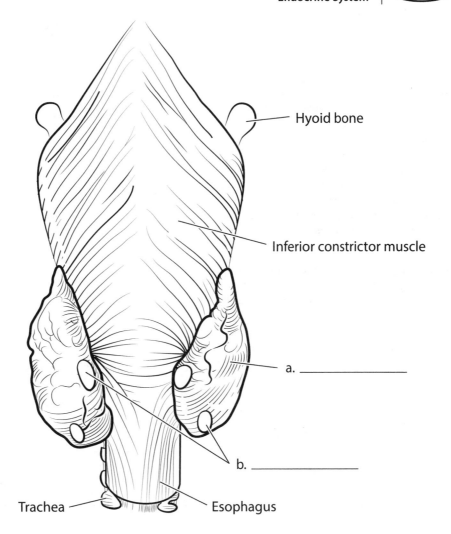

Hyoid bone

Inferior constrictor muscle

a. _____

b. _____

Trachea

Esophagus

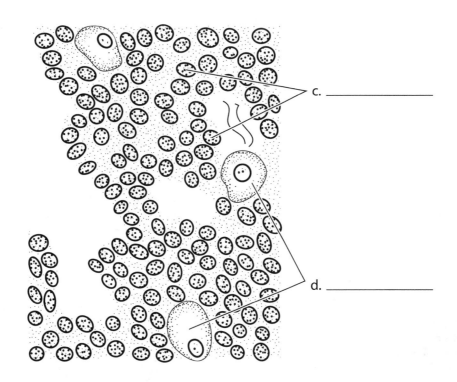

c. _____

d. _____

PANCREAS

The **pancreas** is inferior to the stomach and has several digestive functions. These exocrine secretions are initiated by the **acinar cells**. The endocrine function of the pancreas consists of the secretion of insulin, glucagon, and somatostatin from the **pancreatic islets**. These islets are microscopic collections of cells that have specialized cells for the secretion of hormones. Insulin lowers blood glucose levels while glucagon does the reverse. Somatostatin moderates some of the pancreatic cells that have a role in digestion. Label the illustration.

Color Guide: In the upper figure, make the pancreas yellow or light beige. In the middle figure, use a lighter color for the pancreatic islets (like a light blue) and a deeper color such as red or purple for the acinar cells. Color the gallbladder in green, and use the same color for the pancreas as you did in the upper illustration.

Answer Key

a. Pancreas
b. Pancreatic islets
c. Acinar cells (exocrine)

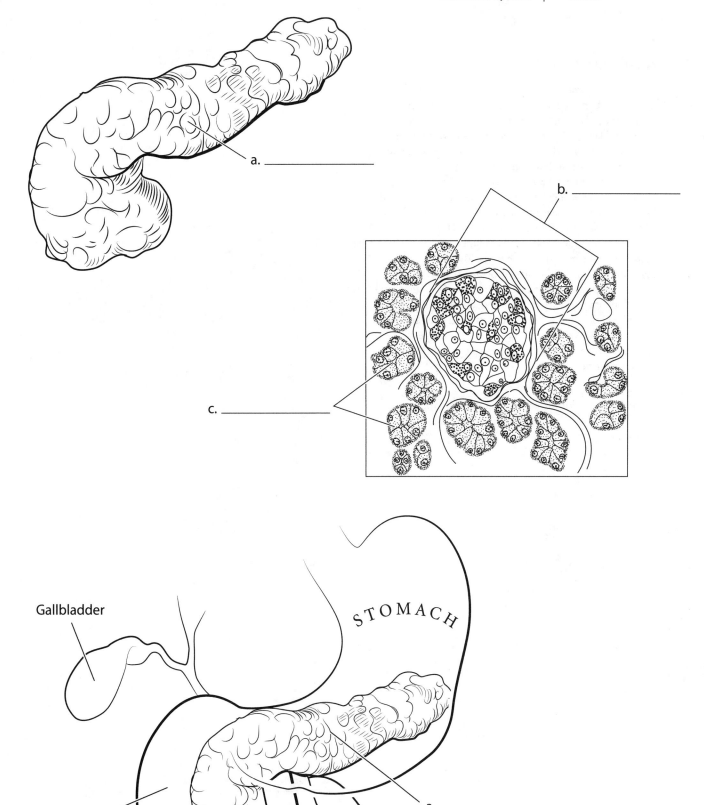

a. _____

b. _____

c. _____

Gallbladder

STOMACH

Duodenum

a. _____

Superior mesenteric artery & vein

ADRENAL GLANDS

The **adrenal glands** are positioned superior to the kidneys and are divided into the adrenal **cortex** and the **medulla**. The cortex has three layers. The most superficial layer is the **zona glomerulosa**, which is deep to the adrenal **capsule** and responsible for the secretion of mineralocorticoid hormones. The next layer is the **zona fasciculata**, which mainly secretes glucocorticoids, hormones responsible for the breakdown of proteins and lipids and the synthesis of glucose. The **zona reticularis** is the deepest layer of the cortex and secretes androgens (male sex hormones) and small amounts of estrogens (female sex hormones) in both sexes. The most prevalent male hormone is DHEA (dehydroepiandrosterone), which is responsible for the development of the sex drive, pubic hair, and axillary hair. The effects of DHEA are minimized in males as the testes secrete greater amounts of testosterone. The adrenal medulla is the deepest part of the adrenal gland and secretes epinephrine and norepinephrine.

Color Guide: Color the adrenal gland beige, and use a different color for each layer of the cortex and another for the medulla.

Answer Key

a. Adrenal gland
b. Cortex
c. Medulla
d. Capsule
e. Zona glomerulosa
f. Zona fasciculata
g. Zona reticularis

LEARNING HINT

The three zones of the adrenal glands resemble their names. The word **glomerulus** means "ball of threads" (like a yarn ball), a **fascicle** is a bundle (like a bundle of sticks), and **reticularis** is "netlike" in appearance.

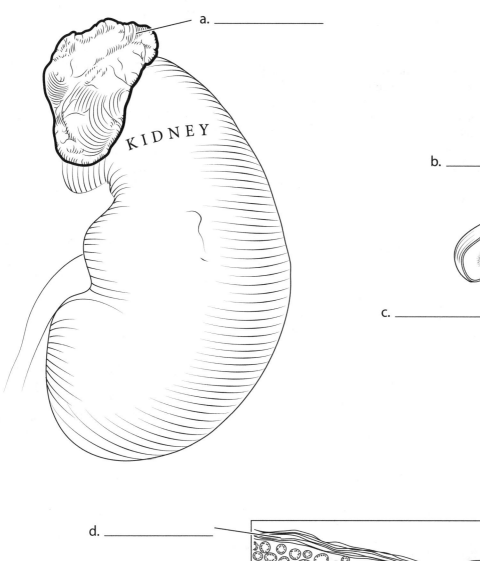

a. _____

KIDNEY

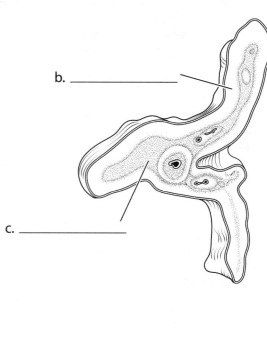

b. _____

c. _____

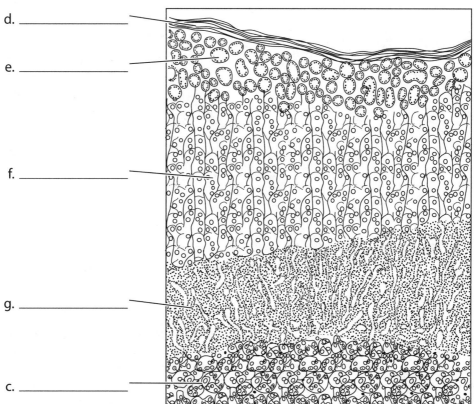

d. _____

e. _____

f. _____

g. _____

c. _____

GONADS

The **ovaries** are mixed glands because they produce the oocytes (egg cells) and have the endocrine function of producing estrogens. Estrogens are a class of female sex hormones that include estradiol and progesterone. Estradiol is produced in the **granulosa cells** of the **ovarian follicles**. These follicles surround the oocytes. Progesterone is produced by the **corpus luteum** after the oocyte has been ovulated.

The **testes** are also mixed glands. As exocrine glands, they produce sperm cells, and as endocrine glands, the **interstitial cells** produce testosterone. Label the interstitial cells and **seminiferous tubules** in the microscopic view of the testes.

Color Guide: Use beige or yellow to color the ovary in the upper illustration. Use reds and blues for the outer layers of "b," "c," and "d," and color the interior blue. Use yellow for the outer part of "e." Select different colors for the lower illustration.

Answer Key

a. Ovary
b. Granulosa cells
c. Ovarian follicles
d. Oocytes
e. Corpus luteum
f. Interstitial cells
g. Testis
h. Seminiferous tubules

LEARNING HINT

The term **corpus luteum** translates to "yellow body."

Interstices are the spaces between other structures. The **interstitial cells** lie in the spaces between the seminiferous tubules.

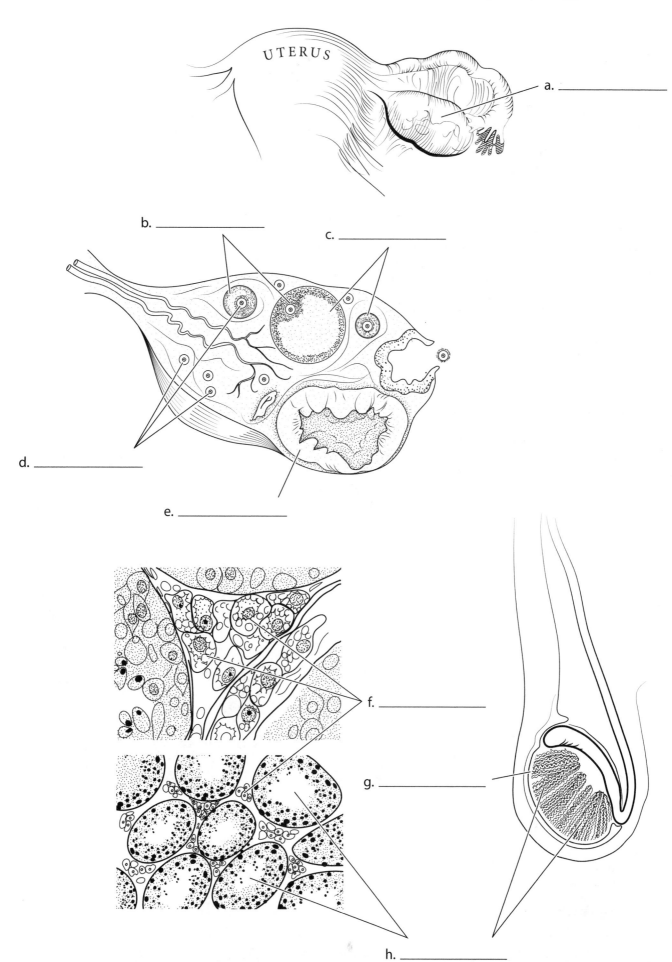

UTERUS

a. _____

b. _____

c. _____

d. _____

e. _____

f. _____

g. _____

h. _____

Chapter Nine: **Cardiovascular System**

OVERVIEW OF THE CARDIOVASCULAR SYSTEM

The cardiovascular system consists of the heart as a pump, blood vessels that take blood away from the heart (arteries), and blood vessels that take blood back to the heart (veins). Locate the **heart** on the illustration. Label the **common carotid artery** and the **internal jugular vein**. The internal jugular vein takes blood to the **superior vena cava**, which takes blood to the heart. Label the **aortic arch**, and find the continuation of the **aorta** that travels down the left side of the body, splits, and takes blood to the **femoral artery**. The vessel parallel to the femoral artery is the **femoral vein**. The femoral vein eventually takes blood to the **inferior vena cava** before it goes to the heart. Blood travels to the arm by the **brachial artery** and deoxygenated blood travels to the lungs in the **pulmonary trunk**.

Color Guide: Most of the arteries in the illustration should be colored red, as they carry oxygenated blood. The exception is the pulmonary trunk, which should be colored blue as it carries deoxygenated blood to the lungs. Trace all the veins that take blood to the superior vena cava, and color them in blue. Do the same for all of the veins that take blood to the inferior vena cava. Color the heart in purple.

Answer Key

a. Internal jugular vein
b. Common carotid artery
c. Superior vena cava
d. Brachial artery
e. Inferior vena cava
f. Aortic arch
g. Pulmonary trunk
h. Heart
i. Aorta
j. Femoral artery
k. Femoral vein

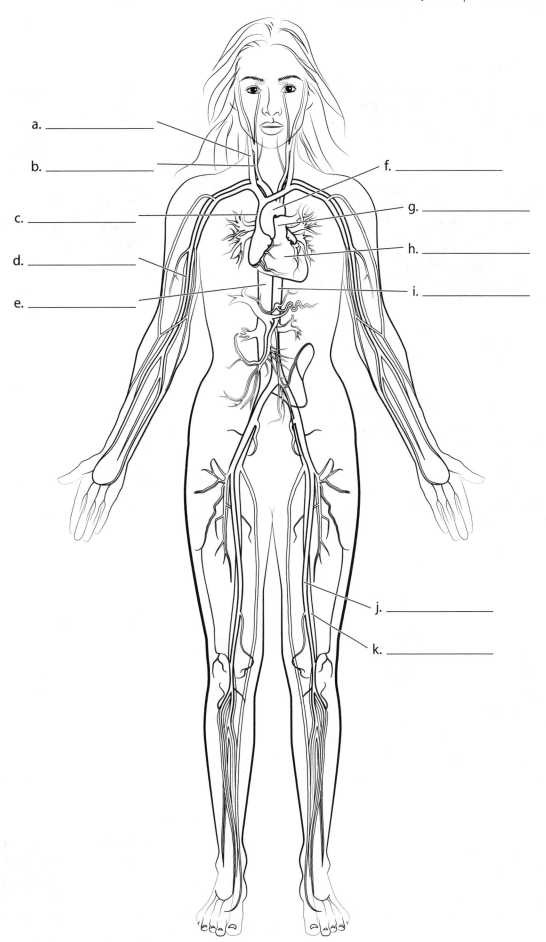

a. _____

b. _____

c. _____

d. _____

e. _____

f. _____

g. _____

h. _____

i. _____

j. _____

k. _____

CIRCULATION

The heart has four chambers including the superior atria and the inferior ventricles. Label the **right atrium**, **right ventricle**, **left atrium**, and **left ventricle**. Remember the heart is in anatomical position, so the right atrium is on the left in the illustration.

There are two major circulations in the body. One goes to the lungs and is called the **pulmonary circulation**. Deoxygenated blood leaves the right ventricle of the heart and travels through the **pulmonary artery** to the lungs, where the blood is oxygenated. Blood returns from the lungs to the left atrium of the heart by the **pulmonary veins**. The other main circulation in the body is called the **systemic circulation**, where blood travels from the left ventricle of the heart and goes to the other regions of the body. Arteries are defined as vascular tubes that take blood away from the heart, while veins are vessels that return blood to the heart. Most arteries carry oxygenated blood, and most veins carry deoxygenated blood, but there are a few exceptions.

The first vessel that leaves the heart is the **aorta**, which is part of the arterial system. **Arteries** receive blood from the aorta and take blood throughout the body. They branch and become smaller until they become **arterioles**. The arterioles are the structures that control blood pressure in the body. As they get smaller, they become capillaries. The **capillaries** are the site of exchange with the cells of the body. On the return flow, the capillaries enlarge and turn into **venules**, which take blood to the veins. Blood from the inferior portion of the heart returns to the heart by the **inferior vena cava**.

Color Guide: There is a conventional coloring pattern for the cardiovascular system. Blue is used to indicate vessels or chambers that carry deoxygenated blood, while red indicates vessels that carry oxygenated blood. Use blue for the pulmonary artery, which transports deoxygenated blood to the lungs. Color the aorta, the arteries of the body, and the arterioles red. Label and then color the capillaries purple. Purple is a good choice for the capillaries because they are the interchange between the arteries (red) and the veins (blue). Use blue to color the venules and remaining veins of the body.

Answer Key

a. Superior vena cava
b. Pulmonary artery
c. Pulmonary vein
d. Pulmonary capillary bed
e. Right atrium
f. Right ventricle
g. Inferior vena cava
h. Vein
i. Venule
j. Aorta
k. Left atrium
l. Left ventricle
m. Descending aorta
n. Artery
o. Arteriole
p. Systemic capillary bed

LEARNING HINT

Atrium is the Latin word for "entry hall." The atria of the heart are the chambers that first receive blood.

Pulmonary derives from another Latin word, *pulmo*, meaning "lung."

Systemic circulation:
head, neck, and arms

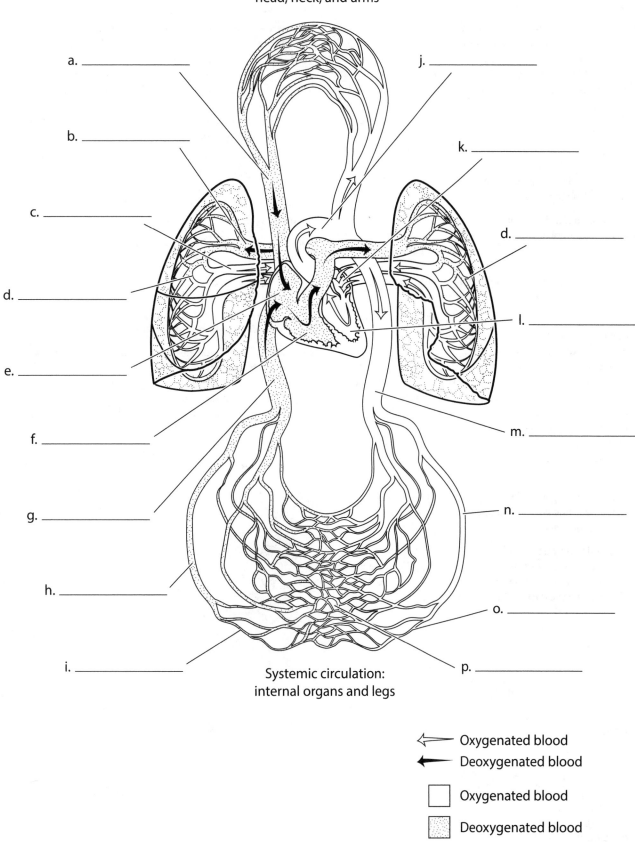

a. _____

b. _____

c. _____

d. _____

e. _____

f. _____

g. _____

h. _____

i. _____

j. _____

k. _____

d. _____

l. _____

m. _____

n. _____

o. _____

p. _____

Systemic circulation:
internal organs and legs

⇐— Oxygenated blood

⬅— Deoxygenated blood

☐ Oxygenated blood

▨ Deoxygenated blood

BLOOD

Blood consists of **plasma** and **formed elements**. The plasma is the fluid portion of the blood and consists of water, proteins, and dissolved materials such as oxygen, carbon dioxide, electrolytes (ionic particles), and other materials. Plasma makes up about 55 percent of the blood volume. Formed elements make up about 45 percent of the blood volume and consist of **erythrocytes** (red blood cells), **leukocytes** (white blood cells), and **thrombocytes** (platelets). There are about 200,000–450,000 thrombocytes per cubic millimeter of blood. They assist the body in clotting to prevent blood from flowing out of small ruptures in blood vessels.

There are about 5 million erythrocytes per cubic millimeter of blood. The erythrocytes do not have a nucleus, and they appear like a donut with a thin spot instead of the donut hole. About a third of the weight of a red blood cell is due to **hemoglobin**, which makes the cells red. Note also the size of the thrombocyte.

There are about 7,000 leukocytes per cubic millimeter of blood. There are two main types of leukocytes: **granulocytes** and **agranulocytes**. The granulocytes have cytoplasmic granules that either stain pink or dark purple or do not stain much at all. The granulocytes that do not stain much at all are called **neutrophils** because the granules are neutral to the stains. They are the most numerous of the leukocytes, making up 60–70 percent of the leukocytes. Neutrophils have a three- to five-lobed nucleus.

The **eosinophils** are granulocytes that have pink or orange staining granules. The nucleus is generally two-lobed. Eosinophils make up about 3 percent of the white blood cells.

Basophils are rare granulocytes in that they make up less than 1 percent of the white blood cells. The nucleus is S-shaped but is frequently difficult to see because it is obscured by the dark-staining cytoplasmic granules.

The two kinds of agranulocytes are the **lymphocytes** and the **monocytes**. The lymphocytes can be large or small, and they make up 20–30 percent of the leukocytes. The cytoplasm is light blue, and the nucleus is purple. The nucleus of the lymphocyte is dented or flattened. Lymphocytes come in two kinds. **B cells** secrete antibodies (antibody-mediated immunity), and **T cells** are involved in cell-mediated immunity.

The monocytes are large cells (about three times the size of a red blood cell) and have a strongly lobed nucleus. Some people say this looks like a kidney bean or a horseshoe. They represent only about 5 percent of the leukocytes.

Label the blood cells on the facing page, and follow the coloring directions below.

Color Guide: At the top of the illustration, use a light red to color in the surface view and cross section of the red blood cell. Color the thrombocyte purple.

Color in the red blood cells in the central part of the illustration with a light red color. Color in the eosinophil ("e") starting with the nucleus using purple, and then using orange for the granules in the cytoplasm. For the basophil ("d"), color in the granules a dark purple so that they almost obscure the nucleus.

For the lymphocytes at the bottom of the page, color in the nucleus with purple and the cytoplasm with light blue.

Color in the nucleus of the monocyte with a purple and the cytoplasm a light blue.

Answer Key

a. Erythrocyte
b. Thrombocyte
c. Leukocytes
d. Basophil
e. Eosinophil
f. Neutrophil
g. Lymphocyte
h. Monocyte

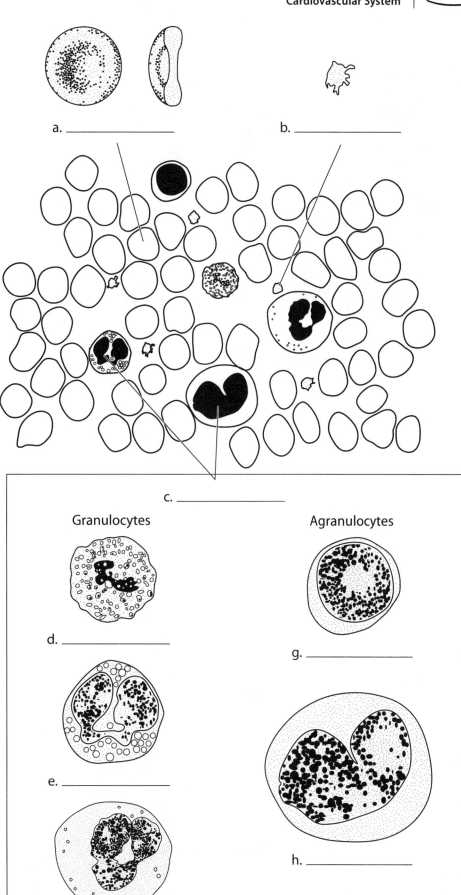

a. _____

b. _____

c. _____

Granulocytes

Agranulocytes

d. _____

g. _____

e. _____

f. _____

h. _____

ANTERIOR SURFACE VIEW OF THE HEART

The **apex** of the heart is inferior, and the **base** is superior. Label each chamber of the heart. Locate the **right coronary artery**. The right coronary artery leads to the **right marginal artery**. The **left coronary artery** (not shown) takes blood to the **anterior interventricular artery** and the **circumflex artery**. The **cardiac veins** can also be seen on the anterior side. The **great cardiac vein** runs in the interventricular sulcus on the anterior side. Label all of the major vessels entering and exiting the heart.

Color Guide: Use red for "a," "f," "j," "m," and "o" as these are arteries carrying oxygenated blood. Use blue for "b," "g," "k," and "p." Color the walls of the heart in light red or pink.

Answer Key

a. Aortic arch
b. Pulmonary trunk
c. Base of heart
d. Left atrium
e. Circumflex artery
f. Anterior interventricular artery
g. Great cardiac vein
h. Left ventricle
i. Apex of heart
j. Descending aorta
k. Inferior vena cava
l. Right ventricle
m. Right marginal artery
n. Right atrium
o. Right coronary artery
p. Superior vena cava

LEARNING HINT

The **coronary arteries** are so named because they form a *corona* (Latin for "crown") around the heart.

The **right marginal artery** is found on the right margin of the heart.

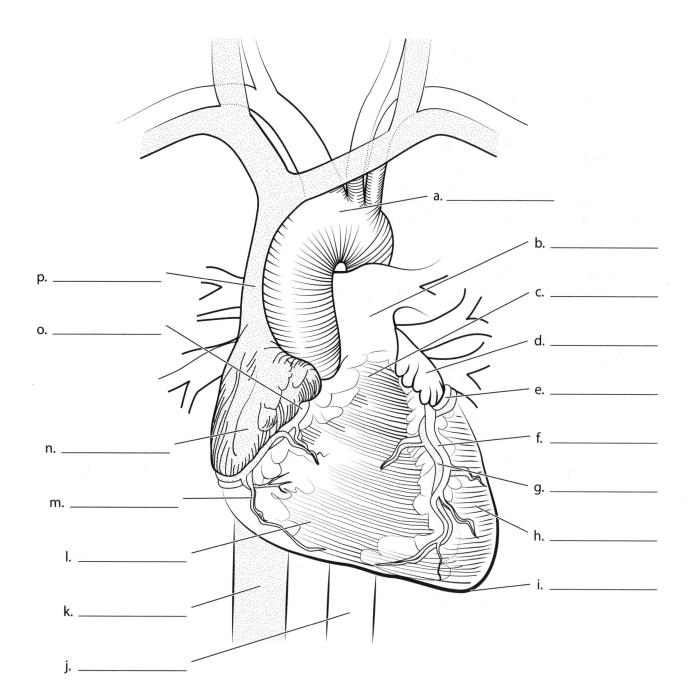

a. _____

b. _____

c. _____

d. _____

e. _____

f. _____

g. _____

h. _____

i. _____

p. _____

o. _____

n. _____

m. _____

l. _____

k. _____

j. _____

POSTERIOR SURFACE OF THE HEART

On the posterior side of the heart are additional arteries and veins. The **posterior interventricular artery** occurs between the ventricles on the posterior surface. It receives blood from the **right coronary artery**. The **middle cardiac vein** runs in the opposite direction and takes blood into the **coronary sinus**. A *sinus* is a space. In the heart, the coronary sinus is a more expanded space than the cardiac veins, which are smaller in diameter. The **small cardiac vein** is also found on the posterior surface of the heart and enters the **coronary sinus** from the opposite direction. Label the posterior features of the heart.

Color Guide: Color the arteries in red (except for the **pulmonary arteries** that carry deoxygenated blood—they should be colored in blue). Color the veins in blue (except for the **pulmonary veins**, which should be colored in red).

Answer Key

a. Aortic arch
b. Left atrium
c. Pulmonary veins
d. Coronary sinus
e. Left ventricle
f. Middle cardiac vein
g. Posterior interventricular artery
h. Right ventricle
i. Inferior vena cava
j. Right coronary artery
k. Right atrium
l. Pulmonary arteries
m. Superior vena cava

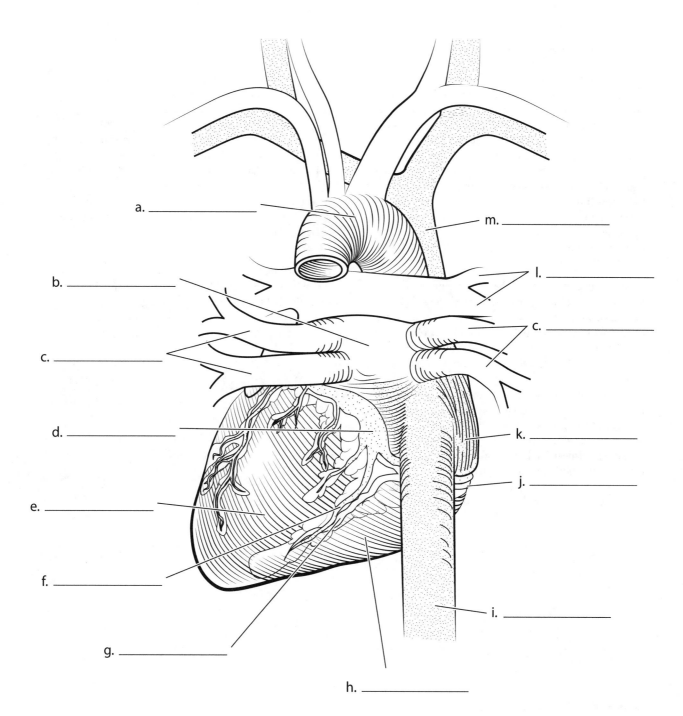

a. _____

b. _____

c. _____

d. _____

e. _____

f. _____

g. _____

h. _____

i. _____

j. _____

k. _____

l. _____

m. _____

c. _____

CORONAL SECTION OF THE HEART

The membranes surrounding the heart, known as the pericardium (*peri-* for "around" and *cardium* for "heart"), are grouped into layers. The outermost layer, the **fibrous pericardium**, surrounds an inner **serous pericardium** that itself consists of two layers. The outer, **parietal layer of the serous pericardium** is attached to the fibrous pericardium, while the inner part touches the heart wall and is called the **visceral layer of the serous pericardium** (or **epicardium**). Between these two layers of serous pericardium is the **pericardial cavity**. The muscular wall of the heart is called the **myocardium**, and the innermost layer of the heart (which is in direct contact with the blood) is the **endocardium**.

Deoxygenated blood enters the **right atrium** of the heart by three vessels: the **superior vena cava**, the **inferior vena cava**, and the **coronary sinus**. The walls of the right atrium are thin as they only have to transfer blood to the **right ventricle**. The blood in the right atrium is in contact with the **fossa ovalis**, which is a thin spot in the interatrial septum. This thin spot is a remnant of a hole in the fetal heart known as the foramen ovale. Blood in the right atrium flows through the cusps of the **tricuspid** or **right atrioventricular valve** into the right ventricle. The tricuspid valve is made of the three cusps, the **chordae tendineae**, and the **papillary muscles** that hold the chordae tendineae to the ventricle wall. The ventricle wall is lined with **trabeculae carneae** that act as struts along the edge of the wall. The wall between the ventricles is known as the **interventricular septum**.

From the right ventricle, blood passes through the **pulmonary semilunar valve** and into the **pulmonary trunk** where the blood goes to the lungs. In the lungs, the blood is oxygenated. From the lungs, the blood returns to the **left atrium** of the heart. Blood in the left atrium moves to the **left ventricle** through the **left atrioventricular valve** or the **biscuspid valve**. This valve has two cusps, chordae tendineae, and papillary muscles. When the left ventricle contracts, the blood moves through the **aortic semilunar valve** and into the **ascending aorta**.

Color Guide: Use red to color in the light arrows indicating oxygenated blood. Color in the small structures first with light colors of your choosing, and shade in the chambers of the heart with darker colors.

Answer Key

a. Pulmonary trunk
b. Pulmonary semilunar valve
c. Left atrium
d. Left atrioventricular valve
e. Aortic semilunar valve
f. Left ventricle
g. Endocardium
h. Fibrous pericardium
i. Parietal layer of serous pericardium
j. Visceral layer of serous pericardium (epicardium)
k. Pericardial cavity

l. Myocardium
m. Interventricular septum
n. Trabeculae carneae
o. Inferior vena cava
p. Papillary muscle
q. Right ventricle
r. Chordae tendineae
s. Right atrioventricular valve
t. Opening of coronary sinus
u. Fossa ovalis
v. Right atrium
w. Superior vena cava
x. Aorta

LEARNING HINT

When learning the anatomy of the heart, it is beneficial to trace blood's path through the heart. Starting with the three vessels that take blood to the right atrium, use your finger to trace the blood flow until you get to the aorta.

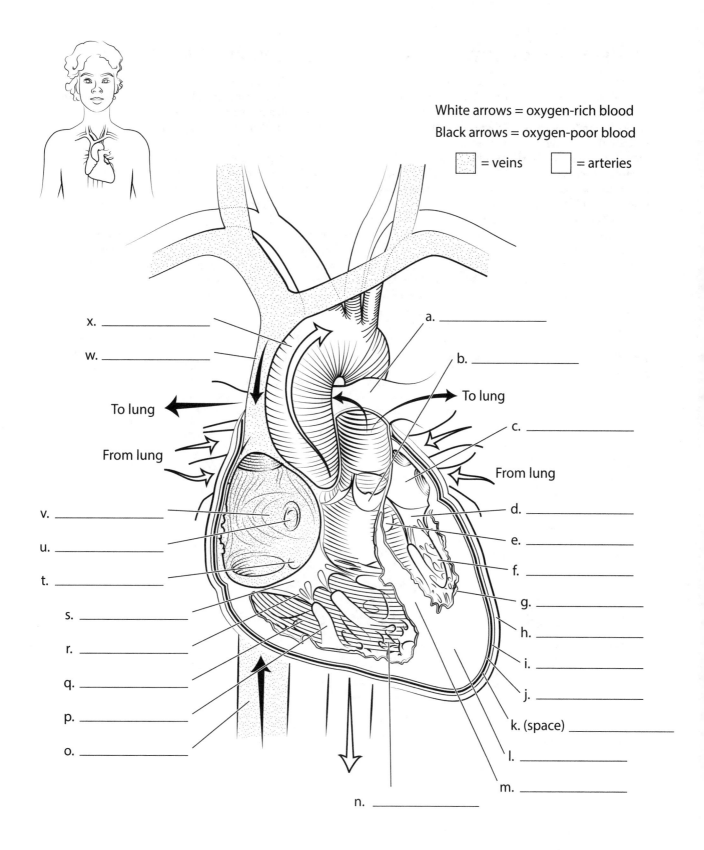

White arrows = oxygen-rich blood

Black arrows = oxygen-poor blood

= veins ☐ = arteries

x. _____

w. _____

To lung

From lung

v. _____

u. _____

t. _____

s. _____

r. _____

q. _____

p. _____

o. _____

a. _____

b. _____

To lung

c. _____

From lung

d. _____

e. _____

f. _____

g. _____

h. _____

i. _____

j. _____

k. (space) _____

l. _____

m. _____

n. _____

SUPERIOR ASPECT OF THE HEART

This view of the heart is seen as if the atria and the major vessels have been removed. You should be able to see all of the major valves of the heart. The most anterior valve is the **pulmonary semilunar valve**, which occurs between the right ventricle and the pulmonary trunk. Posterior to this is the **aortic semilunar valve**, which occurs between the left ventricle and the aorta. When the ventricles contract (ventricular systole), these valves open and let blood flow respectively into the pulmonary trunk or the aorta. When the ventricles relax (ventricular diastole), these valves prevent blood from returning to the ventricles. On the right side of the illustration (and on the right side of the heart) is the **right atrioventricular** (or **tricuspid**) **valve**, so named because it has three flaps or cusps. This valve occurs between the right atrium and the right ventricle. It prevents the blood from returning to the right atrium during ventricular systole. On the left side of the heart is the **left atrioventricular (bicuspid) valve**. It prevents blood from moving back to the left atrium during ventricular systole.

Color Guide: Use blue for "a" and "d"; deoxygenated blood flows through these valves. Color "b" and "c" with red; oxygenated blood flows through these valves.

ECG—CONDUCTION PATHWAY

The heart has specialized cells that initiate an electrical impulse that radiates throughout the heart. The cells are clustered in a particular area known as the **sinoatrial node** or the pacemaker. These cells produce a depolarization that travels across the atria, which depolarize and then contract. Depolarization is an electrical event, while contraction is a mechanical event. Between the wall of the right atrium and the right ventricle is a lump of tissue known as the **atrioventricular (AV) node**. Once the impulse reaches this area, the AV node pauses a moment before sending the impulse to the **atrioventricular bundle**. This bundle divides into the **bundle branches**, and then the impulse travels to the **conduction (Purkinje) fibers**. These fibers reach the muscle of the ventricles and stimulate them to contract.

Color Guide: Use yellow around the arrows to trace the pathway of conductivity in the heart. Color in each chamber of the heart with the same colors that you used on the preceding page.

Answer Key

a. Pulmonary semilunar valve
b. Aortic semilunar valve
c. Left atrioventricular (bicuspid) valve
d. Right atrioventricular (tricuspid) valve
e. Sinoatrial node
f. Atrioventricular node
g. Atrioventricular bundle
h. Bundle branches
i. Purkinje fibers

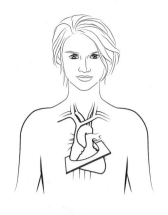

Anterior

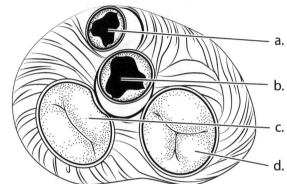

a. _____

b. _____

c. _____

d. _____

Ventricular systole

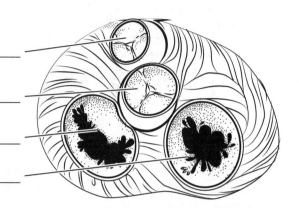

Ventricular diastole

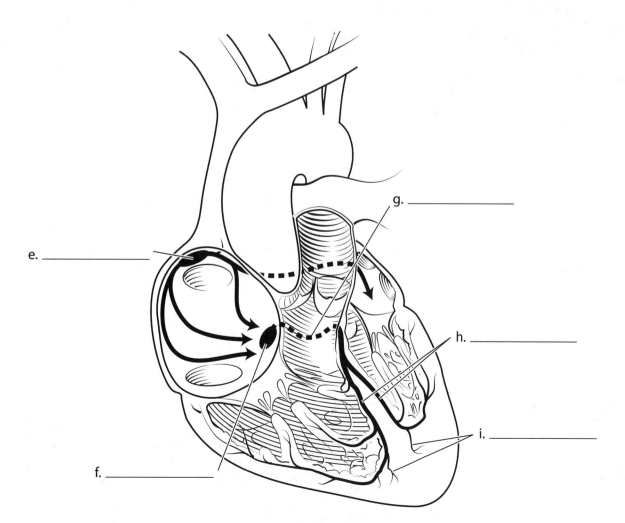

e. _____

g. _____

h. _____

i. _____

f. _____

VESSELS OVERVIEW

The blood vessels have different thicknesses due to the differences in pressure that occur in them or their function with respect to exchanging nutrients with the cells. **Arteries** have thick walls due to the higher pressure found in them. Just as high-pressure hoses have thick walls, so do arteries. The outer layer of the artery is the **tunica externa** (**tunica adventitia**). You should locate the tunica externa and color it in. The middle layer of the artery, the **tunica media**, is the thickest layer and is made of **smooth muscle** and **elastic fibers**. The innermost layer of the artery is the **tunica intima** (**tunica interna**), and it has a special elastic layer called the **internal elastic lamina** (internal elastic membrane). The area in the artery where the blood flows is called the **lumen**. The outer layer of the artery is the **external elastic lamina** (external elastic membrane).

Veins are thinner walled than arteries and do not have the same elastic fibers in the tunica media as arteries. The tunica interna of some veins is folded into valves that allow for the one-way flow of blood through veins.

Capillaries are different from both arteries and veins in that they are composed of only simple squamous epithelium (called **endothelium**). The thin nature of capillaries allows them to exchange nutrients, water, carbon dioxide, and oxygen with the cells.

Color Guide: Use blue to color the tunica externa in both arteries and veins. Color the tunica media red and the tunica intima yellow. Use red to color the smooth muscle ("i"). Color the capillaries yellow.

Answer Key

a. Vein
b. Artery
c. Lumen
d. Tunica intima
e. Tunica media
f. Tunica externa
g. Internal elastic lamina
h. External elastic lamina
i. Smooth muscle
j. Venule
k. Endothelium
l. Arteriole
m. Capillary
n. Venous valve

> **LEARNING HINT**
>
> A layer of the blood vessel is referred to as a **tunica** because it wraps around the vessel like a cloth tunic that wraps around the body.

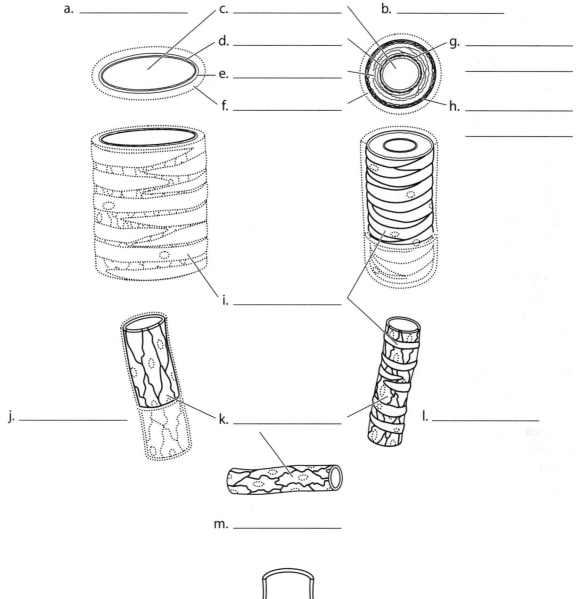

a. _____   c. _____   b. _____

d. _____

g. _____

e. _____

f. _____

h. _____

i. _____

j. _____   k. _____   l. _____

m. _____

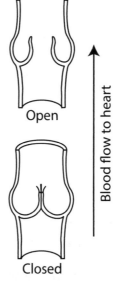

Open

Closed

Blood flow to heart

n. _____

ARTERIES OVERVIEW

One of the ways to study arteries is to draw them as if you were making a street map. Begin with the heart and draw the blood vessels that occur as you take blood to the fingers, toes, or to a particular organ of the body. Use the following artery list, and label the appropriate arteries. The abbreviation for artery is *a*.

Color Guide: Here you will depart from the conventional red coloring of the arteries as you focus on learning the individual arteries of the body. Select any color for the individual arteries, and use a different color for each neighboring artery. You will use these same colors for each artery in the following illustrations.

Ascending aorta

Aortic arch

Thoracic aorta

Abdominal aorta

Brachiocephalic trunk

Common carotid artery

Subclavian artery

Axillary artery

Brachial artery

Radial artery

Ulnar artery

Common iliac artery

Femoral artery

Anterior tibial artery

Fibular artery

Answer Key

a. Common carotid a.
b. Brachiocephalic trunk
c. Ascending aorta
d. Brachial a.
e. Ulnar a.
f. Radial a.
g. Subclavian a.
h. Aortic arch
i. Axillary a.
j. Thoracic aorta
k. Abdominal aorta
l. Common iliac a.
m. Femoral a.
n. Anterior tibial a.
o. Fibular a.

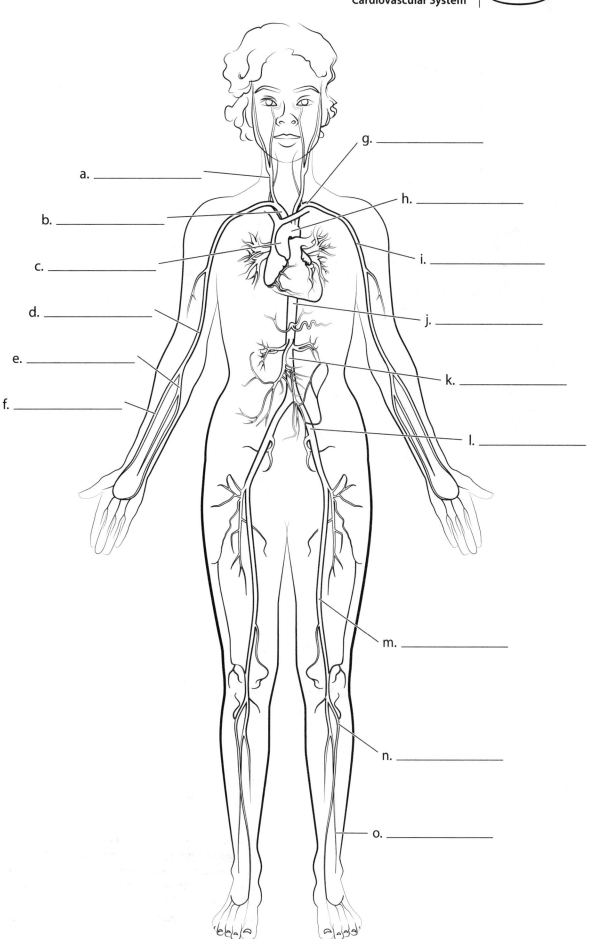

a. _____

b. _____

c. _____

d. _____

e. _____

f. _____

g. _____

h. _____

i. _____

j. _____

k. _____

l. _____

m. _____

n. _____

o. _____

HEAD AND AORTIC ARTERIES

Blood from the heart exits the **brachiocephalic artery** and takes two main pathways to the right side of the head. One of these is the **right common carotid artery**, which exits the brachiocephalic artery and then splits into the **external carotid artery** and the **internal carotid artery**. The external carotid artery has several branches, among them the **facial artery**, the **superficial temporal artery**, the **maxillary artery**, and the **occipital artery**. The internal carotid artery takes blood through the carotid canal of the skull and into the brain. The other main pathway of blood to the right side of the head is the **vertebral artery**, which arises from the **subclavian artery**. The left side of the head has a similar pathway except that the **left common carotid artery** and the **left subclavian artery** arise from the **aortic arch** and not from the brachiocephalic artery. Label these vessels.

Color Guide: Using the same color for the arteries that you chose in previous pages, color in each section of the arterial flow in the illustration. Be sure to use different colors for neighboring arteries.

Answer Key

a. Superficial temporal a.
b. Occipital a.
c. Internal carotid a.
d. Vertebral a.
e. Subclavian a.
f. Brachiocephalic a.
g. Thoracic aorta
h. Facial a.
i. Maxillary a.
j. External carotid a.
k. Common carotid a.
l. Aortic arch
m. Ascending aorta

LEARNING HINT

Most arteries are named for either where they lie (*subclavian* = "under the clavicle") or where they bring blood (renal artery takes blood to the kidney). One exception to this is the **carotid artery**. The word *carotid* means "stupefy," as closing off this artery will cause a person to faint.

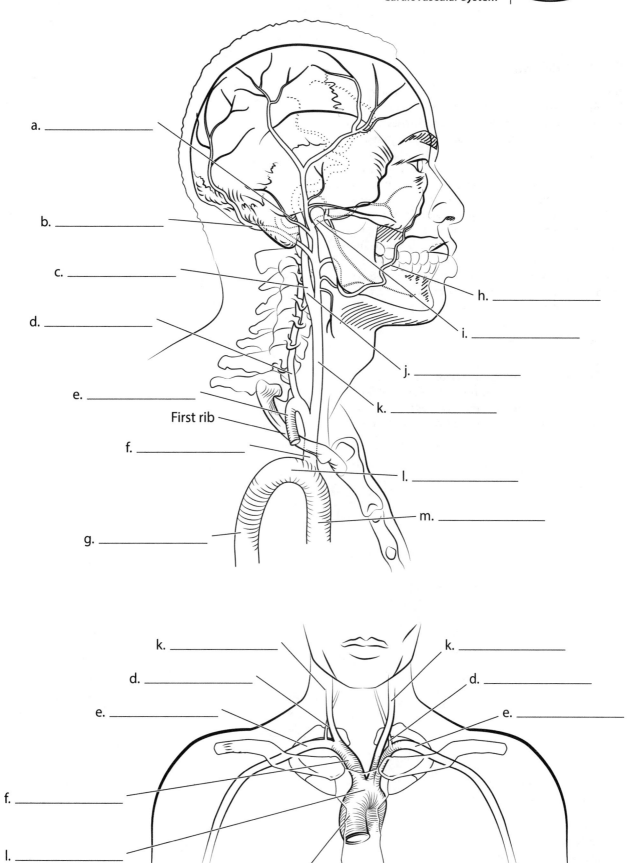

a. _____

b. _____

c. _____

d. _____

e. _____

First rib

f. _____

g. _____

h. _____

i. _____

j. _____

k. _____

l. _____

m. _____

k. _____

d. _____

e. _____

f. _____

l. _____

m. _____

k. _____

d. _____

e. _____

BRAIN ARTERIES

The brain is nourished by two main arterial conduits. The first of these is the flow from the **internal carotid arteries**. Blood from the internal carotid arteries comes from the neck and enters a circular pathway known as the **arterial circle (circle of Willis)**. The other conduit comes from the vertebrae, and these are the **vertebral arteries**. These arteries connect at a vessel called the **basilar artery**, and it leads to the arterial circle. The arterial circle consists of the **anterior communicating arteries** and the **posterior communicating arteries**. From this circle, blood then moves into one of many arteries that feed the brain. The cerebrum is fed by the **anterior, middle**, and **posterior cerebral arteries**. The cerebellum is fed by the **cerebellar arteries**. If there is a blockage in any of these vessels, then blood does not reach the affected part of the brain, and this produces a stroke. Label the illustration. Arteries (plural) are abbreviated *aa*.

Color Guide: Select dark tones to color in the arteries so that they contrast with the tissue of the brain. Use the same color for the pairs of arteries, such as the internal carotid arteries; otherwise, use a different color for each artery.

Answer Key

a. Anterior cerebral a.
b. Middle cerebral a.
c. Internal carotid a.
d. Posterior cerebral a.
e. Basilar a.
f. Anterior communicating a.
g. Arterial circle
h. Posterior communicating a.
i. Cerebellar aa.
j. Vertebral a.

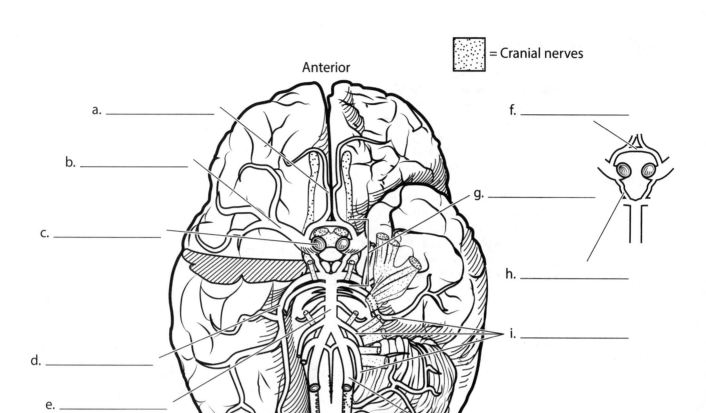

Anterior

a. _____

b. _____

c. _____

d. _____

e. _____

[ ] = Cranial nerves

f. _____

g. _____

h. _____

i. _____

j. _____

Posterior

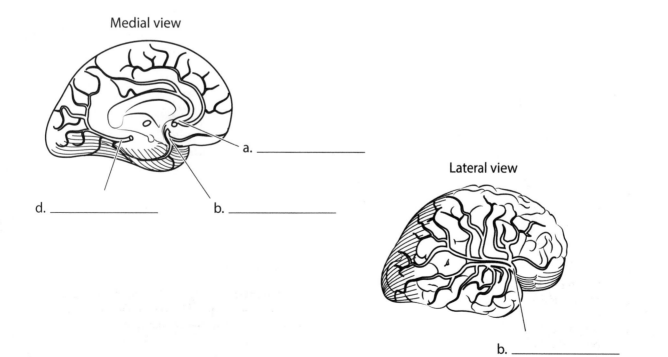

Medial view

a. _____

d. _____

b. _____

Lateral view

b. _____

UPPER LIMB ARTERIES

The arteries of the upper limb receive blood from the **subclavian artery**, which takes blood to the **axillary artery**. Blood in the axillary artery travels to the anterior scapula by the **subscapular artery**, to the external chest wall by the **lateral thoracic artery**, to the upper humeral region by the **posterior circumflex humeral artery**, and to the distal regions of the arm by the **brachial artery**. The brachial artery is the major artery of the arm, and it divides distally to form the **radial** and **ulnar arteries**. The radial artery is frequently palpated at the wrist to determine the pulse rate. The radial and ulnar arteries rejoin (called collateral circulation) in the hand as the **superficial** and **deep palmar arch arteries**. These arteries take blood to the fingers as **digital arteries**. Label these blood vessels.

Color Guide: Select a different color for each section of the arterial flow in the illustration. Use the same color for the arteries that you chose in previous illustrations, and be sure to use different colors for adjacent arteries.

Answer Key

a. Subclavian a.
b. Axillary a.
c. Posterior circumflex humeral a.
d. Brachial a.
e. Radial a.
f. Lateral thoracic a.
g. Subscapular a.
h. Ulnar a.
i. Deep palmar arch
j. Superficial palmar arch
k. Digital a.

LEARNING HINT

The **subclavian, axillary,** and **brachial arteries** are all connected end to end and have separate names simply to reflect the regions this continuous artery passes through.

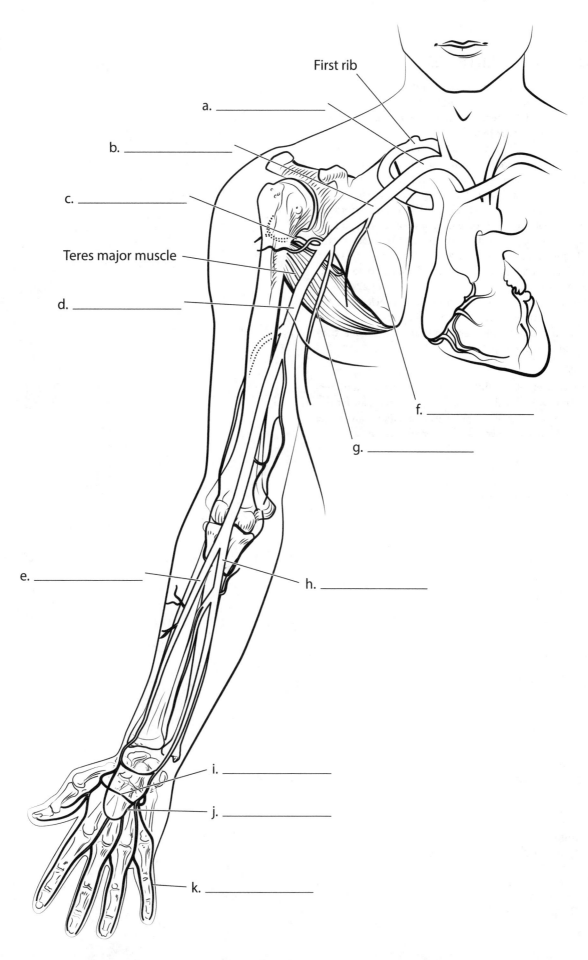

First rib

a. _____

b. _____

c. _____

Teres major muscle ___

d. _____

f. _____

g. _____

e. _____

h. _____

i. _____

j. _____

k. _____

LOWER LIMB ARTERIES

Blood in the lower limb comes from the branches of the iliac arteries. Blood in the **common iliac artery** flows into the **internal iliac artery** and into the **external iliac artery**. Once it passes by the inguinal ligament (a connective tissue band that stretches from the ilium to the pubis), the external iliac artery becomes the **femoral artery**. The femoral artery takes blood down the anterior thigh, but there is a branch called the **deep femoral artery** that takes blood closer to the bone. The femoral artery moves posteriorly to become the **popliteal artery**, and branches of the popliteal artery become the **anterior** and **posterior tibial arteries** and the **fibular (peroneal) artery**. The tibial arteries take blood to the **dorsal arcuate artery**, the **dorsalis pedis artery**, and the **dorsal metatarsal arteries**, which take blood to the **digital arteries**. Arteries that go behind the bone are indicated by dotted outlines, while those in front are drawn with solid lines. Label the lower limb arteries.

Color Guide: Select a different color for each section of the arterial flow in the illustration. Use the same color for the arteries that you chose in previous illustrations, and make sure that you use different colors for adjacent arteries.

Answer Key

a. Common iliac a.
b. Internal iliac a.
c. External iliac a.
d. Femoral a.
e. Deep femoral a.
f. Popliteal a.
g. Anterior tibial a.
h. Posterior tibial a.
i. Fibular a.
j. Dorsalis pedis a.
k. Arcuate a.
l. Dorsal metatarsal a.

a. _____

b. _____

c. _____

d. _____

e. _____

f. _____

g. _____

h. _____

i. _____

j. _____

k. _____

l. _____

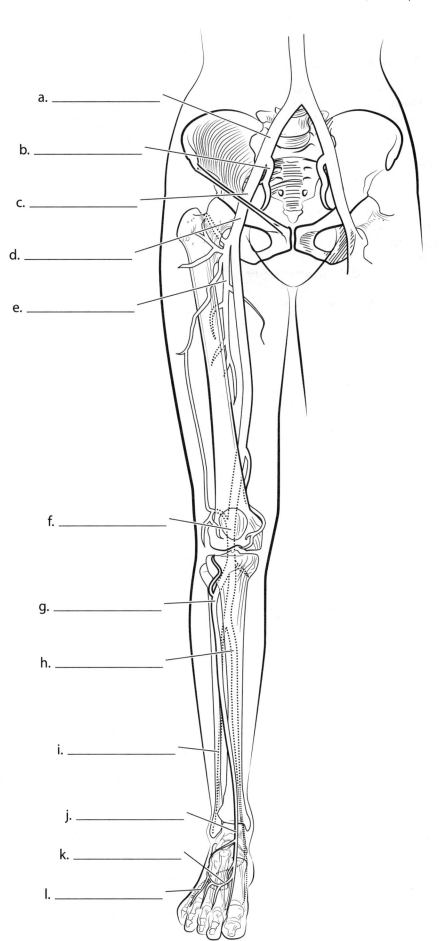

ABDOMINAL/THORACIC ARTERIES

The aorta starts at the **ascending aorta** and curves via the **aortic arch**. The **thoracic aorta** is a portion of the descending aorta. It has several branches that take blood to most of the ribs and intercostal muscles. These are the **posterior intercostal arteries**. Below the diaphragm, the descending aorta is known as the **abdominal aorta** and has several branches. The first of these is the **celiac trunk**, and it branches to take blood to the stomach, spleen, and liver. The next branch is the **superior mesenteric artery**. Below this are the **renal arteries** that take blood to the kidneys. The **gonadal arteries** are found inferior to the renal arteries, and they take blood to the testes in males or the ovaries in females. A single **inferior mesenteric artery** is found below the gonadal arteries. The aorta terminates as it divides into the **common iliac arteries**. Label these vessels.

Color Guide: Select a different color for each section of the arterial flow in the illustration. Use the same color for the arteries that you chose in previous illustrations, and make sure that you use different colors for adjacent arteries.

Answer Key
a. Aortic arch
b. Ascending aorta
c. Thoracic aorta
d. Posterior intercostal arteries
e. Celiac trunk
f. Superior mesenteric artery
g. Renal artery
h. Abdominal aorta
i. Gonadal artery
j. Inferior mesenteric artery
k. Common iliac artery

LEARNING HINT

The **mesentery** is a flat sheet of tissue in the abdominal cavity, and the superior and inferior mesenteric arteries pass through this tissue.

Some of the arteries in the abdomen and thorax are named for where they can be found, such as the **thoracic aorta**, while others are named for the destination of the blood they carry, such as the **gonadal arteries**.

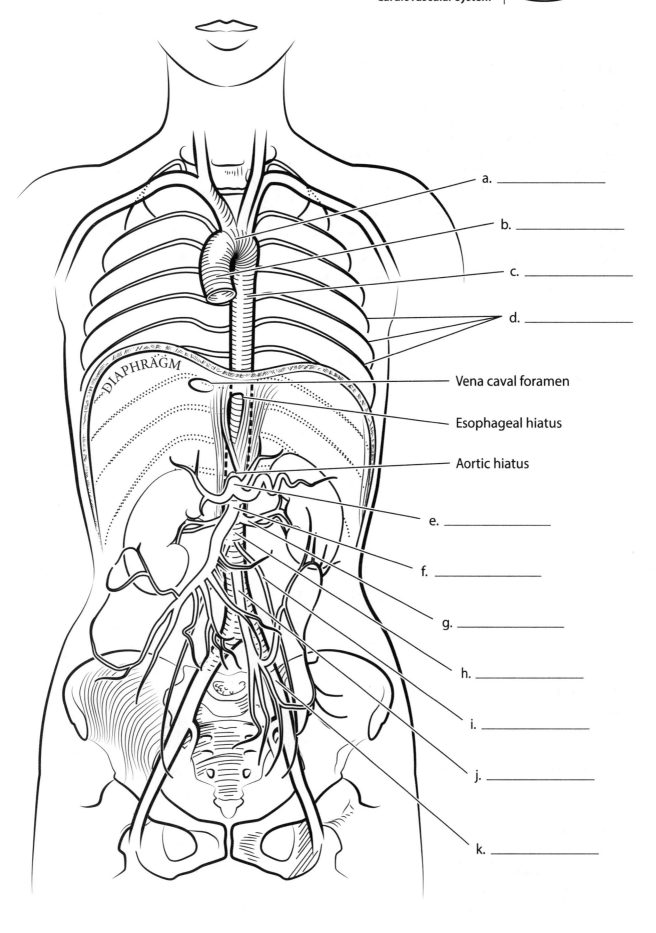

a. _____

b. _____

c. _____

d. _____

DIAPHRAGM

Vena caval foramen

Esophageal hiatus

Aortic hiatus

e. _____

f. _____

g. _____

h. _____

i. _____

j. _____

k. _____

ARTERIES OF THE DIGESTIVE SYSTEM

The **celiac trunk** splits into three branches, the **common hepatic artery**, the left **gastric artery**, and the **splenic artery**. There are other branches to the stomach that have collateral circulation (two or more arteries taking blood to one area). One of these is the **right gastroepiploic artery**, and another is the **left gastroepiploic artery**. Inferior to the celiac trunk is the **superior mesenteric artery**, which takes blood to the small intestine and to several of the colic arteries that supply blood to the proximal portion of the large intestine. These are the **middle colic artery**, the **intestinal branches**, the **right colic artery**, and the **ileocolic artery**. The **inferior mesenteric artery** takes blood to the distal portion of the large intestine via the **left colic artery**, **sigmoid artery superior**, and **rectal artery**.

Color Guide: Select a different color for each section of the arterial flow in the illustration. Use the same color for the arteries that you chose in previous illustrations, and make sure that you use different colors for adjacent arteries.

Answer Key

a. Celiac trunk
b. Common hepatic a.
c. Left gastric a.
d. Splenic a.
e. Right gastroepiploic a.
f. Left gastroepiploic a.
g. Superior mesenteric a.
h. Middle colic a.
i. Intestinal branches
j. Right colic a.
k. Ileocolic a.
l. Inferior mesenteric a.
m. Left colic a.
n. Sigmoid a.
o. Superior rectal a.

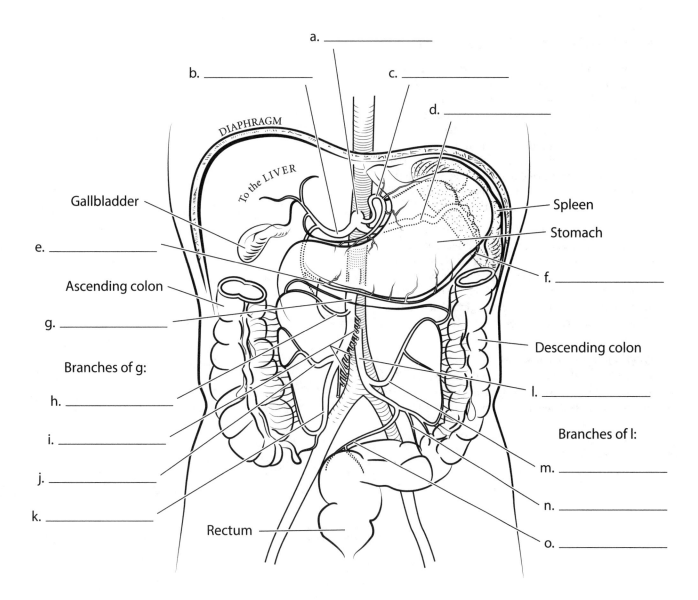

a. _____

b. _____

c. _____

d. _____

DIAPHRAGM

To the LIVER

Gallbladder

Spleen

Stomach

e. _____

Ascending colon

f. _____

g. _____

Descending colon

Branches of g:

h. _____

l. _____

i. _____

Branches of l:

j. _____

m. _____

k. _____

n. _____

Rectum

o. _____

MALE AND FEMALE PELVIC ARTERIES

The **common iliac artery** takes blood to the **external iliac artery**, and the **internal iliac artery** takes blood to the pelvis. In females, branches of the internal iliac artery take blood to the inner pelvis. The **vesical arteries** take blood to the bladder, the **uterine arteries** take blood to the uterus, the **vaginal arteries** feed the vagina, the **rectal arteries** feed the rectum, and the sacral arteries go to the sacrum. The **pudendal artery** takes blood to the external regions where it supplies blood to the pelvic floor, the labia majora and minora, and the clitoris.

In males, the internal iliac artery takes blood to the bladder, rectum, sacrum, prostate, and seminal vesicles on the inside. The pudendal artery takes blood to the scrotum, penis, and external pelvic floor. In both sexes, the **obturator artery** takes blood from the internal iliac artery to the medial thigh while the **gluteal arteries** take blood to the muscles posterior to the pelvic cavity.

Color Guide: Select a different color for each section of the arterial flow in the illustration. Use the same color for the arteries that you chose in previous illustrations, and make sure that you use different colors for adjacent arteries.

Answer Key

a. Common iliac a.
b. Internal iliac a.
c. External iliac a.
d. Obturator a.
e. Superior vesical aa.
f. Lateral sacral a.
g. Gluteal aa.
h. Superior gluteal a.
i. Inferior gluteal a.
j. Uterine a.
k. Pudendal a.
l. Middle rectal a.
m. Vaginal a.
n. Inferior vesical a.

LEARNING HINT

While most of the pelvic arteries are named for where they take blood (e.g., uterine, vaginal, and rectal arteries), the **pudendal artery** has a more generic name. This is because it takes blood to a number of different areas.

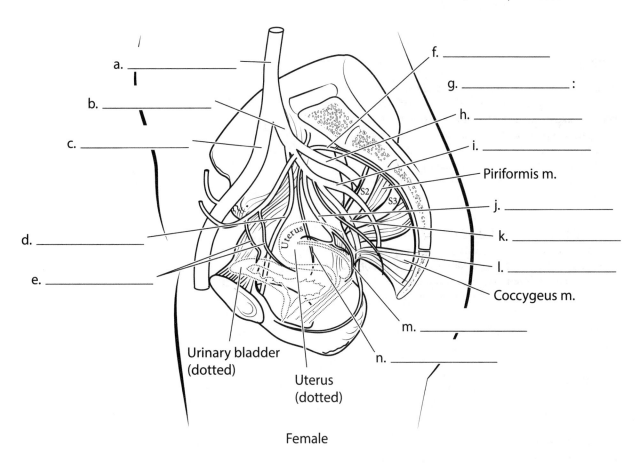

a. _____

b. _____

c. _____

d. _____

e. _____

f. _____

g. _____ :

h. _____

i. _____

Piriformis m.

j. _____

k. _____

l. _____

Coccygeus m.

m. _____

n. _____

Urinary bladder
(dotted)

Uterus
(dotted)

S2

S3

Uterus

Female

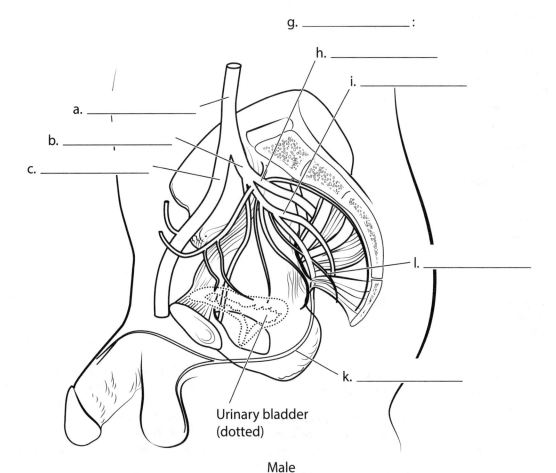

g. _____ :

h. _____

i. _____

a. _____

b. _____

c. _____

l. _____

k. _____

Urinary bladder
(dotted)

Male

VEINS

Veins are blood vessels that return blood to the heart. They are characteristically colored blue on illustrations. The deep veins typically take the name of the artery next to them or the name of the organ that provides them with blood. Therefore, the femoral vein runs next to the femoral artery, and the splenic vein receives blood from the spleen. Some veins have names unique to them; these are typically the superficial veins. Use the following list and label the major veins of the body.

Color Guide: Here you will depart from the conventional blue coloring of the veins as you focus on learning the individual veins of the body. Select a different color for each section of the venous system so that each vein has its own color. You will use these same colors for each vein in the following illustrations.

Cephalic vein

Basilic vein

Radial veins

Ulnar veins

Brachial veins

Axillary vein

Subclavian vein

Brachiocephalic vein

Superior vena cava

Vertebral vein

Internal jugular vein

External jugular vein

Femoral vein

Great saphenous vein

Small saphenous vein

External iliac vein

Internal iliac vein

Common iliac vein

Inferior vena cava

Renal vein

Gonadal vein

Answer Key

a. Internal jugular vein
b. Brachiocephalic vein
c. Superior vena cava
d. Brachial veins
e. Ulnar veins
f. Radial veins
g. Internal iliac vein
h. External iliac vein
i. Femoral vein
j. Vertebral vein
k. External jugular vein
l. Subclavian vein
m. Axillary vein
n. Cephalic vein
o. Basilic vein
p. Inferior vena cava
q. Renal vein
r. Gonadal vein
s. Common iliac vein
t. Great saphenous vein
u. Small saphenous vein

> **LEARNING HINT**
>
> When learning the veins, it is beneficial to trace the blood's path through them. Direction of flow in the veins is generally the reverse of the arteries, because blood flow in the veins goes *toward* the heart. So ulnar veins lead to the brachial veins, which lead to the axillary vein.

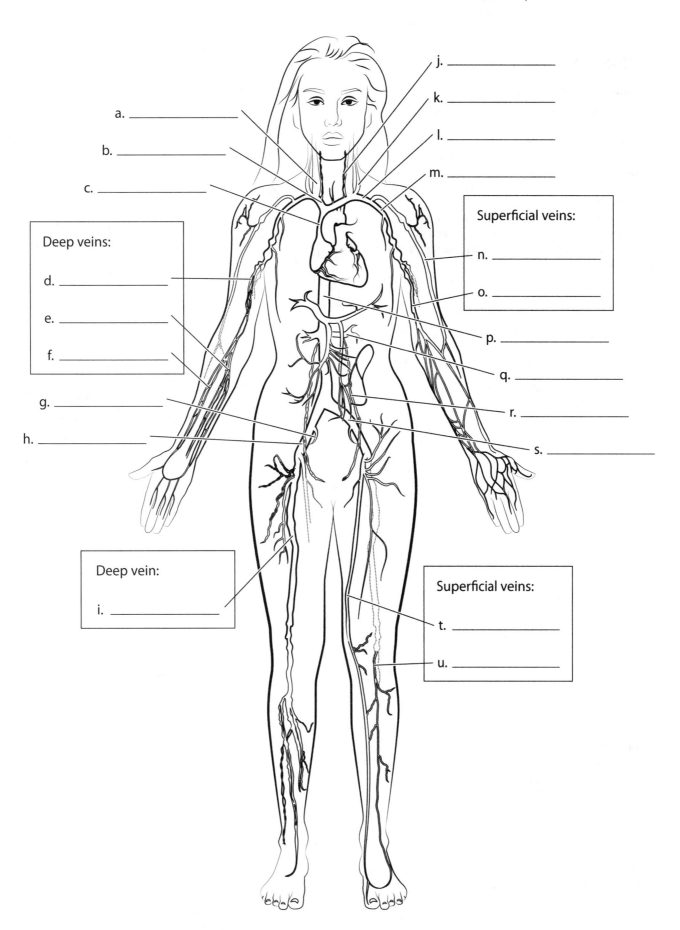

a. _____

b. _____

c. _____

j. _____

k. _____

l. _____

m. _____

Deep veins:

d. _____

e. _____

f. _____

g. _____

h. _____

Superficial veins:

n. _____

o. _____

p. _____

q. _____

r. _____

s. _____

Deep vein:

i. _____

Superficial veins:

t. _____

u. _____

HEAD AND NECK VEINS

Superior Vena Cava Veins

The drainage of the head occurs by the **jugular veins**. The posterior neck muscles are drained by the **vertebral veins**. Some of the blood coming from the brain travels down the **superior sagittal sinus** and through the large **internal jugular veins**. These veins take blood down both sides of the neck and enter the **brachiocephalic veins**. The external portion of the head is drained by several veins. The **facial vein** and the **maxillary vein** take blood to the internal jugular vein while the **superficial temporal vein** and the **posterior auricular vein** take blood to the **external jugular vein**, which then flows into the **subclavian vein** before reaching the brachiocephalic vein. A vein is abbreviated as *v.*

Color Guide: Use the same colors as you did in the previous illustration for the same veins. Make sure that you have a different color for each particular vein.

Answer Key

a. Sagittal sinus
b. Superficial temporal v.
c. Posterior auricular v.
d. External jugular v.
e. Vertebral v. (plexus)
f. Subclavian v.
g. Maxillary v.
h. Facial v.
i. Internal jugular v.
j. Brachiocephalic v.
k. Superior vena cava

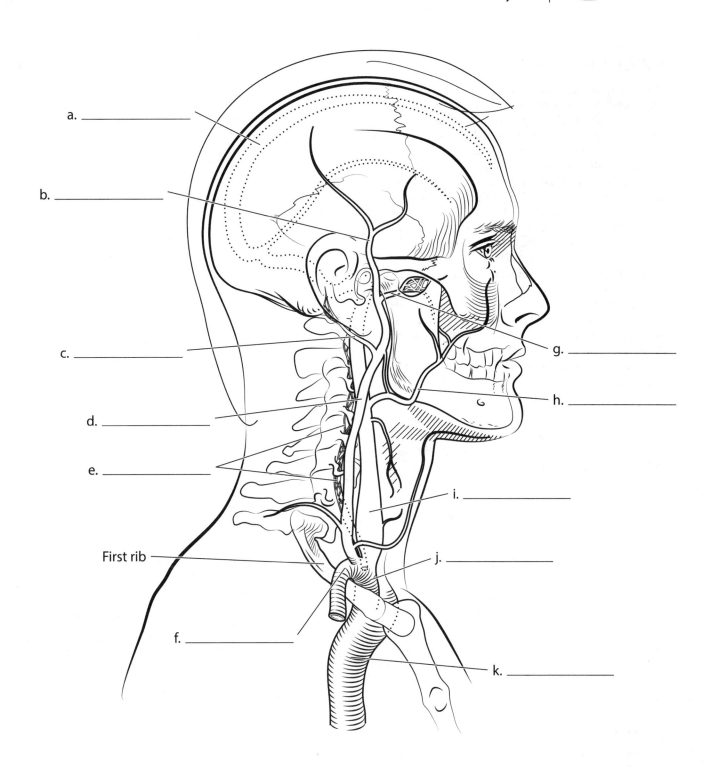

a. _____

b. _____

c. _____

d. _____

e. _____

First rib _____

f. _____

g. _____

h. _____

i. _____

j. _____

k. _____

UPPER LIMB VEINS

The veins of the upper limb are somewhat variable and have many cross connections between them, but they can be divided into the deep veins and the superficial veins. The deep veins of the upper limb frequently form a meshwork around the arteries (venae comitantes), which allows for a great amount of heat transfer. Cool blood from the limbs is warmed by the arterial blood moving in a countercurrent flow. Blood in the fingers returns to the forearm by the **digital veins** and then the **superficial** and **deep palmar arch veins**. The deep veins of the upper limb are the **radial veins**, the **ulnar veins**, and the **brachial veins**. The brachial veins lead to the **axillary vein**, which takes blood to the **subclavian vein**. The superficial veins of the upper limb are the **basilic vein**, found on the medial aspect of the forearm and arm; the **median antebrachial vein**, on the anterior aspect of the forearm; the **cephalic vein**, found on the lateral aspect of the forearm and arm; and a small vein that connects the basilic vein with the cephalic vein called the **median cubital vein**. This vein is used frequently to withdraw blood. Label the veins of the upper limb. Veins (plural) are abbreviated as *vv*.

Color Guide: Use the same color for each vein that you used in the overview of the venous system. Use different colors for adjacent veins.

Answer Key

a. Subclavian v.
b. Cephalic v.
c. Axillary v.
d. Radial vv.
e. Median antebrachial v.
f. Deep palmar arch
g. Digital vv.
h. Basilic v.
i. Brachial vv.
j. Median cubital v.
k. Ulnar vv.
l. Superficial palmar arch v.

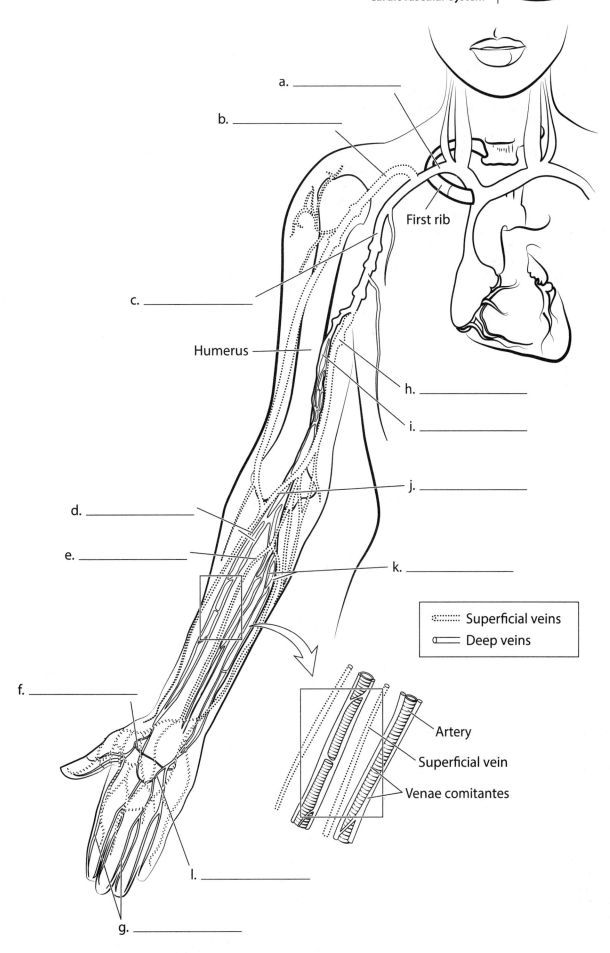

a. _____

b. _____

First rib

c. _____

Humerus

h. _____

i. _____

j. _____

d. _____

e. _____

k. _____

| :::::: Superficial veins |
| o——— Deep veins |

f. _____

Artery

Superficial vein

Venae comitantes

l. _____

g. _____

LOWER LIMB VEINS

Blood in the toes returns by the **digital veins**. These veins take blood to the **dorsal metatarsal veins** and the **dorsal venous arch veins**. On the underside of the foot are the **plantar veins**. Blood moves up the leg by the **posterior** and **anterior tibial veins** and the **great** and **small saphenous veins**. The **anterior** and **posterior tibial veins** join together to form the **popliteal vein** posterior to the knee. The small saphenous vein joins the **popliteal vein**, taking blood to the **femoral vein**. The **great saphenous vein** begins around the medial malleolus and runs the entire length of the medial lower limb when it enters into the femoral vein. Once the femoral vein crosses the inguinal ligament, it becomes the **external iliac vein**.

Color Guide: Use the same color for each vein that you used in the overview of the venous system. Use different colors for adjacent veins.

Answer Key

a. External iliac v.
b. Femoral v.
c. Deep femoral v.
d. Anterior tibial v.
e. Dorsal venous arch
f. Dorsal metatarsal v.
g. Digital v.
h. Great saphenous v.
i. Popliteal v.
j. Small saphenous v.
k. Posterior tibial v.
l. Plantar v.

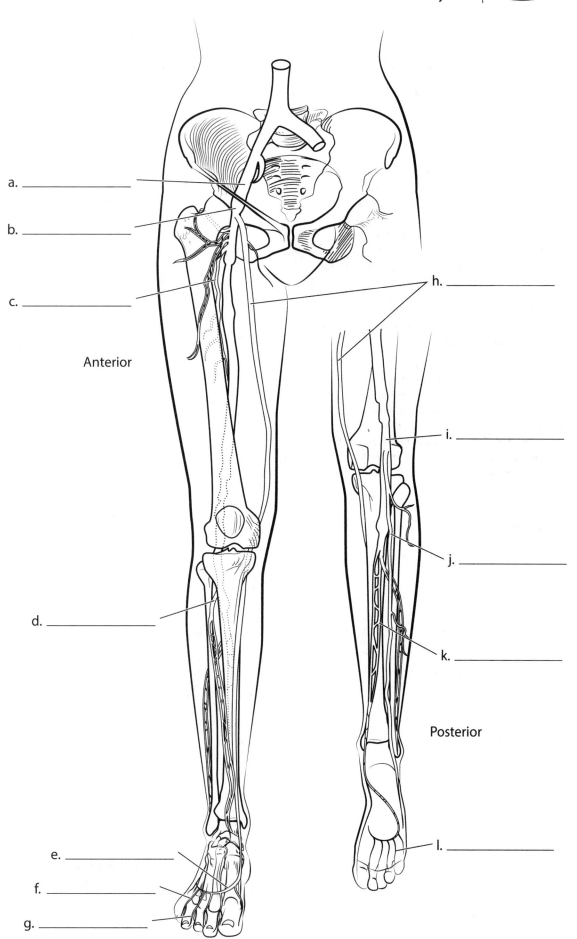

a. _____

b. _____

c. _____

Anterior

d. _____

e. _____

f. _____

g. _____

h. _____

i. _____

j. _____

k. _____

l. _____

Posterior

HEPATIC PORTAL VEINS AND TRUNK VEINS

Most of the blood of the body returns to the heart by capillaries flowing into venules and finally into veins before reaching the heart. In a **portal system**, blood moves from one capillary system to another capillary system before reaching the heart. The **hepatic portal system** takes blood from the capillary beds of many of the abdominal organs and carries it to the liver where metabolic processing takes place. The **gastric veins** take blood to the **hepatic portal vein**. The **inferior mesenteric vein** takes blood primarily from the colon and empties into the **splenic vein**. The splenic vein and the **gastroepiploic vein** flow into the **superior mesenteric vein**, which takes blood from the small intestine and proximal part of the large intestine and empties into the hepatic portal vein. Once the blood is processed in the liver, it enters the systemic circulation by the **hepatic veins**.

The return of blood from other parts of the pelvic and abdominal cavities does not go through the hepatic portal system but enters the inferior vena cava. The **renal veins** take blood from the kidneys to the inferior vena cava. The **gonadal veins** take blood from the testes or the ovaries. The **left gonadal vein** enters **the left renal vein** while the **right gonadal vein** enters the **inferior vena cava**. The **intercostal veins** take blood to the **hemiazygos** and the **azygos veins**.

Color Guide: Use the same color for each vein that you used in the overview of the venous system. Use different colors for adjacent veins.

Answer Key

a. Azygos v.
b. Inferior vena cava
c. Hepatic v.
d. Renal v.
e. Posterior intercostal vv.
f. Hemiazygos v.
g. Gonadal v.
h. Hepatic portal v.
i. Superior mesenteric v.
j. Right colic v.
k. Gastric v.
l. Splenic v.
m. Gastroepiploic v.
n. Inferior mesenteric v.

> **LEARNING HINT**
>
> As with the arteries, a great learning device is to draw a "road map" of the veins so you can see which veins flow into the others, and in what sequence.

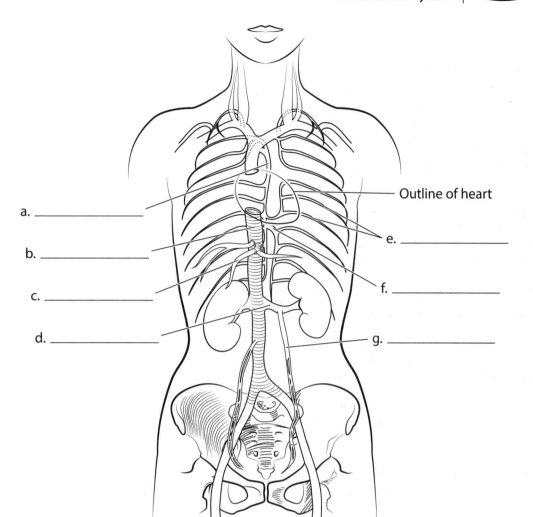

a. _____

b. _____

c. _____

d. _____

Outline of heart

e. _____

f. _____

g. _____

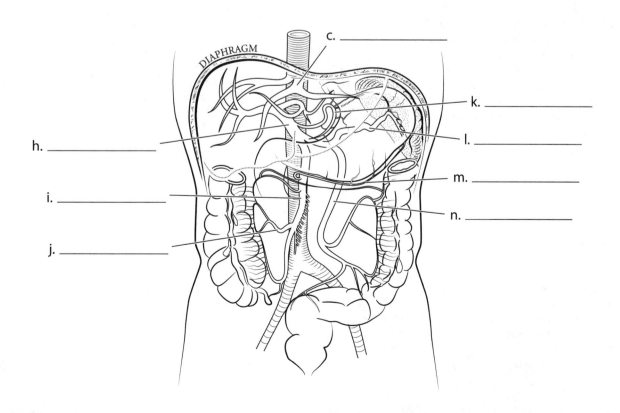

DIAPHRAGM

c. _____

h. _____

i. _____

j. _____

k. _____

l. _____

m. _____

n. _____

FETAL CIRCULATION

The significant difference between fetal circulation and adult circulation lies in the fact that the lungs are nonfunctional in the fetus. The source of oxygen for the fetus is the **placenta**, where maternal blood carries oxygen and nutrients to the fetus. Blood from the placenta travels to the fetus by the **umbilical vein**. It is called a vein because it carries blood to the fetal heart. The blood flowing in the umbilical vein is oxygenated blood, which is not typical of most blood that occurs in veins. From the umbilical vein, the blood passes through a small shunt vessel known as the **ductus venosus** and enters the **inferior vena cava**, where it mixes with blood returning from the lower limbs. The fetus receives a mixture of oxygenated and deoxygenated blood.

This mixed blood reaches the fetal heart and begins the first of two bypass routes. Since the lungs do not oxygenate blood in the fetus, they do not require the entire blood volume to pass through them. The first bypass route is through the **foramen ovale**, a hole between the **right** and **left atria** of the heart. Another bypass route occurs as the blood enters the **pulmonary trunk**. Blood moves from the pulmonary trunk through the **ductus arteriosus** and into the aortic arch.

Blood traveling back from the fetus is not fully deoxygenated but is a mixture of oxygenated and deoxygenated blood. This blood flows from the **internal iliac arteries** of the fetus into the **umbilical arteries**. From the umbilical arteries, the blood flows into the placenta.

Color Guide: Use red for the umbilical vein, which carries oxygenated blood. Use blue for the blood flowing into the **superior vena cava** and the lower part of the inferior vena cava, which is deoxygenated. Use purple to color the umbilical arteries, which contain a mixture of oxygenated and deoxygenated blood. Color the rest of the system purple as well, as these vessels also carry partially oxygenated blood.

Answer Key

a. Superior vena cava
b. Right atrium
c. Foramen ovale
d. Placenta
e. Umbilical cord
f. Ductus arteriosus
g. Right ventricle
h. Ductus venosus

i. Inferior vena cava
j. Umbilical vein
k. Aorta
l. Internal iliac artery
m. Umbilical arteries
n. Pulmonary artery
o. Pulmonary trunk
p. Left atrium

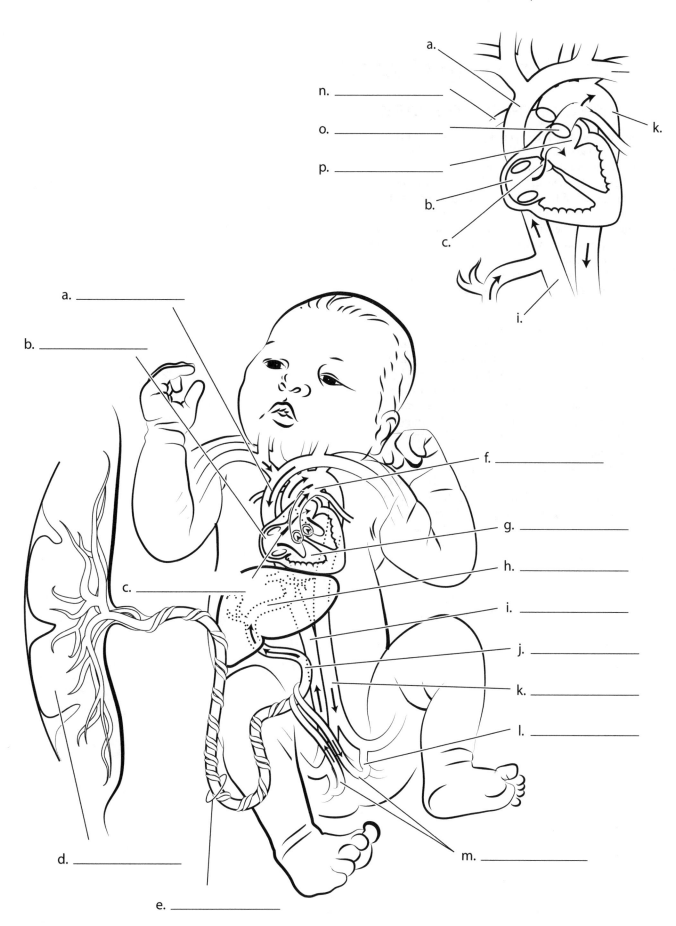

a. _____

n. _____

o. _____

p. _____

b. _____

c. _____

k. _____

i. _____

a. _____

b. _____

f. _____

g. _____

h. _____

c. _____

i. _____

j. _____

k. _____

l. _____

d. _____

m. _____

e. _____

■ Chapter Ten: **Lymph System**

OVERVIEW OF THE LYMPH SYSTEM

The lymph system is composed of **lymphatics** or **lymph vessels** and glands and has many functions. Fluid that bathes the cells (interstitial fluid) is returned to the cardiovascular system, in part, by the lymph system. This fluid, called **lymph**, passes through **lymph nodes** where impurities and foreign microbes are removed. Other parts of the lymph system include lymph organs such as the **spleen**. Lymph nodes and the spleen produce cells that protect the body from foreign compounds and have other immune functions such as cleansing the body of cellular debris and removing old blood cells from circulation.

The main exchange of fluid from the cardiovascular system occurs at the capillary level. **Arterioles** carry blood to the capillary bed, and the **venules** return blood from the capillaries. About 90 percent of the fluid that flows from the blood capillaries to the interstices around the cells is reabsorbed by the capillaries. The remaining 10 percent of the interstitial fluid enters the lymph system by **lymph capillaries** and travels through lymphatics. These lymph capillaries have one-way valves that allow the fluid to enter the lymphatics and not return to the cells. Once the fluid enters the lymphatic system, it is called lymph. The lymph travels through the lymphatics, and some of these vessels merge into a large sac in the abdomen called the **cisterna chyli**. This sac is the beginning of the **thoracic duct**, which returns the lymph to the cardiovascular system. Label the structures of the lymph system.

Color Guide: Use dark brown for the spleen, and color the remainder of the lymph system dark green. Use red for the arteriole in the lower figure, blue for the venule, and green for the lymph capillaries.

Answer Key
a. Thoracic duct
b. Spleen
c. Cisterna chyli
d. Lymphatics
e. Lymph nodes
f. Venule
g. Arteriole
h. Lymph capillaries

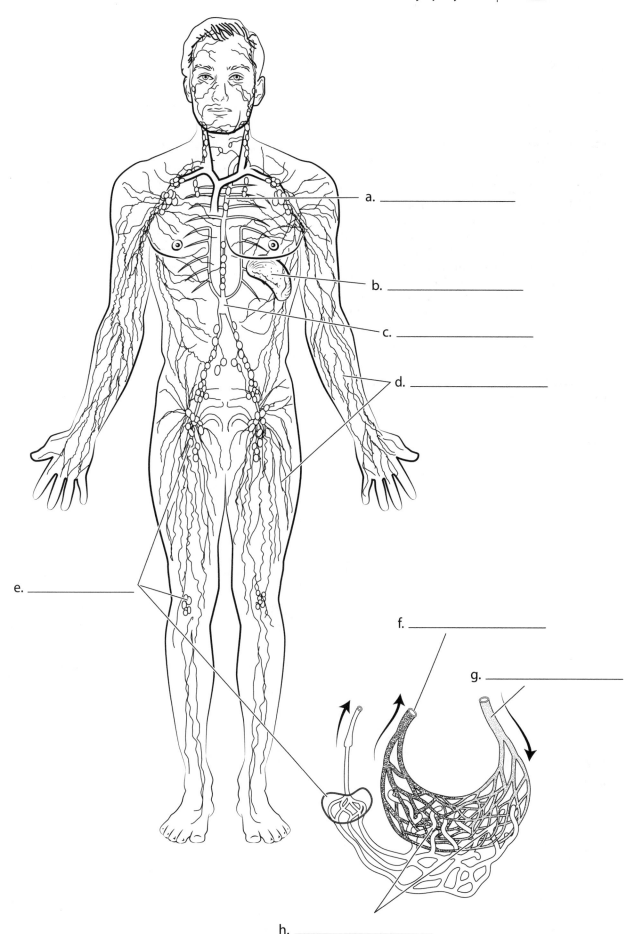

a. _____

b. _____

c. _____

d. _____

e. _____

f. _____

g. _____

h. _____

RETURN DRAINAGE

One of the functions of the lymph system is to return tissue fluid to the cardiovascular system.

The **right lymphatic duct** returns blood to the **right internal jugular vein**. This occurs at the junction where the **right subclavian vein** and the right internal jugular vein reach the right brachiocephalic vein. The **thoracic duct** enters the cardiovascular system at the point where the **left internal jugular vein** and the **left subclavian vein** enter the left brachiocephalic vein. **Lymph nodes** occur along the path and cleanse the lymph. The **thymus** is a lymph organ that occurs near these **drainage areas**. The thoracic duct receives lymph from most of the body while the right lymphatic duct receives lymph from the right side of the head, the right pectoral region, shoulder, and right upper limb. Label the veins of the neck and upper thorax, and label the lymphatic vessels that return fluid to the cardiovascular system.

Color Guide: Use blue for the veins and green for the lymphatic system. In the lower illustration, color the shaded part of the body dark green. Select a pale green tone to color in the unshaded right side of the head, right side of the neck, right thoracic region, and right upper limb to show the drainage of the right lymphatic duct.

Answer Key
a. Right internal jugular vein
b. Right lymphatic duct
c. Right subclavian vein
d. Lymph nodes
e. Left internal jugular vein
f. Thoracic duct
g. Left subclavian vein
h. Thymus
i. Right drainage area
j. Left drainage area

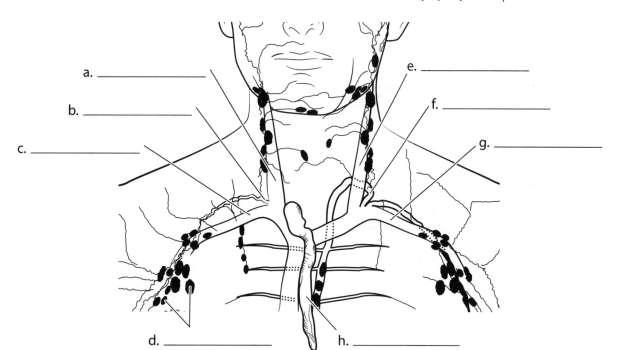

a. _____

b. _____

c. _____

e. _____

f. _____

g. _____

d. _____

h. _____

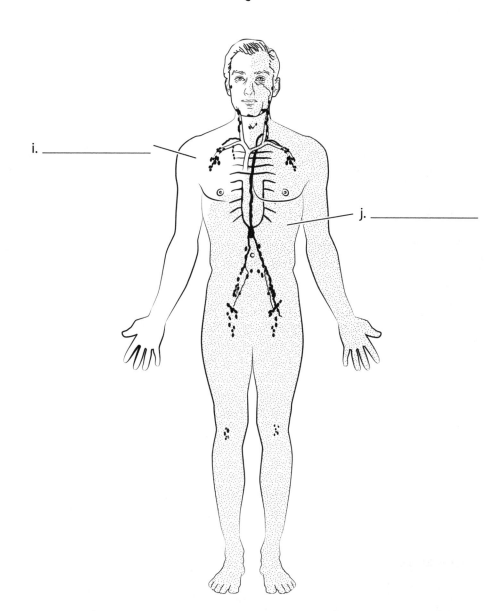

i. _____

j. _____

TONSILS

The tonsils are lymph organs that provide protection against microbes entering the mouth and nose. Tonsils are regions of mucous membrane with lymph tissue. The **pharyngeal tonsils** are located in the nasopharynx (a region posterior to the nasal cavity and superior to the oral cavity) and provide some protection from inhaled material. The **lingual tonsils** are on the posterior part of the **tongue** and, along with the **palatine tonsils** on the side of the oral cavity, they provide protection from material that enters the body by mouth. These tonsils cluster to form a **tonsillar (Waldeyer's) ring** that protects the body from microbial invasion. Label the tonsils and associated structures.

Color Guide: Select one color for the pharyngeal tonsils, a second color for the lingual tonsils, and another color for the palatine tonsils.

Answer Key

a. Pharyngeal tonsil
b. Tongue
c. Palatine tonsil
d. Lingual tonsil
e. Tonsillar (Waldeyer's) ring

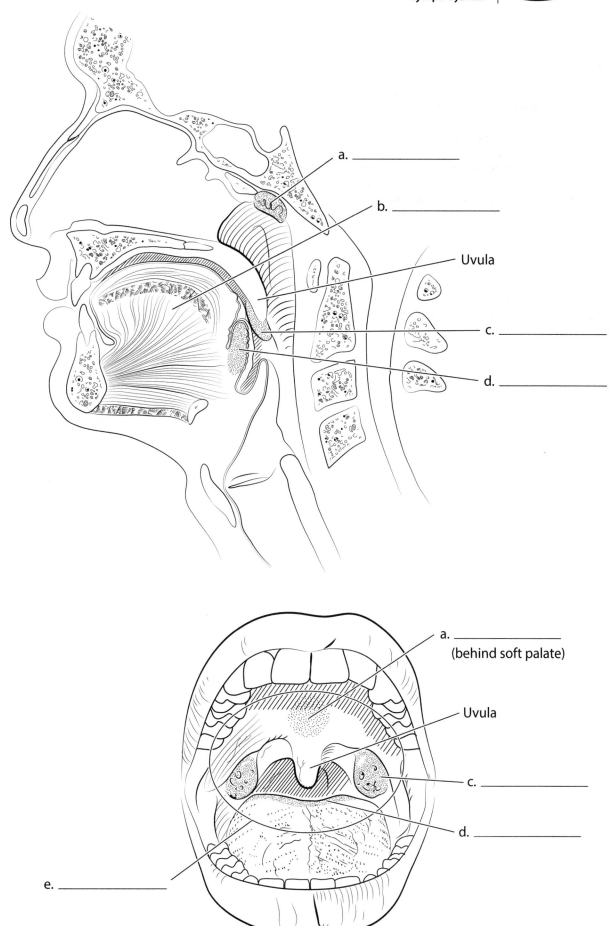

a. _____

b. _____

Uvula

c. _____

d. _____

a. _____
(behind soft palate)

Uvula

c. _____

d. _____

e. _____

SPLEEN

The **spleen** is on the left side of the body close to the pancreas. The **splenic artery** takes blood to the spleen, and the **splenic vein** takes blood from the spleen. The spleen is important in removing aging red blood cells from circulation and recycling them. The spleen has both **red pulp** and **white pulp**. The red pulp is involved in red blood cell removal, and the white pulp produces lymphocytes. The spleen has **splenic cords** that have lymphocytes along their length. Label the parts of the spleen and associated structures.

Color Guide: In the upper illustration, color the spleen a deep shade of purple. In the lower illustration, select red for the red pulp and leave the white pulp white. Color the pancreas in beige and the kidney in brown.

Answer Key

a. Spleen
b. Splenic artery
c. Splenic vein
d. Red pulp
e. Arteriole
f. Sinuses
g. White pulp

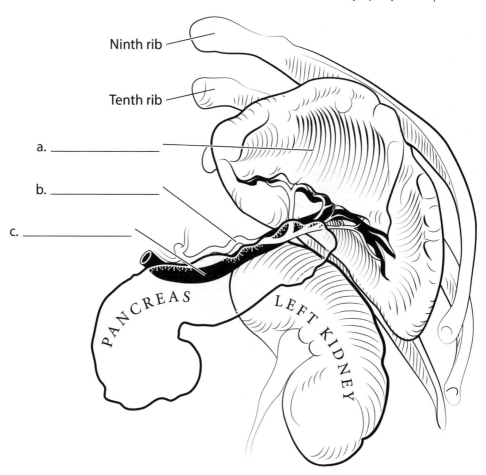

Ninth rib

Tenth rib

a. _____

b. _____

c. _____

PANCREAS

LEFT KIDNEY

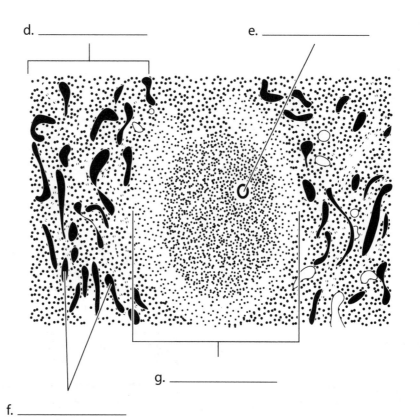

d. _____

e. _____

f. _____

g. _____

(filled with red blood cells)

LYMPH NODES

Lymph nodes are found typically in clusters along the route that **lymphatics** take as lymph is returned to the cardiovascular system. **Afferent lymphatics** bring lymph to the node, and **efferent lymphatics** receive lymph from the node.

Lymph nodes consist of an outer **cortex** with lymphatic nodules and an inner **medulla**. The cortex produces lymphocytes, and the medulla has **medullary cords**, which have clusters of lymph cells that cleanse the lymph passing through the nodes. Label the lymphatics and parts of the lymph node.

Color Guide: Use yellow for the **capsule** and purple for the lymphatic nodules in the cortex and the lymphatic tissue of the medullary cords (stippled in the medulla). Use a darker shade of green for the afferent lymphatics and a lighter shade of green for the efferent lymphatics.

Answer Key

a. Efferent lymphatics
b. Capsule
c. Cortex
d. Medulla with medullary cords
e. Afferent lymphatics
f. Blood vessels

LEARNING HINT

The word **cortex** comes from the Latin for "bark," as in a tree's outer layer. The cortex of the lymph node is the outer "bark" of the node.

Medulla comes from another Latin word, meaning "marrow." Like bone marrow, it is found on the inside.

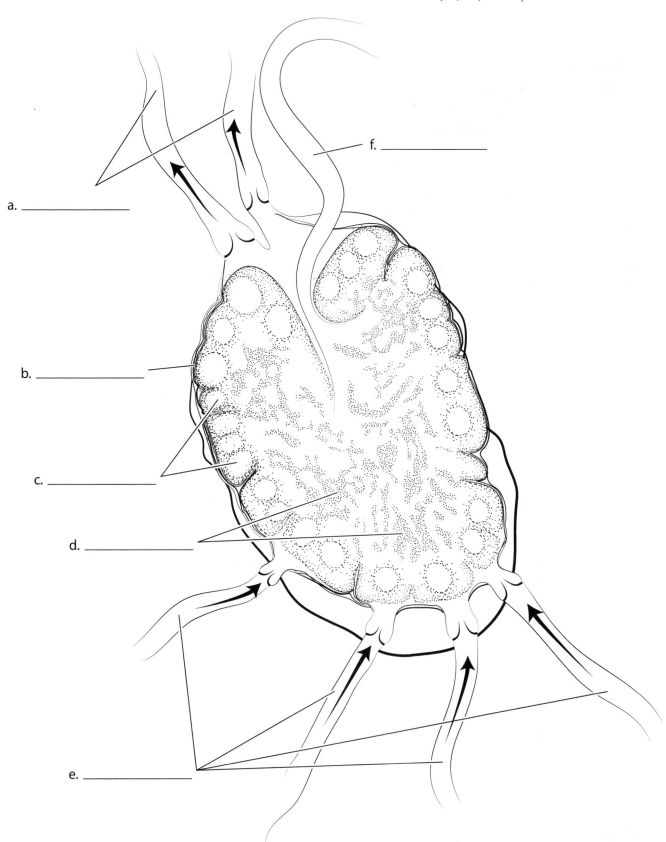

a. _____

b. _____

c. _____

d. _____

e. _____

f. _____

LACTEALS

The lymph system has a special function in digestion. Not only are there lymph nodes along parts of the digestive tract that protect the body from possible invasion from ingested microbes, but fatty acids from the digestion of lipids are absorbed by special vessels called **lacteals**. The fatty acids travel through the **lymphatic vessels** to the cardiovascular system. Lacteals are found in the **small intestine** in fingerlike structures called **villi**. These villi also contain **capillaries**, which absorb sugars and amino acids. Label the villi, capillaries, and lacteals.

Color Guide: Color the small intestine red and the villi pink. Use yellow for the lacteals.

Answer Key

a. Small intestine
b. Lymphatic vessel
c. Villi
d. Capillaries
e. Lacteal

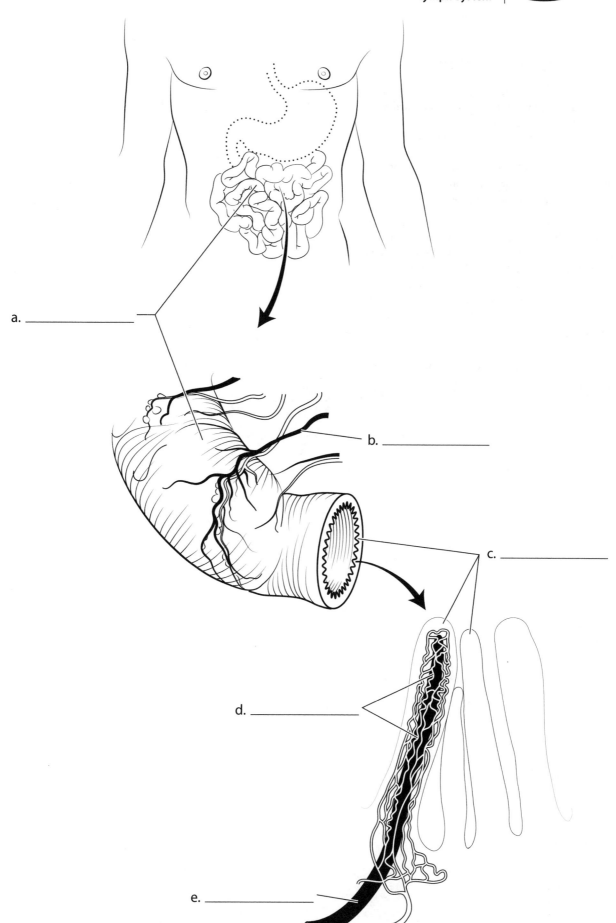

a. _____

b. _____

c. _____

d. _____

e. _____

TWO TYPES OF IMMUNITY

The body can control against foreign particles either by **cell-mediated immunity** or **antibody-mediated immunity**. In antibody-mediated immunity, foreign particles called **antigens** (typically proteins or carbohydrates on the surface of invading cells) stimulate **B cells** to become **plasma cells** and **memory B cells**. The plasma cells produce **antibodies**, and these react with the antigens, stimulating their destruction.

In cell-mediated immunity, the reacting cells are called **helper T cells**, and they cause the activation of and the differentiation of other **T cells** into **memory T cells** and **effector** or **cytotoxic T cells**. The cytotoxic T cells can recognize foreign cells and destroy them. The steps in immune reactions are much more complex than this, but this description provides a general understanding of the process. Fill in the illustration using the terms provided.

Color Guide: Select one color for the different cells and antibodies and another for T cells.

Answer Key

a. Antigens
b. B cell
c. Memory B cell
d. Antibodies
e. Plasma cell
f. Helper T cell
g. Activated T cell
h. Effector (cytotoxic) T cell
i. Memory T cell

Antibody-mediated immunity

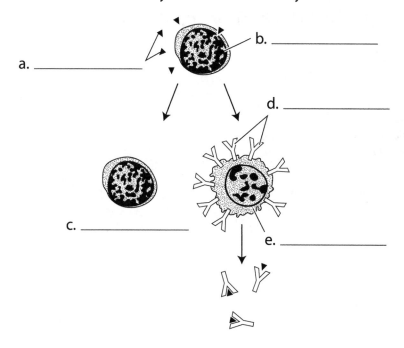

a. _____

b. _____

c. _____

d. _____

e. _____

Cell-mediated immunity

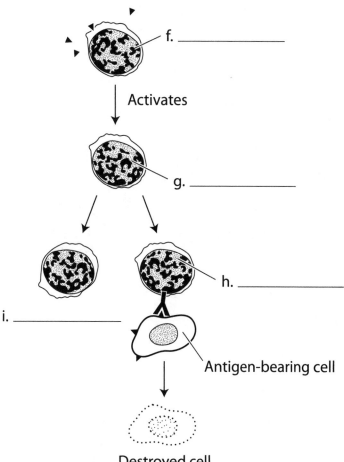

f. _____

Activates

g. _____

h. _____

i. _____

Antigen-bearing cell

Destroyed cell

▪ Chapter Eleven: **Respiratory System**

OVERVIEW OF THE RESPIRATORY SYSTEM

The respiratory system consists of the nose, **nasal cavity**, **pharynx**, **larynx**, **trachea**, **lungs**, linings of the lungs (**pleura**), and respiratory muscles such as the **diaphragm** and intercostal muscles. Label the respiratory figure.

Color Guide: Notice that the right lung has three lobes. Use a different color for each lobe: superior, middle, and inferior. Use different colors for the two lobes of the left lung. Select a separate color each for the nasal cavity, pharynx, and trachea.

Answer Key

a. Pharynx
b. Trachea
c. Right lung
d. Pleura
e. Nasal cavity
f. Larynx
g. Left lung
h. Diaphragm

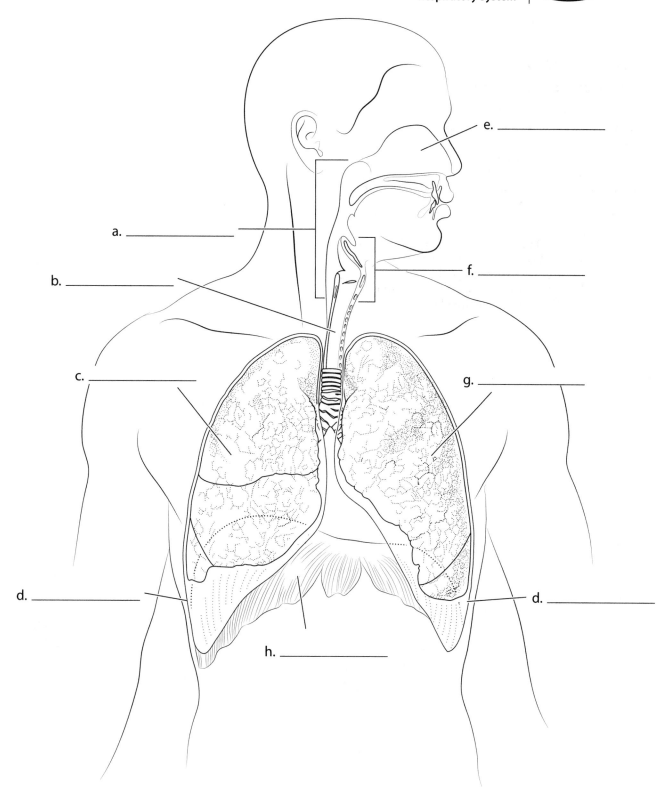

e. _____

a. _____

b. _____

f. _____

c. _____

g. _____

d. _____

d. _____

h. _____

LARYNX, TRACHEA, AND LUNGS OVERVIEW

Two main cartilages of the larynx can be seen from an anterior view. The **thyroid cartilage** is superior to the **cricoid cartilage**. Below the larynx is the **trachea**, which divides into the **right** and **left main bronchi** (primary bronchi). The right main bronchus leads to the **right lung**, and the left main bronchus leads to the **left lung**. Label the parts of the respiratory system illustrated.

Color Guide: Color the two visible cartilages of the larynx different colors and the trachea another color. Color the bronchi in first with a darker color, and then color the lungs in with a lighter color. Select colors that you will use throughout the Larynx, Trachea, and Lungs section.

Answer Key

a. Trachea
b. Right main bronchus
c. Right lung
d. Thyroid cartilage
e. Cricoid cartilage
f. Left main bronchus
g. Left lung

LEARNING HINT

The **thyroid** (THIGH-royd) cartilage is shield-shaped, while the **cricoid** (CRY-koyd) cartilage is shaped like a signet ring (e.g., a class ring).

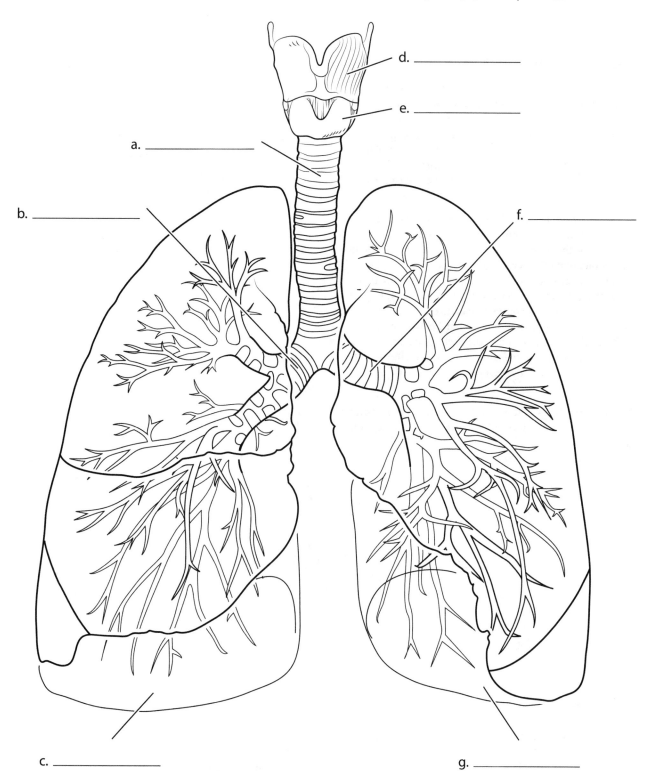

d. _____

e. _____

a. _____

b. _____

f. _____

c. _____

g. _____

NOSE AND NASAL SEPTUM

The nose consists of the **nasal bones**, the **frontal process of the maxilla** at the root of the nose, and a number of cartilages. These nasal cartilages are mostly made of hyaline cartilage. These are the **lateral nasal cartilages**, the **greater alar cartilages**, and the **lesser alar cartilages**. The **septal cartilage** also forms part of these cartilages. The openings of the nose (nostrils) are the **external nares** (**external naris** singular).

The nasal cavity has a wall that runs down the middle of it called the **nasal septum**. The septum consists of three parts, the **perpendicular plate of the ethmoid bone** (a continuation of the **crista galli**), the **vomer**, and the **septal cartilage**. At the end of the nasal septum are two holes that separate the nasal cavity from the **nasopharynx**. These are the **choanae** or **nasal apertures**. The floor of the nasal cavity is bordered by the **hard palate** and the **soft palate**. At the junction of the crista galli and the perpendicular plate of the ethmoid is the **cribriform plate** of the ethmoid. Label the various structures of the nose.

Color Guide: Use a different color to color in each separate cartilage of the nose. Use a blue tone for the nasal septum and different shades of yellow for the perpendicular plate of the ethmoid and vomer bones.

Answer Key

a. Nasal bone
b. Frontal process of maxilla
c. Septal cartilage
d. Lateral nasal cartilage
e. Lesser alar cartilages
f. Greater alar cartilage
g. External naris
h. Crista galli
i. Cribriform plate
j. Perpendicular plate of ethmoid bone
k. Vomer
l. Hard palate
m. Soft palate
n. Choana

LEARNING HINT

The word **alar** (plural *alae*) is Latin for "wing," and the alae flank the nostrils like wings. The **septum** is the "fence" between the nostrils.

The nasal cartilages provide structure to the nose but remain bendable. Imagine if these structures were made of bone: Any trauma to the face—such as a simple trip and fall—would break them.

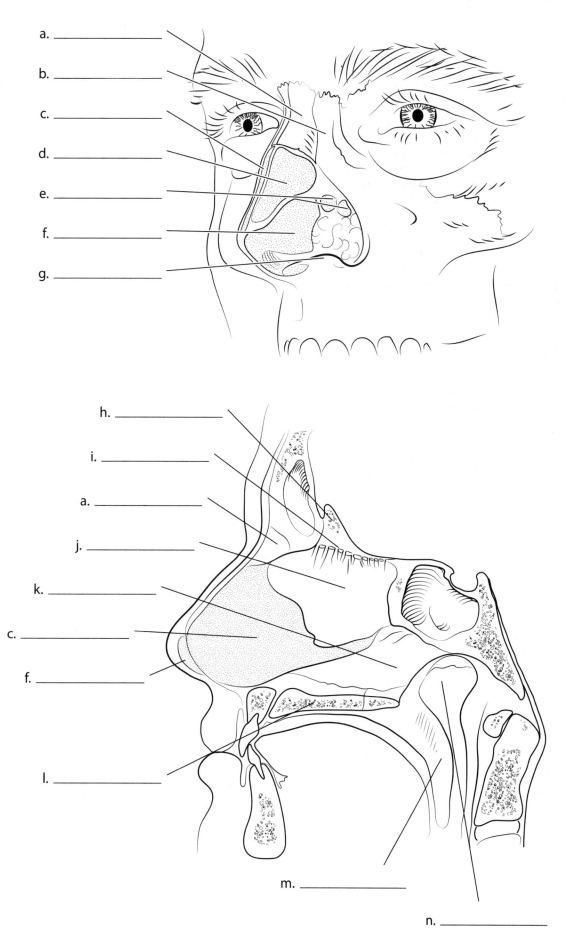

a. _____

b. _____

c. _____

d. _____

e. _____

f. _____

g. _____

h. _____

i. _____

a. _____

j. _____

k. _____

c. _____

f. _____

l. _____

m. _____

n. _____

LATERAL WALL OF NASAL CAVITY AND RESPIRATORY EPITHELIUM

When looking at the nasal cavity, if the septal cartilage is removed, you can see the **nasal conchae**. These structures force the inhaled air to come into contact with the wall of the nasal cavity where the air is warmed and moistened. There are three nasal conchae, the **superior nasal concha**, the **middle nasal concha**, and the **inferior nasal concha**. Note the position of the conchae with the **nasal bone**, the **hard palate**, and the **soft palate**. Label the nasal cavity and the structures that are associated with the cavity.

The nasal cavity is lined with **respiratory epithelium**, which is **pseudostratified ciliated columnar epithelium** with **goblet cells**. Respiratory epithelium is found in the nasal cavity, the lower larynx, trachea, and bronchi. The goblet cells secrete **mucus**, which forms a film over the epithelial surface. Dust and other particulate matter stick to the **mucous sheet**, which is moved by the **cilia**. This provides a protective function, preventing particulate matter from entering the lungs where it might do damage. Label the various parts of respiratory epithelium, such as the **nucleus, cilia, mucous sheet, goblet cells**, and **basement membrane**.

Color Guide: In the upper illustration, color the nasal bone and the hard palate in yellow. Use a different color for each of the nasal conchae.

In the lower illustration, use light tones such as pale blue or yellow for the goblet cells and the mucous sheet. Color the remaining epithelial cells pink or purple. Select any color for the cilia.

Answer Key
a. Nasal bone
b. Superior nasal concha
c. Middle nasal concha
d. Inferior nasal concha
e. Hard palate
f. Soft palate
g. Mucous sheet
h. Cilia
i. Goblet cells
j. Nuclei
k. Basement membrane

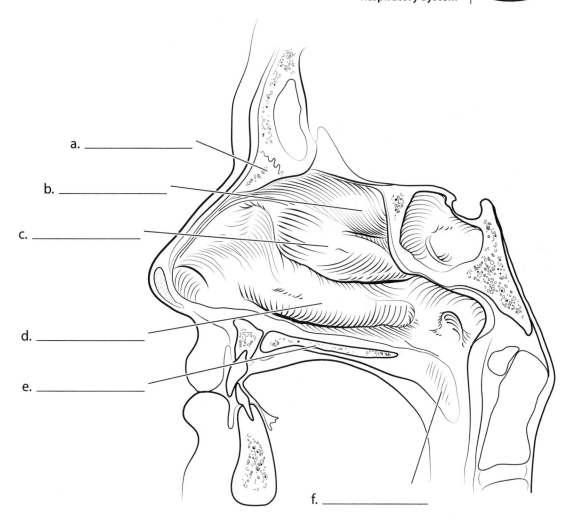

a. _____

b. _____

c. _____

d. _____

e. _____

f. _____

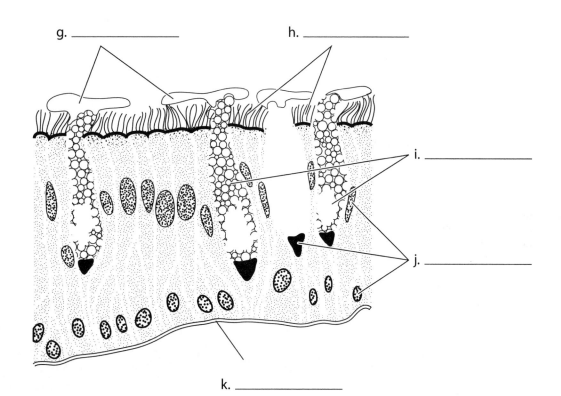

g. _____

h. _____

i. _____

j. _____

k. _____

CORONAL VIEW OF THE NASAL CONCHAE AND LARYNX

The nasal cavity is more than a hole behind the nose. Inhaled air swirls around the conchae and is warmed and moistened in the process. Label the **septal cartilage** in a coronal section of the nose. Label each of the conchae. The **frontal** and **ethmoid sinuses** can also be seen in this illustration. They give resonance to the voice. Note the location of the **hard palate** and the **external naris** in this coronal section. The larynx is also sectioned in this plane, and the position of the **thyroid cartilage**, the **vocal fold**, the **cricoid cartilage**, and the **trachea** are seen in this view. Label the rest of the structures in this illustration.

Color Guide: Color the **superior nasal concha**, **middle nasal concha**, and **inferior nasal concha** using the same colors that you chose in the previous illustration. Use light colors for the sinuses and yellow for the hard palate. Select your preferred colors for the cartilages of the larynx.

Answer Key

a. Sinuses
b. Superior nasal concha
c. Middle nasal concha
d. Septal cartilage
e. Inferior nasal concha
f. Hard palate
g. External naris
h. Thyroid cartilage
i. Vocal fold
j. Cricoid cartilage
k. Trachea
l. Upper respiratory tract

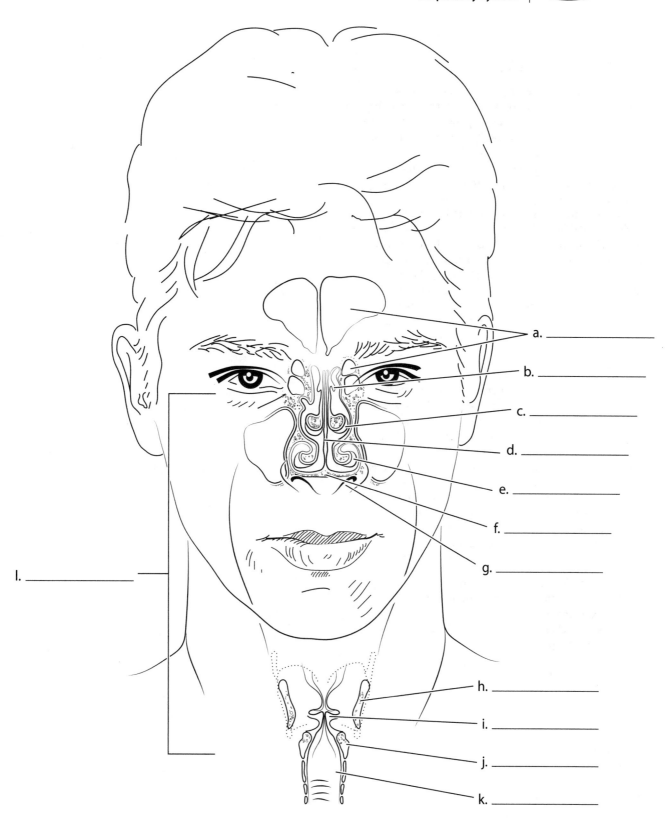

a. _____

b. _____

c. _____

d. _____

e. _____

f. _____

g. _____

l. _____

h. _____

i. _____

j. _____

k. _____

LARYNX AND TRACHEA

The **larynx** is the "voice box," and it not only produces sound for speech but also separates the flow of air to the lungs from the flow of foods and liquids that go down the esophagus. The **thyroid cartilage** is the largest cartilage of the larynx and is easily seen from the anterior aspect. The thyroid cartilage is inferior to the **hyoid bone**. Behind the thyroid cartilage is the **epiglottis**, which is the only laryngeal structure made of elastic cartilage. Inferior to the thyroid cartilage is the **cricoid cartilage**, and it is the inferior border of the larynx. The **cricothyroid ligament** joins these anterior structures together. Above the cricoid cartilage are the paired **arytenoid cartilages**. These attach to the vocal folds and tighten them, causing the voice to increase in pitch. Superior to the arytenoid cartilages are the **corniculate cartilages** that are shaped like small horns. The glottis is the opening into the larynx, and the **epiglottis** is the flap that folds over the glottis during swallowing.

In the midsagittal section of the larynx, you can see that the **cricoid cartilage** is larger on the posterior aspect. The **thyroid cartilage** is prominent on the anterior side. The **arytenoid** and **corniculate cartilages** are prominent on the posterior side, along with the **epiglottis** and the vocal folds. The **vestibular fold (false vocal cord)** is superior and is found on the lateral wall of the larynx. Below this is the **vocal cord (vocal fold)** that produces sound. The **conus elasticus** consists of elastic tissue and connects the vocal folds to the cartilages. Below the larynx is the **trachea**, which leads from the larynx to the lungs. Label the structures of the larynx and the trachea.

Color Guide: Color in both the anterior view of the larynx on the left side of the page and the midsaggital section of the larynx on the right side of the page using the same colors that you chose for the larynx and trachea in the previous illustration.

Answer Key

a. Epiglottis
b. Hyoid bone
c. Thyroid cartilage
d. Corniculate cartilage
e. Vestibular fold
f. Vocal fold
g. Arytenoid cartilage
h. Conus elasticus
i. Cricothyroid ligament
j. Cricoid cartilage
k. Trachea

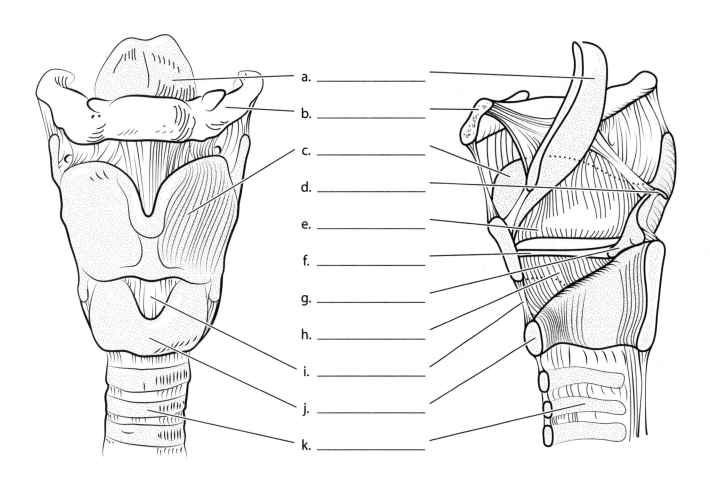

a. _____

b. _____

c. _____

d. _____

e. _____

f. _____

g. _____

h. _____

i. _____

j. _____

k. _____

TRACHEA AND BRONCHIAL TREE

The **trachea** connects to the larynx superiorly and ends inferiorly in a keel-shaped structure called the **carina**. The trachea is composed of the **tracheal rings**, which are hyaline cartilage. The posterior surface of the trachea has smooth muscle called the **trachealis muscle**, which allows for the food in the esophagus to bulge into the trachea. The trachea branches into the **right main** (primary) **bronchus** and the **left main** (primary) **bronchus**, which form part of the lungs. Label the structures in the upper diagram, which shows the **bronchial tree** in anatomical position.

Color Guide: Use blue to color the tracheal rings and pink to color the walls of the trachea. Color the carina a different color from the rings and use separate colors for the right main bronchus and the left main bronchus. Use different shades of these colors for the bronchial tree.

Color the lower figure, which is a cross section of the trachea. Use the same color for the tracheal rings in both illustrations. Use pink for the trachealis muscle.

Answer Key

a. Trachea
b. Right main bronchus
c. Tracheal ring
d. Left main bronchus
e. Carina
f. Trachealis muscle

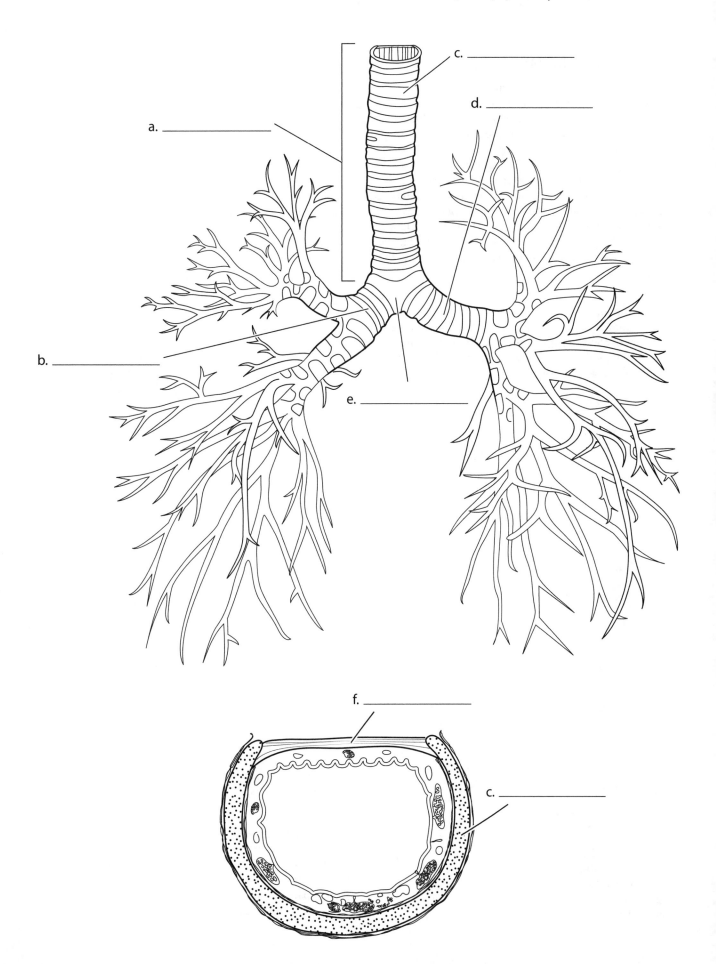

a. _____

b. _____

c. _____

d. _____

e. _____

f. _____

c. _____

LUNGS AND MEMBRANES

The lungs are in the **thoracic cavity** on either side of the mediastinum. The membrane that occurs on the inside of the ribs and on the superior aspect of the diaphragm is known as the **parietal pleura**. The space inside of this is the **pleural cavity**, and the lungs occupy most of the space in the pleural cavities. The innermost membrane is the **visceral pleura**, and it is attached to the surface of the lung. The right lung has three lobes: a **superior lobe**, a **middle lobe**, and an **inferior lobe**. The left lung has two lobes: a **superior lobe** and an **inferior lobe**. The left lung also has an indentation where the heart protrudes into the left lung, the **cardiac notch**. Label the membranes and the parts of the lungs.

Color Guide: Color in each lobe of the lung a different color, using the colors you selected on the Overview of the Respiratory System page. In the lower illustration, use a light color for the pleural cavity and darker colors for the parietal pleura and visceral pleura.

Answer Key

a. Parietal pleura
b. Visceral pleura
c. Superior lobe
d. Middle lobe
e. Inferior lobe
f. Cardiac notch
g. Pleural cavity
h. Trachea

LEARNING HINT

The pleura are linings in the chest cavity. The **parietal pleura** line the inner wall of the thorax (*parietal* pertains to "a wall"), while the **visceral pleura** line the outer surface of the lungs (*visceral* pertains to "internal organs"). The **pleural cavity** is the space between the pleura.

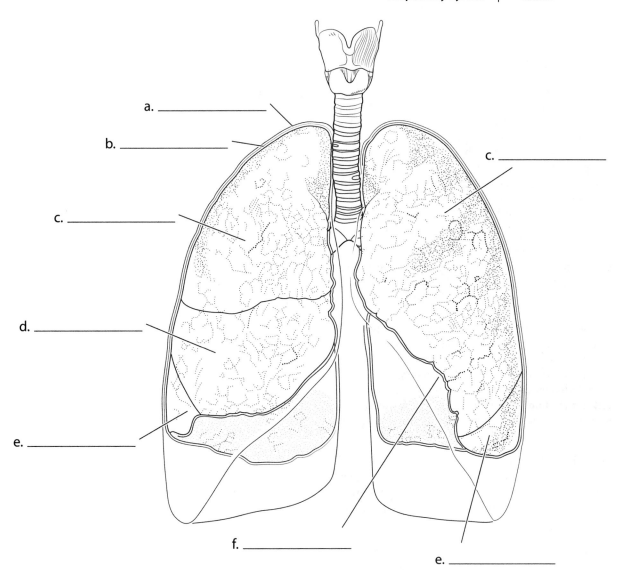

a. _____

b. _____

c. _____

c. _____

d. _____

e. _____

f. _____

e. _____

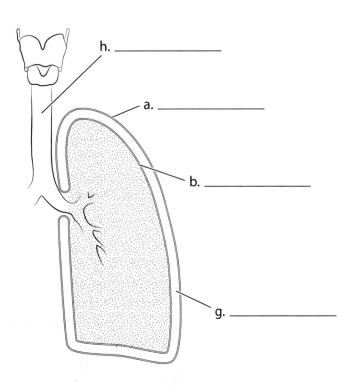

h. _____

a. _____

b. _____

g. _____

PATHWAY OF AIR

The lungs are like large sponges filled with microscopic spaces. Air travels to these spaces by the **bronchial tree**. The trachea splits at the level of the lungs into two **main (primary) bronchi**. Each lung has a main bronchus that divides to **lobar (secondary) bronchi**. These divide further to **segmental (tertiary) bronchi**, which divide into smaller branches. Finally bronchi become **bronchioles**, and these lead to smaller sacs where the exchange of oxygen and carbon dioxide occurs between the lungs and blood. Shade the major segments of the bronchial tree.

The air from the bronchioles moves into the **alveolar ducts**, which are part of the clusters called **alveolar sacs**. The alveolar duct is a conduit to the individual **alveoli** (**alveolus** singular), and these are the areas where there is an exchange of oxygen and carbon dioxide between the air and blood. **Capillaries** are situated next to the alveoli, and there are two thin sets of membranes—one of the alveolus and one of the capillary—that allow the exchange of oxygen and carbon dioxide. Additionally, there are **type II alveolar cells (septal cells)** that secrete a material called **surfactant**. This substance reduces the surface tension of the lungs, allowing them to expand more easily.

Color Guide: Color each part of the bronchus, bronchioles, and alveoli with different colors of your choosing. Color in the structures of the alveolar sacs and the associated structures. Use red for the red blood cells and purple for the type II alveolar cells.

Answer Key

a. Main bronchus
b. Lobar bronchus
c. Segmental bronchus
d. Bronchi
e. Bronchioles
f. Alveoli
g. Capillaries
h. Type II alveolar cell (septal cell)
i. Surfactant
j. Red blood cell
k. Alveolus
l. Pulmonary artery
m. Alveolar ducts
n. Pulmonary vein
o. Alveolar sac

LEARNING HINT

The word **alveolus** is from Latin, meaning "a basin." The alveoli of the lungs are little "basins" that exchange gases between the lungs and the blood.

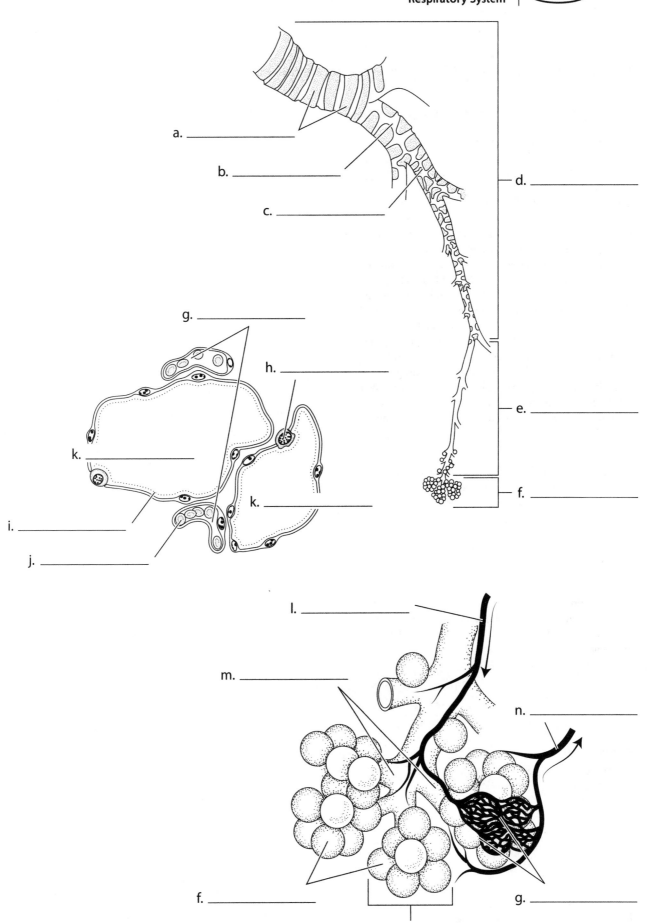

a. _____

b. _____

c. _____

d. _____

g. _____

h. _____

e. _____

f. _____

k. _____

i. _____

j. _____

k. _____

l. _____

m. _____

n. _____

f. _____

g. _____

o. _____

Chapter Twelve: **Digestive System**

OVERVIEW OF THE DIGESTIVE SYSTEM

The digestive system is composed of a long tube called the **alimentary canal** (gastrointestinal tract) and the **accessory organs** including the liver, pancreas, and gall bladder. The alimentary canal starts at the mouth and can be defined as the tube through which ingested products move. The accessory organs have digestive functions but do not come into contact with material passing through the digestive tract. The alimentary canal consists of numerous organs including the **mouth**, which is the opening to the system and is directly anterior to the oral cavity. Posterior to the oral cavity is the **oropharynx**. This chamber receives food and liquid from the mouth and air from both the mouth and nasal cavity. The oropharynx leads to the **esophagus**, which is a muscular tube that takes ingested material to the **stomach**. The stomach is a storage organ leading to the **small intestine** where material is digested and absorbed. The **large intestine** receives material from the small intestine, removes a significant amount of water, and stores the fecal material prior to defecation through the rectum and anus.

The **salivary glands** are the most superior accessory glands. They lubricate food and add digestive enzymes to material that is swallowed. The **liver**, **pancreas**, and **gallbladder** all add secretions to the ingested material and aid in the digestive process. Label the parts of the digestive system, including the alimentary canal and the accessory organs.

Color Guide: Color each of the digestive structures in the illustration in a different color. Conventionally, yellow is used to identify the salivary glands, brown for the liver, and beige for the pancreas.

Answer Key
a. Mouth
b. Esophagus
c. Stomach
d. Small intestine
e. Large intestine
f. Rectum
g. Anus
h. Salivary glands
i. Liver
j. Pancreas
k. Gallbladder

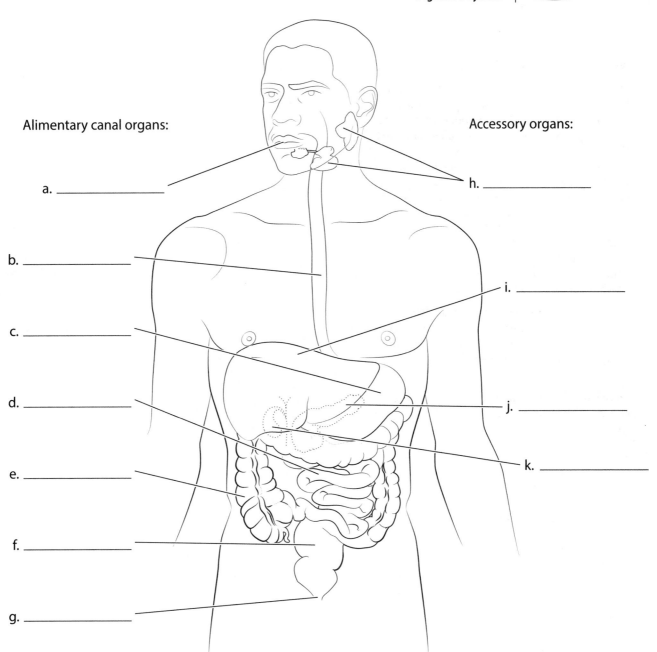

Alimentary canal organs:

a. _____

b. _____

c. _____

d. _____

e. _____

f. _____

g. _____

Accessory organs:

h. _____

i. _____

j. _____

k. _____

MOUTH AND ORAL CAVITY

The mouth is the entrance to the digestive system. It is bordered by the two **labia** or lips. Each labium has a **labial frenulum** (**superior** and **inferior**) that holds the lip to the **gingiva**. If you bend your upper or lower lip back you will see a thin piece of tissue that attaches the lip to the gums. This is the labial frenulum. The gingiva (gums) have a surface tissue of stratified squamous epithelium, which is the cell type that lines the entire oral cavity. The oral cavity encloses the teeth and the **tongue**. It is bordered by the **hard palate**, the **soft palate**, the **uvula** (pronounced YOO-vyuh-luh), the cheek walls, the muscles, and associated tissue that spans across the bodies of the mandible. The oral cavity leads to the **oropharynx**, which in turn leads to the **esophagus**.

The tongue is a large muscle in the oral cavity that pushes food to the posterior part of the oral cavity for swallowing and helps form speech. It is held to the floor of the oral cavity by the **lingual frenulum**.

Color Guide: Select your preferred colors for the structures of the mouth and oral cavity.

Answer Key

a. Superior labial frenulum
b. Gingiva
c. Hard palate
d. Soft palate
e. Uvula
f. Oropharynx
g. Tongue
h. Inferior labial frenulum
i. Esophagus

LEARNING HINT

The **uvula** (from the Latin, meaning "little grape") is visible as the little "punching bag" at the back of your throat.

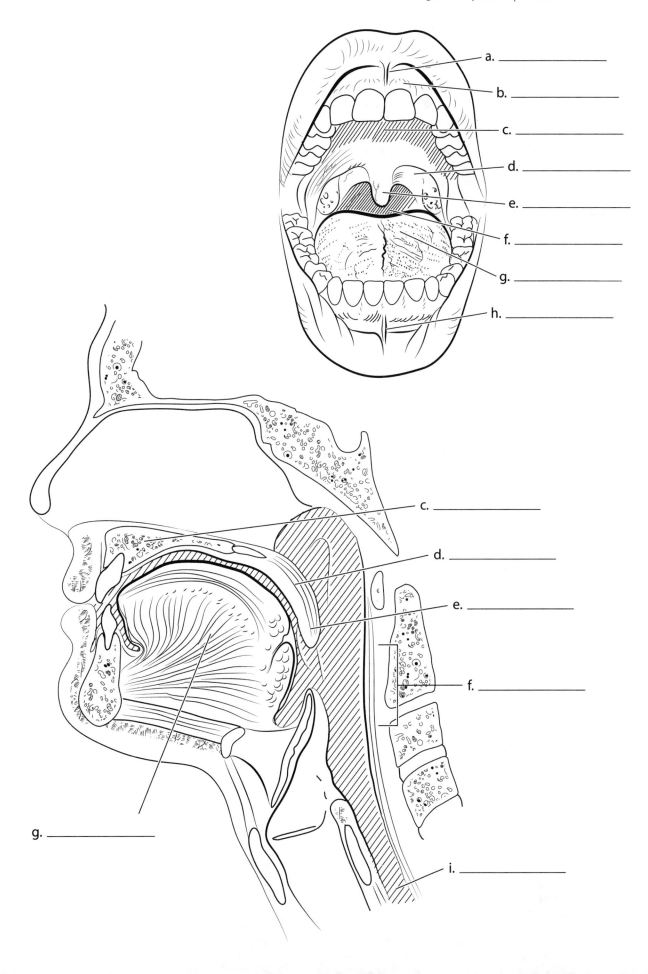

a. _____

b. _____

c. _____

d. _____

e. _____

f. _____

g. _____

h. _____

c. _____

d. _____

e. _____

f. _____

g. _____

i. _____

SALIVARY GLANDS

The three pairs of salivary glands secrete saliva inside
the oral cavity. The largest pair consists of the **parotid
glands** located just anterior to the ears. The **parotid duct**
leads from the gland to posterior to the upper second
molar. The **submandibular glands** are located inferior
to the mandible and take secretions to either side of the
lingual frenulum. The **sublingual glands** are inferior to
the tongue and have many tubes that lead to the lower
oral cavity. Label the salivary glands and the parotid duct.

Color Guide: Color the muscles in red. Color each salivary
gland a different color.

Answer Key
a. Sublingual gland
b. Submandibular gland
c. Parotid gland
d. Parotid duct

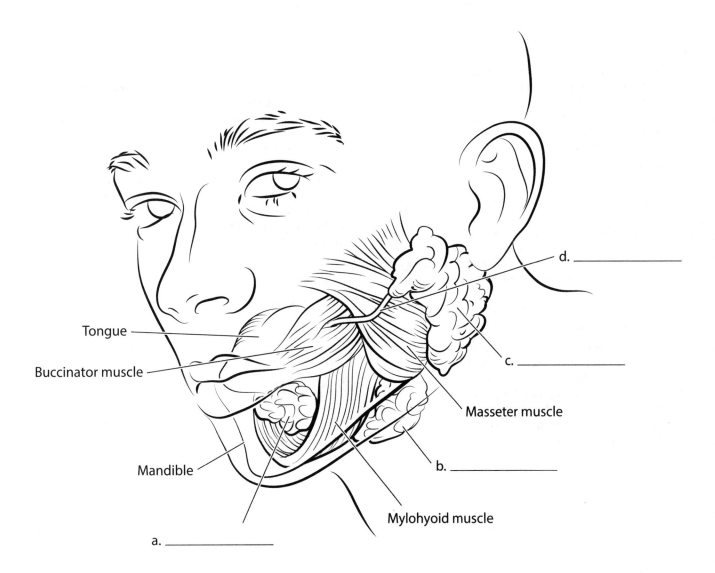

Tongue

Buccinator muscle

Mandible

a. _____

d. _____

c. _____

Masseter muscle

b. _____

Mylohyoid muscle

TEETH

The tooth has three general regions: the crown, the neck, and the root. The **crown** is the part of the tooth that erupts from the gums into the oral cavity. The **neck** is normally at the level of the gingiva, and the **root** is imbedded into the bone. The tooth fits into the alveolar socket of the maxilla or the mandible and is held there by the **periodontal ligaments**.

The internal anatomy of the tooth reveals the hard **enamel**, which is an extremely dense material that resists wear and abrasion. Deep to this is the **dentin**, a material similar to bone that provides the major structure of the tooth. In the root, the dentin is coated with **cementum**, which helps fix the tooth in the alveolar socket. Inside of the dentin is the **pulp cavity** that houses **nerves** and **blood vessels**. These structures enter the tooth by the **apical foramen** and make their way to the pulp cavity by the **root canal**.

Humans have two series of teeth. Early in development come the **deciduous (milk) teeth**. The **permanent teeth** emerge as the skull increases in size. In deciduous teeth, there are **incisors, cuspids (canines)**, and **molar teeth**, but there are no premolars. In adults, there are the **incisor teeth**, the **cuspids, premolars (bicuspids)**, and **molar teeth**. Label the parts of the tooth.

Color Guide: Leave the enamel white, and color the dentin a pale beige. Use red and blue for the blood vessels and bright yellow for the nerves, then color the pulp cavity pale pink. Use pale yellow for the bone and shades of pink and red for the periodontal ligaments. Shade the brackets as you color in the regions of the tooth on one side of the illustration and the enamel, dentin, and other features on the other part of the illustration. For the deciduous and permanent teeth, use the same color for the incisors on both illustrations. Use another color for the cuspids, another color for the premolars, and still another color for the molars.

Answer Key

a. Crown
b. Neck
c. Root
d. Enamel
e. Dentin
f. Pulp cavity
g. Periodontal ligament
h. Root canal
i. Cementum
j. Apical foramen
k. Blood vessels and nerves
l. Incisors
m. Cuspids (canines)
n. Premolars (bicuspids)
o. Molars

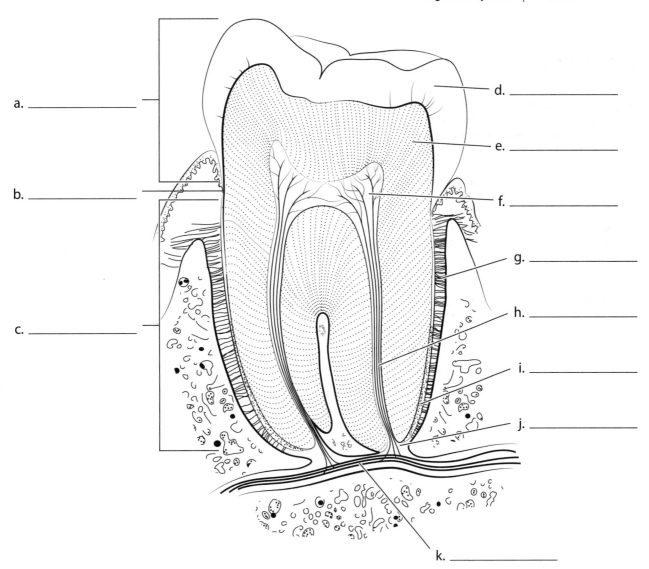

a. _____

b. _____

c. _____

d. _____

e. _____

f. _____

g. _____

h. _____

i. _____

j. _____

k. _____

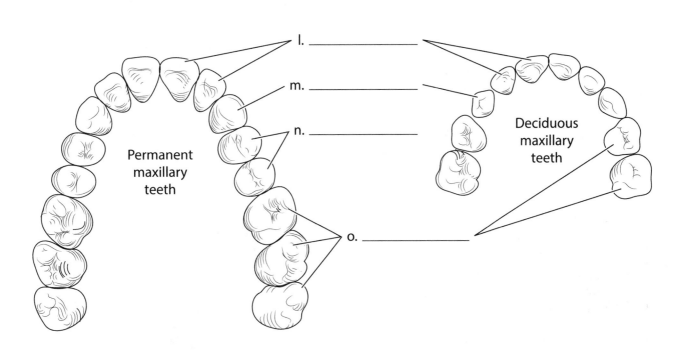

l. _____

m. _____

n. _____

o. _____

Permanent maxillary teeth

Deciduous maxillary teeth

ESOPHAGUS

In swallowing, food moves from the **oral cavity** to the **oropharynx** by action of the tongue. The **uvula** flips upward at this time, keeping the food from entering the nasal cavity. Food passes from the oropharynx into the **laryngopharynx** before moving to the esophagus. The food enters the **esophagus** as a lump or **bolus** and passes through the **esophageal sphincter** to the **stomach**. The stomach contents are restricted from flowing back into the esophagus by the esophageal sphincter. Once it enters the stomach, the **bolus** mixes with stomach fluid and becomes a liquid called **chyme**. Label the structures from the oral cavity to the stomach.

Color Guide: Use a different color for each section of the digestive tract illustrated.

Answer Key

a. Oropharynx
b. Laryngopharynx
c. Esophagus
d. Uvula
e. Oral cavity
f. Stomach
g. Esophageal sphincter

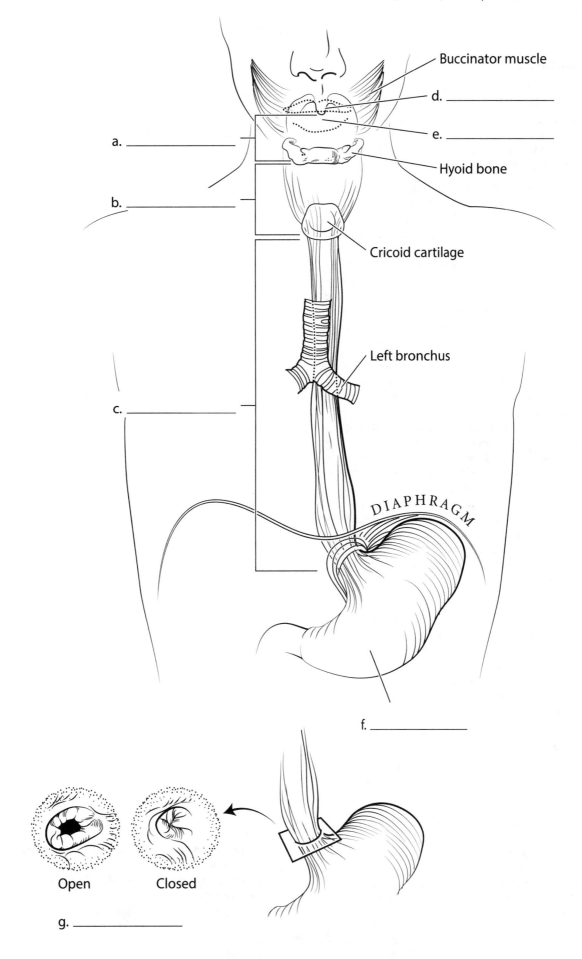

Buccinator muscle

d. _____

e. _____

Hyoid bone

a. _____

b. _____

Cricoid cartilage

Left bronchus

c. _____

DIAPHRAGM

f. _____

Open   Closed

g. _____

STOMACH

The stomach is located on the left side of the body, just inferior to the diaphragm. It is the part of the alimentary canal located between the esophagus and the small intestine. The stomach has an upper **cardia** and a small domed portion called the **fundus**. If stomach fluid refluxes into the esophagus, it is felt as heartburn.

The main portion of the stomach is the **body**. The narrow region of the stomach leading to the **duodenum** is the **pyloric region**, which includes the **pyloric canal, pyloric sphincter**, and **antrum**. The antrum is the wider part of the pyloric region, the pyloric canal is the narrowest part, and the pyloric sphincter is the ring of muscle that controls outflow to the duodenum. The **greater curvature** is located on the left edge of the stomach, and the **lesser curvature** is on the right side. The stomach has inner ridges called **rugae**, which allow for expansion of the stomach.

The stomach has many layers. The inner layer, called the **mucosa**, is rich in glands that secrete acids and inactive enzymes such as pepsinogen into the stomach cavity. Pepsinogen is activated by hydrochloric acid. The mucosa has **gastric pits** with **parietal cells** and **chief cells** emptying into the pits. The parietal cells secrete hydrochloric acid, and the chief cells secrete pepsinogen. External to the mucosa is the **submucosa**, and this layer has many blood vessels embedded in connective tissue. Beyond this is the **muscularis**. In the stomach, there are three layers of the muscularis. These are the **oblique layer, circular layer**, and **longitudinal layer**. The **serosa** (also known as the **visceral peritoneum**) is superficial to the muscularis (next to the abdominal cavity). Label the parts of the stomach.

Color Guide: Color the layers of the muscularis using a different shade of red or pink for each layer. Color the general regions of the stomach different colors along with the separate sphincters. In the lower illustration, use pink for the mucosa, yellow for the submucosa, and different shades of red for the muscularis.

Answer Key

a. Fundus
b. Cardia
c. Lesser curvature
d. Longitudinal layer (of muscularis)
e. Circular layer (of muscularis)
f. Oblique layer (of muscularis)
g. Body
h. Rugae
i. Greater curvature
j. Pyloric canal
k. Pyloric sphincter
l. Antrum
m. Gastric pit
n. Chief cell
o. Parietal cell
p. Mucosa
q. Submucosa
r. Serosa

LEARNING HINT

The term *pylorus* is Greek for "gatekeeper." The **pyloric sphincter** holds material in the stomach prior to emptying the contents into the small intestine. The **rugae** ("ridges") allow for expansion of the stomach.

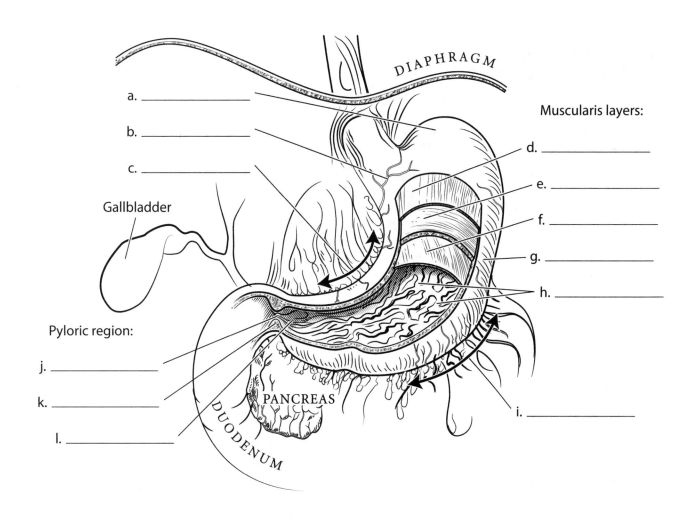

DIAPHRAGM

a. _____

b. _____

c. _____

Gallbladder

Pyloric region:

j. _____

k. _____

l. _____

PANCREAS

DUODENUM

Muscularis layers:

d. _____

e. _____

f. _____

g. _____

h. _____

i. _____

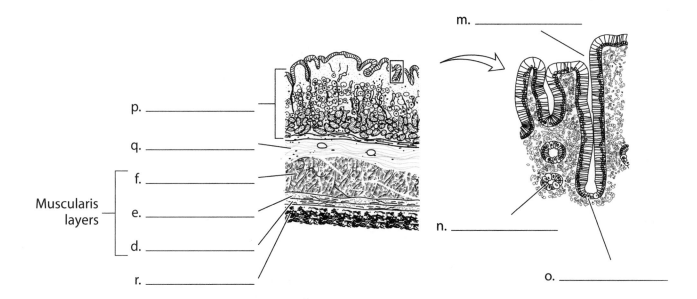

m. _____

p. _____

q. _____

Muscularis layers

f. _____

e. _____

d. _____

r. _____

n. _____

o. _____

SMALL INTESTINE AND ASSOCIATED ORGANS

The small intestine receives the contents of the stomach, continues the process of digestion, and absorbs nutrients. The first part of the small intestine is the **duodenum**, a short tube of about 12 inches (30 cm) in length that receives material from the stomach, enzymes and buffers from the **pancreas**, and bile from the **gallbladder**. The duodenum has **circular folds** in the wall that increase the surface area. The **jejunum** is the next section of the small intestine, and it makes up about 40 percent of the small intestine. There are **circular folds** in the jejunum as well. The **ileum** is the terminal portion of the small intestine and represents about 60 percent of the small intestine. The small intestine is small in diameter— and thus, its name.

The small intestine is distinguished from the rest of the alimentary canal by the presence of **villi**. These small structures in the mucosa increase the surface area of the small intestine and house blood capillaries and lacteals for the absorption of nutrients. The small intestine has the four layers typical of the other organs of the gastrointestinal tract: the **mucosa**, **submucosa**, **muscularis**, and **serosa**. Label the parts of the small intestine.

Color Guide: Color the villi and circular fold in pink as you did for the mucosa in the previous illustration. Use yellow for the submucosa and red for the muscularis in the various regions and layers of the small intestine.

Answer Key

a. Gallbladder
b. Pancreas
c. Duodenum
d. Jejunum
e. Ileum
f. Circular fold
g. Villi
h. Submucosa
i. Muscularis

LEARNING HINT

The **duodenum** (from the Latin for "twelve") is about 12 inches long.

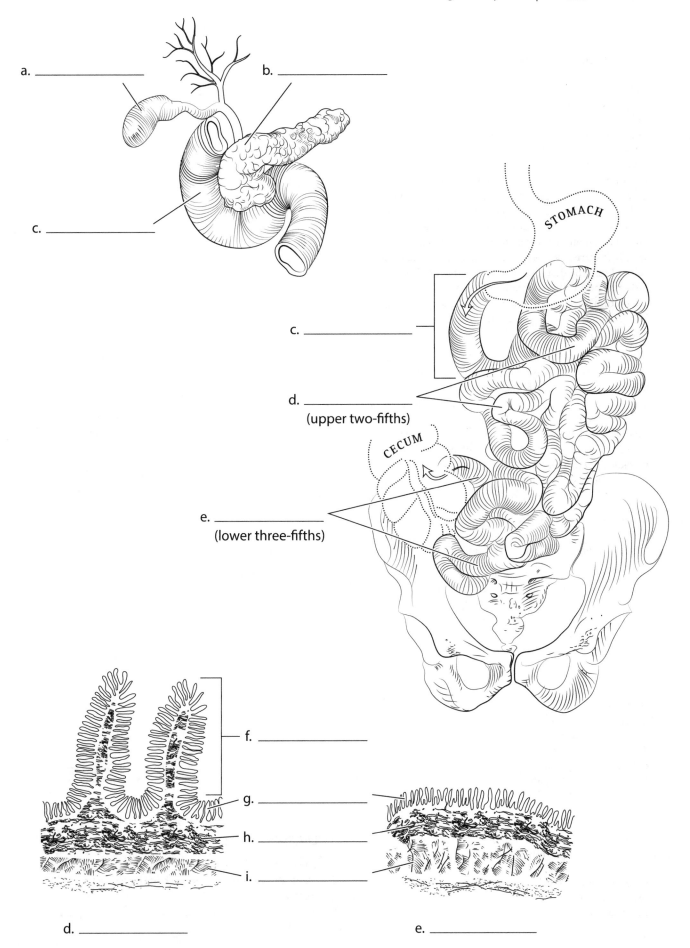

a. _____

b. _____

c. _____

STOMACH

c. _____

d. _____
(upper two-fifths)

CECUM

e. _____
(lower three-fifths)

f. _____

g. _____

h. _____

i. _____

d. _____

e. _____

LARGE INTESTINE

The large intestine is shorter than the small intestine but has greater width. The large intestine begins in the lower right quadrant of the abdomen with a saclike structure called the **cecum**. The ileocecal valve is a muscular sphincter that prevents the fecal material in the cecum from flowing back into the ileum. At this junction is the **vermiform appendix**. Material in the large intestine moves from the cecum to the **ascending colon** and then makes a sharp turn at the **hepatic flexure**. Once this turn is accomplished, the material is in the **transverse colon**. From here, there is a sharp downward angle called the **splenic flexure**, and the material enters the **descending colon**. From the descending colon, the material enters an S-shaped tube called the **sigmoid colon** and then enters the **rectum**. The rectum is the end of the large intestine. The rectum leads to the **anal canal**, which is a short tube leading to the **anus**.

There are several anatomical features that separate the large intestine from the small intestine. The large intestine has long strips of smooth muscle that run its length. These are called the **teniae coli**. These muscles pull the intestine into small compartments called **haustra** (**haustrum** singular). Another distinguishing feature of the large intestine is the presence of small fat globules called **epiploic appendages** (omental appendices). Label the parts of the large intestine.

Color Guide: Color in each region of the large intestine with a different color. Color the haustra light red and the teniae coli pink. Color the epiploic appendages yellow.

Answer Key
a. Hepatic flexure
b. Splenic flexure
c. Transverse colon
d. Descending colon
e. Epiploic appendages
f. Sigmoid colon
g. Rectum
h. Anal canal
i. Anus
j. Vermiform appendix
k. Cecum
l. Ascending colon
m. Teniae coli
n. Haustra

LEARNING HINT

The Latin word *vermis* means "worm." True to this name, the **vermiform appendix** is shaped like a worm.

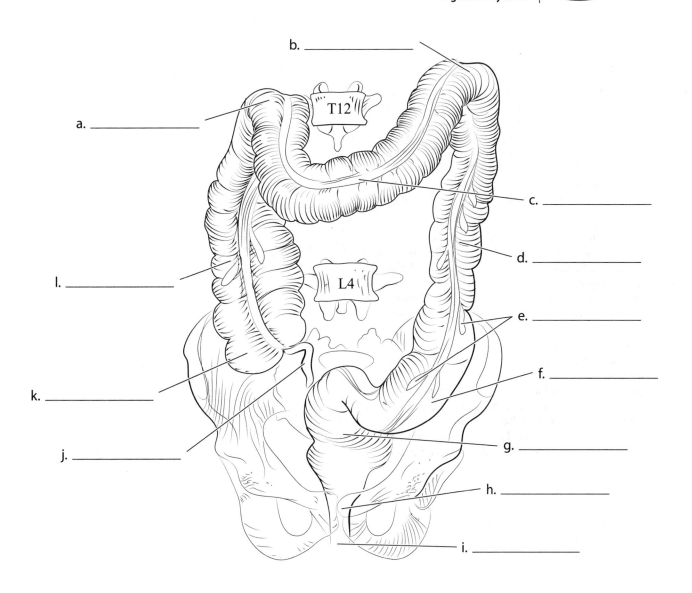

b. _____

a. _____

c. _____

d. _____

l. _____

e. _____

f. _____

k. _____

g. _____

j. _____

h. _____

i. _____

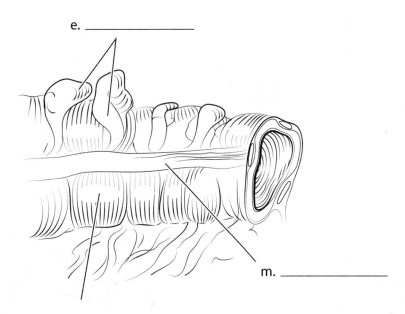

e. _____

m. _____

n. _____

LIVER

The liver is the largest internal organ of the body. It is on the right side of the body and plays a major metabolic function in digestion and in processing material from the blood. The liver has four lobes in humans and is held to the diaphragm by the **falciform ligament**. The **right lobe** is the largest of the lobes. The **left lobe** is also reasonably large. The **quadrate lobe** is anterior and is rectangular in shape when seen from the inferior view. The **caudate lobe** is a posterior lobe of the liver.

The blood flows into the liver from two sources. The **hepatic portal vein** takes blood to the liver from the digestive tract and some abdominal organs. The **hepatic artery** brings oxygenated blood to the liver. The liver is composed of microscopic sections called **liver lobules**. These are typically hexagonal columns that have a **central vein** that takes blood back to the heart via the hepatic vein. Blood travels to the central vein by **sinusoids**, canals that are lined by **hepatocytes** (liver cells). Hepatocytes clean the blood or process material in the blood. Old blood pigments are recycled by the liver and converted to bile. The bile moves through **bile canaliculi** and eventually is stored in the gallbladder. The branches of the hepatic artery, portal vein, and **bile duct** are clustered together and form the **portal triad**. Label the liver structures on the illustrations.

Color Guide: Color in the lobes of the liver using different colors for each lobe. Color the hepatic portal vein blue, the hepatic artery red, and the bile ducts green.

Answer Key

a. Right lobe
b. Left lobe
c. Falciform ligament
d. Portal vein
e. Hepatic artery
f. Caudate lobe
g. Quadrate lobe
h. Portal triad
i. Central vein
j. Bile duct
k. Hepatic artery branch
l. Bile canaliculus
m. Portal vein branch
n. Sinusoids
o. Hepatocytes

LEARNING HINT

Falciform means "sickle-shaped" in Latin, and this describes the **falciform ligament**.

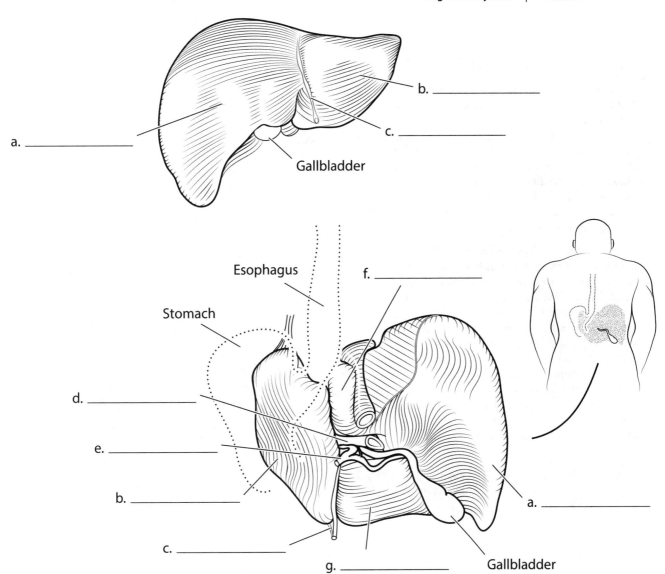

a. _____

b. _____

c. _____

Gallbladder

Esophagus

Stomach

f. _____

d. _____

e. _____

b. _____

c. _____

g. _____

a. _____

Gallbladder

Liver lobule

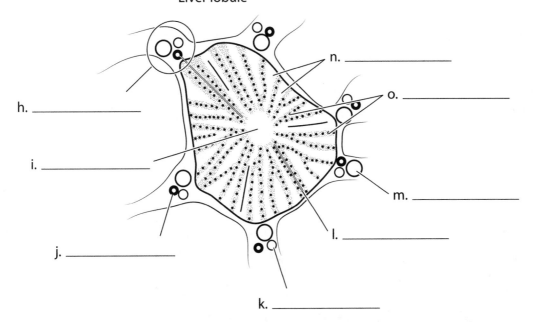

h. _____

i. _____

j. _____

k. _____

l. _____

m. _____

n. _____

o. _____

PANCREAS AND GALLBLADDER

The **pancreas** is a complex organ that has both a digestive function and an endocrine function. The digestive function of the pancreas consists of producing enzymes for the digestion of materials in the small intestine and the secretion of buffers to increase the pH of the fluid secreted from the stomach. The pancreas has a **head** next to the **duodenum**, a main **body**, and a **tail** near the spleen. The enzymes and buffers secreted into the small intestine flow into the **pancreatic duct** before entering the small intestine.

The **gallbladder** receives bile from the **liver**, storing and condensing it prior to secreting it into the small intestine. Bile is an emulsifier of fats, making them disperse in the liquid chyme of the digestive tract. Bile flows from the **left** and **right hepatic ducts**, into the **common hepatic duct**, into the **cystic duct**, and finally enters the gallbladder. When the gallbladder contracts, bile moves back out the cystic duct and into the **common bile duct** before entering the small intestine. Usually the common bile duct and the pancreatic duct join before they enter the small intestine. In this case, the tube is called the **hepatopancreatic ampulla**, and it leads to the **duodenal papilla**. Label the parts of the pancreas, gallbladder, and ducts.

Color Guide: Color the gallbladder green and the pancreas beige. Use your preferred color for the ducts that lead from the liver to the duodenum.

Answer Key

a. Gallbladder
b. Pancreas
c. Duodenum
d. Head
e. Body
f. Tail
g. Right hepatic duct
h. Cystic duct
i. Duodenal papilla
j. Left hepatic duct
k. Common hepatic duct
l. Common bile duct
m. Pancreatic duct

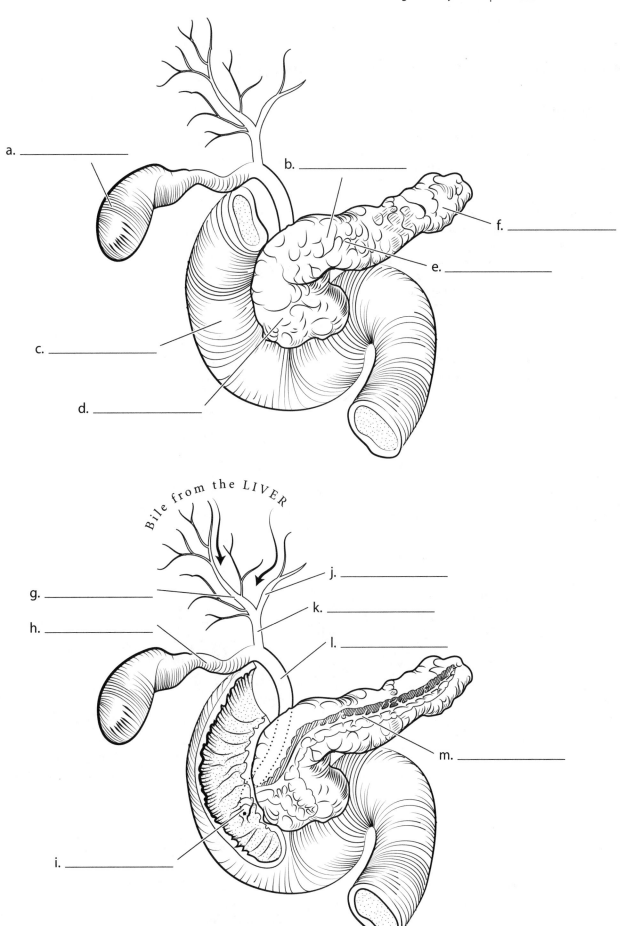

a. _____

b. _____

f. _____

e. _____

c. _____

d. _____

Bile from the LIVER

g. _____

h. _____

j. _____

k. _____

l. _____

m. _____

i. _____

Chapter Thirteen: **Urinary System**

OVERVIEW OF THE URINARY SYSTEM

The urinary system consists of two **kidneys**, two **ureters**, a **urinary bladder**, and a **urethra**. The right kidney is a little more inferior than the left kidney due to the presence of the liver on the right side of the body. The kidneys are located near the 12th vertebra and extend to the 3rd lumbar vertebra. They receive blood from the **renal artery**. The kidneys are **retroperitoneal**, meaning that they are posterior to the parietal peritoneum. The ureters are also retroperitoneal and take urine to the bladder. Since the urinary bladder is located anterior to the parietal peritoneum, it is described as **anteperitoneal**. Label the organs of the urinary system.

Color Guide: Use separate colors for the kidneys, ureters, urinary bladder, and urethra. In the lower illustration, color the bones yellow and the muscles and the aorta red.

Answer Key

a. Kidney
b. Ureter
c. Urinary bladder
d. Urethra
e. Renal artery

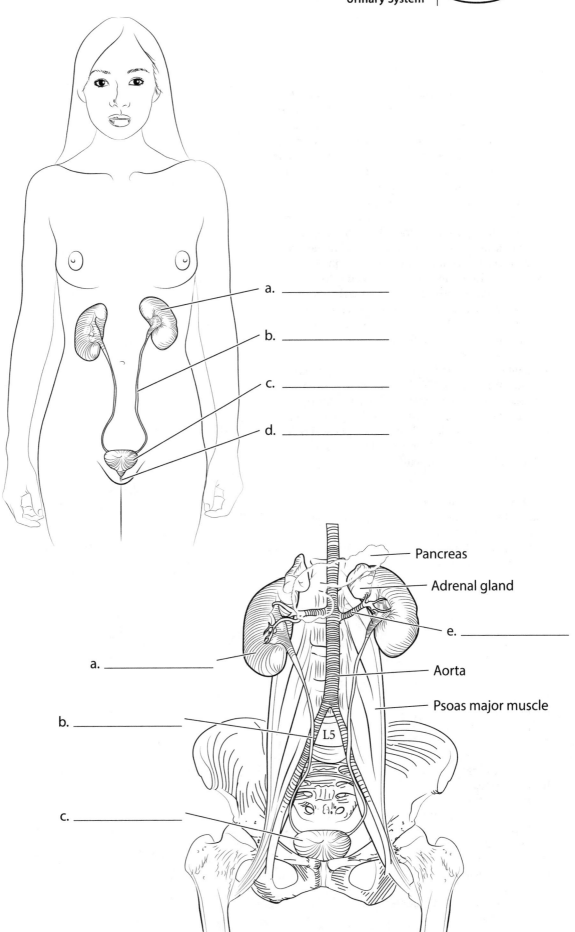

a. _____

b. _____

c. _____

d. _____

Pancreas

Adrenal gland

e. _____

Aorta

Psoas major muscle

a. _____

b. _____

c. _____

L5

KIDNEY

The kidney is a bean-shaped organ. The outer surface of the kidney is covered by the **renal capsule**. The depression on the medial side is the **hilum** where the **renal artery** enters the kidney and the **renal vein** and the **ureter** exit. The kidney is sectioned in the coronal plane to study the internal anatomy. The renal capsule is a thin membrane on the exterior of the kidney. Deep to the capsule is the **renal cortex** where filtration takes place in the kidney. The **renal medulla** is deep to the cortex and is divided into **renal columns** and **renal pyramids**. Each pyramid ends in a **papilla** and this drips urine into small funnel-shaped structures called the **minor calyces** (*calyx* singular). The minor calyces join to form the **major calyces**, and these, in turn, take urine to the **renal pelvis**. The renal pelvis occupies most of the **renal sinus**, a space in the kidney. The renal pelvis takes urine to the ureter on the medial side of the kidney. Blood travels to the kidney by the **renal artery**. From there, the blood moves into **segmental arteries** and then **interlobar arteries**. From the interlobar arteries, the blood travels to the **arcuate arteries**. These arteries are the dividing structures between the renal cortex and the renal medulla. From the arcuate arteries, blood flows into the **cortical radiate arteries** (interlobular arteries). Label the parts of the kidney and associated structures.

Color Guide: Use one color for the cortex and different shades of another color for the renal pyramids and columns. Color the renal artery and the arterial system in the kidney red, and color the renal vein blue. Use yellow for the pelvis and ureter.

Answer Key

a. Renal artery
b. Hilum
c. Renal vein
d. Renal pelvis
e. Ureter
f. Renal capsule
g. Major calyces
h. Renal sinus
i. Renal cortex
j. Renal pyramid (in renal medulla)
k. Papilla
l. Renal column
m. Minor calyces
n. Segmental arteries
o. Interlobar artery
p. Cortical radiate (interlobular) artery
q. Arcuate arteries

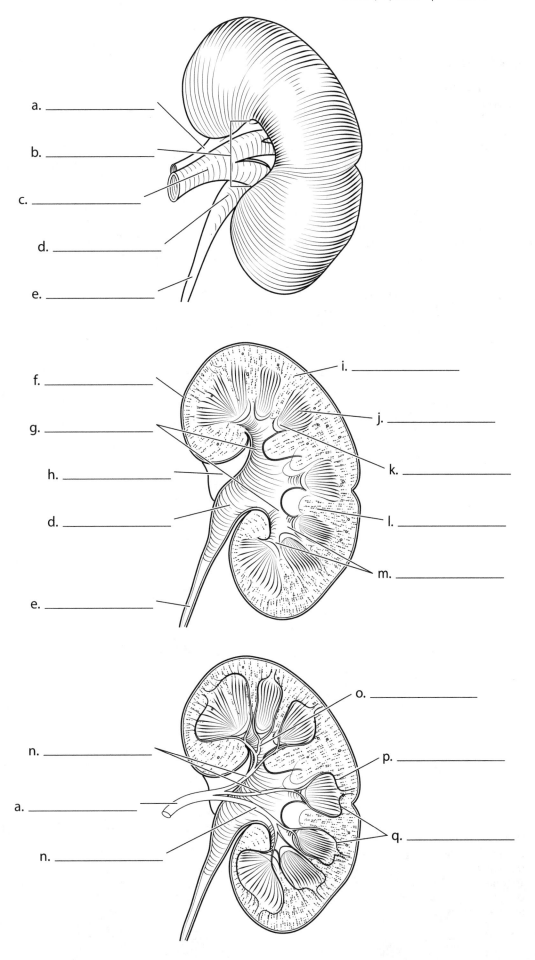

a. _____

b. _____

c. _____

d. _____

e. _____

f. _____

g. _____

h. _____

d. _____

e. _____

i. _____

j. _____

k. _____

l. _____

m. _____

n. _____

a. _____

n. _____

o. _____

p. _____

q. _____

URINARY BLADDER

The **urinary bladder** is a storage organ for holding urine. The **ureters** enter the bladder at the **ureteral orifices**, and the urethra exits the bladder inferiorly. These three openings make a triangular region known as the **trigone** at the posterior wall of the bladder. The **urethra** is the external tube that takes urine voided from the urinary bladder to outside the body. The urethra in the female is much shorter than in the male, which makes females more susceptible to bladder infections. The wall of the bladder consists of **smooth muscle** called the **detrusor muscle** and an inner lining of transitional epithelium. Label the features of the bladder, urethra, and associated structures.

Color Guide: Use the same colors that you chose for the Overview of the Urinary System for the structures in this figure.

Answer Key

a. Ureter
b. Urinary bladder
c. Detrusor muscle
d. Ureteral orifice
e. Trigone
f. Urethra
g. Right kidney

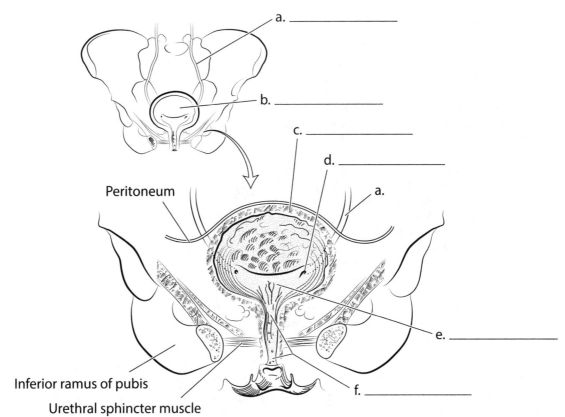

a. _____

b. _____

c. _____

d. _____

a. _____

Peritoneum

e. _____

f. _____

Inferior ramus of pubis

Urethral sphincter muscle

Female urinary system

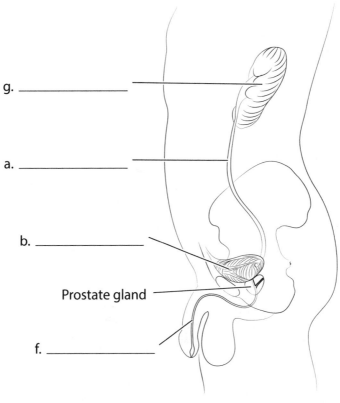

g. _____

a. _____

b. _____

Prostate gland

f. _____

Male urinary system

NEPHRON

The functional unit of the kidney is the **nephron**. It is here that material is filtered from the blood; some material is lost in the urine while other material is reabsorbed back into the cardiovascular system. The **renal corpuscle** of the nephron includes the **glomerulus** and the **glomerular (Bowman's) capsule**. The lining of the capsule wraps around the glomerulus, and filtered material enters the nephron at this point. The glomerular capsule leads to the **proximal convoluted tubule**. This tubule has many microvilli that provide for a great surface area for reabsorption of materials. Most of the reabsorption of material in the nephron occurs here. The **peritubular capillaries** wrap around the kidney tubules and reabsorb the filtered material. From the proximal convoluted tubule, the fluid flows into the **nephron loop (loop of Henle)**. The nephron loop takes fluid to the **distal convoluted tubule**. From here, the filtrate flows into a **collecting duct**. Collecting ducts receive fluid from many nephrons. Label the parts of the nephron and associated structures.

Color Guide: Color the collecting duct yellow. Use red for the arterioles. Each part of the nephron should be colored a different color.

Answer Key

a. Renal corpuscle
b. Distal convoluted tubule
c. Proximal convoluted tubule
d. Cortex
e. Medulla
f. Arcuate vein
g. Arcuate artery
h. Nephron loop (loop of Henle)
i. Nephron
j. Collecting duct
k. Afferent arteriole
l. Efferent arteriole
m. Glomerular (Bowman's) capsule

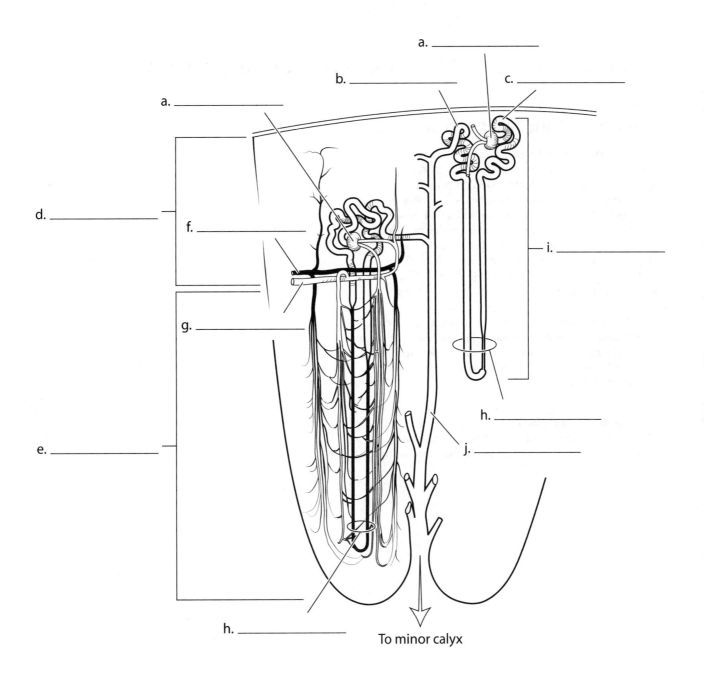

a. _____

b. _____   c. _____

a. _____

d. _____

f. _____

i. _____

g. _____

h. _____

e. _____

j. _____

h. _____

To minor calyx

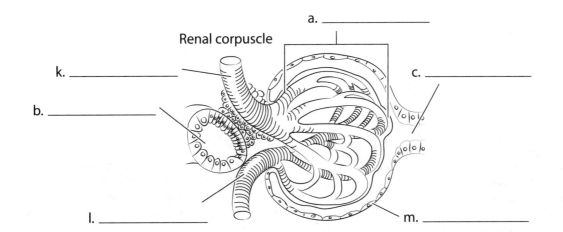

Renal corpuscle

a. _____

k. _____

b. _____

c. _____

l. _____

m. _____

▪ Chapter Fourteen: **Male Reproductive System**

OVERVIEW OF THE MALE REPRODUCTIVE SYSTEM

The male reproductive system consists of the two **testes**, the **epididymis**, the **ductus deferens** enclosed in the **spermatic cord**, the **seminal vesicles**, the **prostate** gland, the **bulbourethral glands**, and the **penis**. The testes are the glands that produce testosterone and sperm cells. Sperm cells travel from the testes to the epididymis where they are stored and mature. From the epididymis, sperm cells move into the ductus deferens, which enters the body and travels to the posterior bladder. From here, the ductus deferens turns into the ejaculatory duct, which receives fluid from the seminal vesicles. The ejaculatory duct leads to the **urethra** where secretions from the prostate and bulbourethral glands are added. Finally the sperm cells and seminal fluid (together these make **semen**) are ejaculated from the penis. Label the parts of the male reproductive system.

Color Guide: Color the various structures in the illustration. Use darker colors for the organs or glands that are shaded in and lighter colors for those that are not.

Answer Key

a. Ductus deferens
b. Seminal vesicle
c. Prostate
d. Bulbourethral gland
e. Epididymis
f. Testis
g. Uncircumcised penis
h. Circumcised penis
i. Urethra

LEARNING HINT

The term **epididymis** (plural *epididymides*) comes from the Greek, meaning "on the twins." These curved structures lie on both testes.

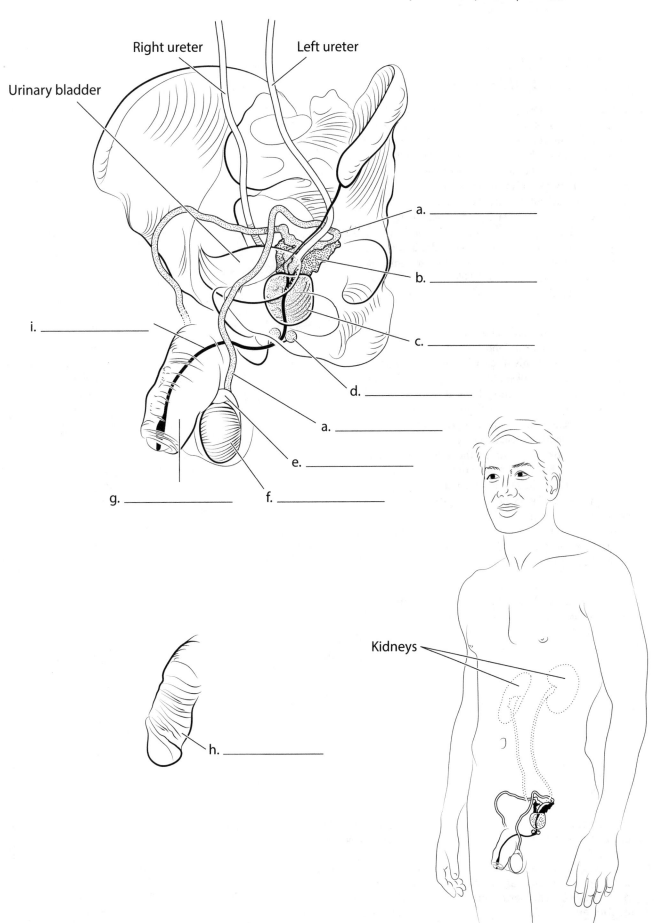

Right ureter

Left ureter

Urinary bladder

a. _____

b. _____

c. _____

d. _____

i. _____

a. _____

e. _____

g. _____ f. _____

h. _____

Kidneys

ORGANS OF THE MALE REPRODUCTIVE SYSTEM

The **testes** are enclosed in the **scrotal sac**, which is lined with a smooth muscle layer called the **dartos muscle**. This muscle contracts when the temperature drops near the testes, causing them to withdraw closer to the body where it is warmer. Another muscle of the region is the **cremaster muscle**. It also contracts when it is cold, but it is made of skeletal muscle. The **epididymis** sits on top of the testis like a small cap and is a place where sperm cells mature. The **spermatic cord** consists of the cremaster muscle, the **ductus deferens**, the **testicular artery**, and a complex meshwork of veins called the **pampiniform plexus**. This plexus cools arterial blood flowing to the testes, maintaining the testes at about 35 degrees C, which is important for proper sperm maturation.

The sperm are produced in the seminiferous tubules of the testis. This occurs in **lobules of the testis** before they move to the epididymis. The epididymis has a series of long coiled tubules called the **ductus epididymis**, and the sperm cells slowly pass through this ductwork. After the sperm cells mature in the epididymis, they travel to the **ductus deferens**, which loops around the **ureters** before reaching the **seminal vesicles** located on the posterior surface of the **urinary bladder**. The seminal vesicles add a fluid that has buffers and that provides fructose to the sperm cells. From the seminal vesicles, the fluid passes through the **ejaculatory duct** to the **prostate**. The prostate adds further fluid that is rich in buffers. This fluid passes into the **urethra**. The **bulbourethral glands** add a protein lubricant to the fluid. Label the organs and their features in the illustration.

Color Guide: Use the same colors for the structures in this illustration as you did for the same structures in the preceding illustration.

Answer Key

a. Ductus deferens
b. Pampiniform plexus
c. Testicular artery
d. Epididymis
e. Testis
f. Cremaster muscle and fascia
g. Scrotal skin and dartos muscle
h. Ureter
i. Urinary bladder
j. Seminal vesicle
k. Ejaculatory duct
l. Prostate
m. Bulbourethral gland
n. Urethra
o. Ductus epididymis
p. Lobules of testis

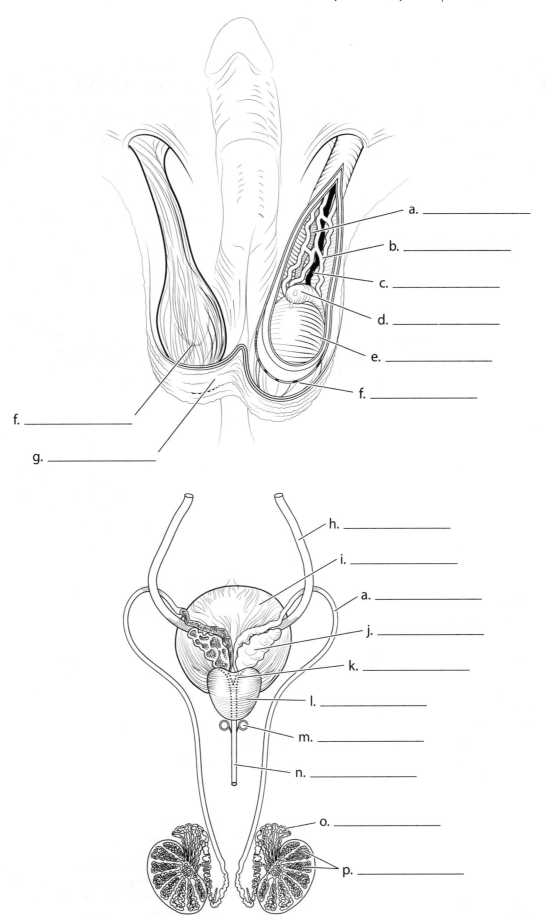

a. _____

b. _____

c. _____

d. _____

e. _____

f. _____

f. _____

g. _____

h. _____

i. _____

a. _____

j. _____

k. _____

l. _____

m. _____

n. _____

o. _____

p. _____

Posterior view

MIDSAGITTAL SECTION OF MALE PELVIS

When seen in a midsagittal section, the relationship of the glands that produce seminal fluid can easily be seen. The **prostate** is approximately the size of a golf ball and is located inferior to the **urinary bladder**. The **prostatic urethra** is the portion of the urethra that is enclosed in the prostate. The **bulbourethral glands** are located in the wall of the pelvic floor, and the **seminal vesicles** are posterior to the urinary bladder. Exterior to the body wall are the testes, and these are enclosed in the **scrotal sac**. The **epididymis** receives sperm from the testis and has three parts, a **head**, a **body**, and a **tail**. The **symphysis pubis** is an important reference point in the midsagittal section. In males, there is a flap of tissue encircling the **glans penis**. This is the **prepuce** (foreskin), and it is sometimes removed at birth in a procedure called a circumcision. The **corpus cavernosum** can be seen in this section along with the **corpus spongiosum** and the **spongy urethra**.

CROSS SECTION OF PENIS AND SEMINIFEROUS TUBULES

The cross section of the penis illustrates the relative position of the erectile tissue in the male. On the dorsal aspect of the penis are the paired **corpora cavernosa** (corpus cavernosum singular). These cylinders fill with blood and produce an increase in length and diameter of the penis. These, along with the **corpus spongiosum**, are involved in making the penis erect. The corpus spongiosum contains the **spongy urethra**. The **deep dorsal vein** of the penis is also seen in cross section. Label the structures seen in a cross section of the penis.

The formation of sperm is known as spermatogenesis and begins with **spermatogonia** on the superficial wall of the seminiferous tubules. These produce cells called **primary spermatocytes**, which in turn mature into **secondary spermatocytes**. **Spermatids** derive from secondary spermatocytes, and they, in turn, become **spermatozoa** (sperm cells). **Sertoli cells** (sustenocytes) assist in the process. Label the cells.

Color Guide: Use the same colors on this page that you chose for the same structures in the preceding illustrations. Use two different colors, one for the corpus spongiosum and another for the corpora cavernosa; these are seen in the top and middle illustrations. For the cells in the seminiferous tubule at the bottom of the page, use a different color for each stage of the production of sperm from the spermatogonia to the spermatozoa.

Answer Key
a. Urinary bladder
b. Symphysis pubis
c. Corpus cavernosum
d. Corpus spongiosum
e. Glans penis
f. Prepuce
g. Testis
h. Tail of epididymis
i. Body of epididymis
j. Head of epididymis
k. Spongy urethra
l. Bulbourethral gland
m. Prostate
n. Seminal vesicle
o. Deep dorsal vein
p. Spermatozoa
q. Spermatids
r. Secondary spermatocytes
s. Primary spermatocytes
t. Sertoli cell
u. Spermatogonia

LEARNING HINT

The word *corpus* is Latin for "body." From it come the names **corpus spongiosum** (a "spongy body") and **corpora cavernosa** (the "cavernous bodies").

a. _____

b. _____

c. _____

d. _____

e. _____

f. _____

g. _____

n. _____

m. _____

l. _____

k. _____

j. _____

i. _____

h. _____

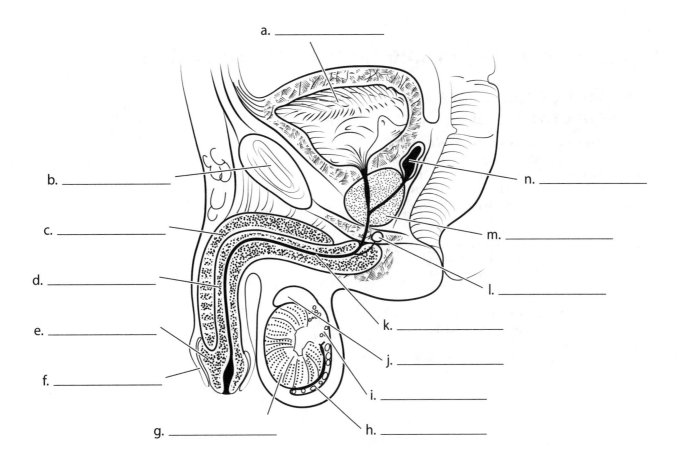

o. _____

c. _____

d. _____

k. _____

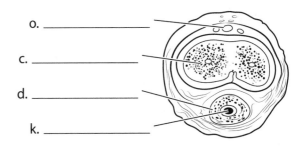

p. _____

q. _____

r. _____

u. _____

t. _____

s. _____

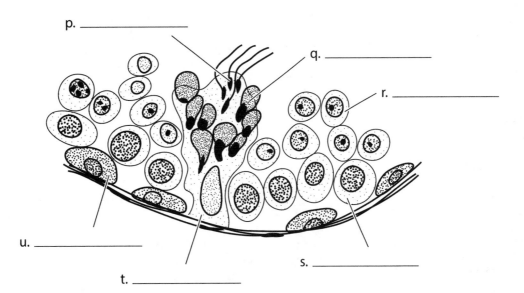

▪ Chapter Fifteen: **Female Reproductive System**

OVERVIEW OF THE FEMALE REPRODUCTIVE SYSTEM

The female reproductive system consists of the two **ovaries**, the **uterine tubes**, a single **uterus**, **vagina**, and the **vaginal orifice**. The uterus is held to the anterior body by the **round ligaments** and held to the pelvic wall by the suspensory ligaments. Blood flows to the ovaries by the **gonadal arteries**.

The breasts are integumentary structures, and each one has **mammary glands**, an **areola**, and a **nipple**. Label the structures of the female reproductive system.

Color Guide: Use a different color for each organ of the female reproductive system. You will use these colors for the same structures on subsequent pages. In the lower figure, color the aorta and the associated arteries red and the inferior vena cava and associated veins blue.

Answer Key

a. Areola
b. Nipple
c. Mammary glands
d. Ovary
e. Uterine tube
f. Round ligament
g. Uterus
h. Vagina
i. Labium minus
j. Ovarian vessels

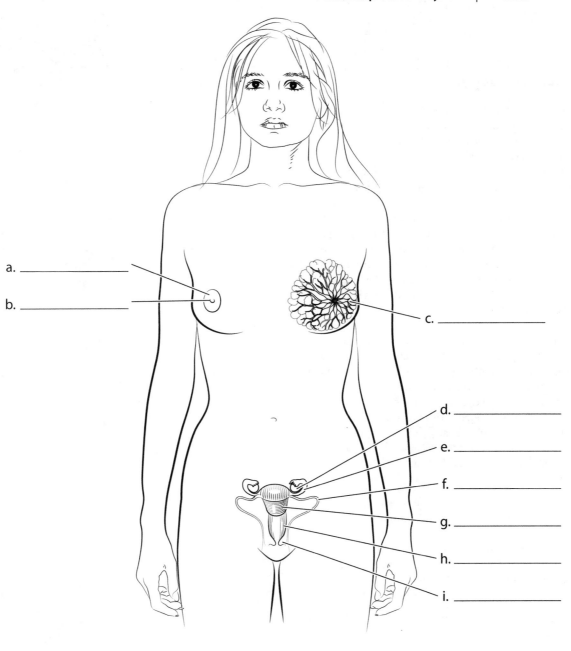

a. _____

b. _____

c. _____

d. _____

e. _____

f. _____

g. _____

h. _____

i. _____

Aorta

Ureter

j. _____

L5

External iliac vessels

e. _____

g. _____

f. _____

Urinary bladder

h. _____

MIDSAGITTAL SECTION OF FEMALE PELVIS

The **ovaries** produce the oocytes that are released into the pelvic cavity. Locate the **suspensory ligaments** that attach the ovaries to the pelvic wall. The **round ligament** attaches the uterus anteriorly. The oocytes travel into the **uterine tubes** and then pass into the **uterus**. The uterus has a domed **fundus** near the entrance of the uterine tubes and a **cervix** that inserts into the vagina. The depression between the uterus and the rectum is the **rectouterine pouch**. The **vagina** is inferior to the uterus and terminates with the **vaginal orifice**. Anterior to the vaginal orifice is the **urethral orifice**, the external opening of the urethra. In this section, you can see the **fornix** of the vagina, a pocket that surrounds the cervix of the uterus. You can also see the relationship of the **labium minus** and the **labium majus** in this section. The labia minora are the inner vaginal lips and the labia majora are the outer vaginal lips. These are part of the vulva or external genitalia. Another part of the vulva is the **clitoris**, which consists of the external glans and the body of the clitoris. The body of the clitoris is imbedded in the body tissue. The glans is covered with a prepuce. Anterior to the clitoris is the **mons pubis,** a fatty pad of tissue overlying the symphysis pubis. Label the organs and other structures in the midsagittal section of the female pelvis.

Color Guide: Use the same colors for the individual organs in this illustration as you did in the preceding illustration. For the uterus, use different shades for the fundus and cervix, and use a different shade from both for the body of the uterus, which lies between them. Select new colors for structures that are unique to this page.

Answer Key

a. Suspensory ligaments
b. Ovary
c. Uterine tube
d. Round ligament
e. Uterus
f. Fundus
g. Cervix
h. Clitoris
i. Labium majus
j. Labium minus
k. Urethral orifice
l. Vaginal orifice
m. Vagina
n. Fornix
o. Rectouterine pouch

LEARNING HINT

The word **fundus** is Latin for the "base" or "depth." In the context of the uterus, it is the part farthest away from the vagina (the depth of the uterus). The **cervix** (Latin for "neck") of the uterus is the part closest to the vagina.

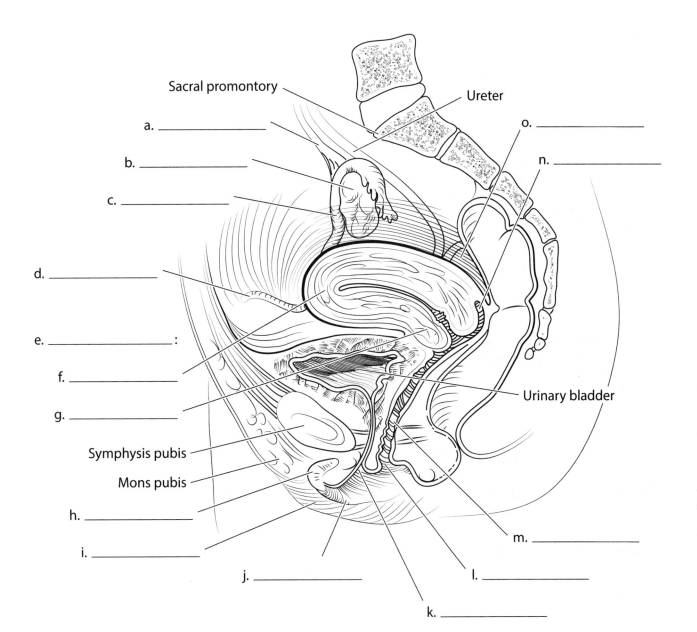

Sacral promontory

Ureter

a. _____

o. _____

b. _____

n. _____

c. _____

d. _____

e. _____ :

f. _____

g. _____

Urinary bladder

Symphysis pubis

Mons pubis

h. _____

i. _____

j. _____

k. _____

l. _____

m. _____

OVARY

The **ovary** is the gonad of the female reproductive system. It produces **oocytes** in a process known as oogenesis, and when they are mature they are released from the ovary by **ovulation**. Development of all the oocytes begins during fetal development of the female, but they remain as **primary oocytes** until puberty. Each month, during a woman's reproductive span, a group of primary oocytes (located in enclosures known as **primary follicles**) begins to mature. Usually only one of the primary oocytes matures to a **secondary oocyte**, which is located in a **secondary follicle**. The secondary oocyte is ovulated and, if it is fertilized, it becomes an **ovum**. The remaining follicle cells become the **corpus luteum**, which secretes hormones. If fertilization does not occur, the corpus luteum develops into the **corpus albicans**.

The two cycles that occur in the female reproductive system are the **ovarian cycle**, which involves changes in the ovary with a **preovulatory**, **ovulatory**, and **postovulatory** phase, and the **menstrual cycle**, which reflects changes in the endometrium. The endometrium has a **basal layer** that stays the same thickness throughout the menstrual cycle and a **functional layer** that fluctuates in thickness and composition during the cycle. The menstrual cycle has a **proliferative**, **secretory**, and **menstrual phase**. The proliferative phase prepares the endometrium for implantation. The secretory phase provides glycogen as a food source for the developing conceptus, and the functional layer is shed during the menstrual phase, which occurs if there is no implantation.

Color Guide: Use a different color for each stage of oocyte maturation in both the top and lower illustrations. Select other colors for the phases of the menstrual cycle.

Answer Key

a. Primary oocytes
b. Ovarian follicles
c. Ovulated secondary oocyte
d. Corpus luteum
e. Corpus albicans
f. Preovulatory phase
g. Ovulation
h. Postovulatory phase
i. Uterine gland
j. Functional layer
k. Basal layer
l. Proliferative stage
m. Secretory stage
n. Menstrual stage

LEARNING HINT

The term **oocytes** (pronounced OH-oh-sites) literally means "egg cells." If they develop completely, oocytes become **ova** (eggs).

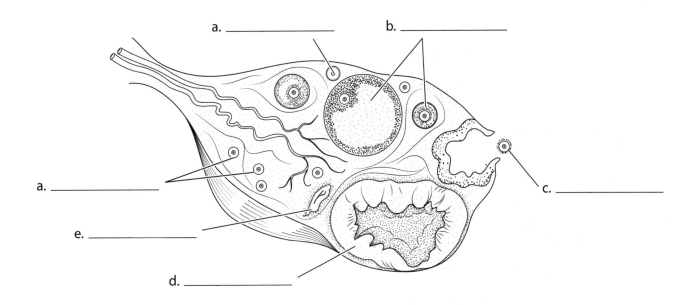

a. _____   b. _____

a. _____

e. _____

c. _____

d. _____

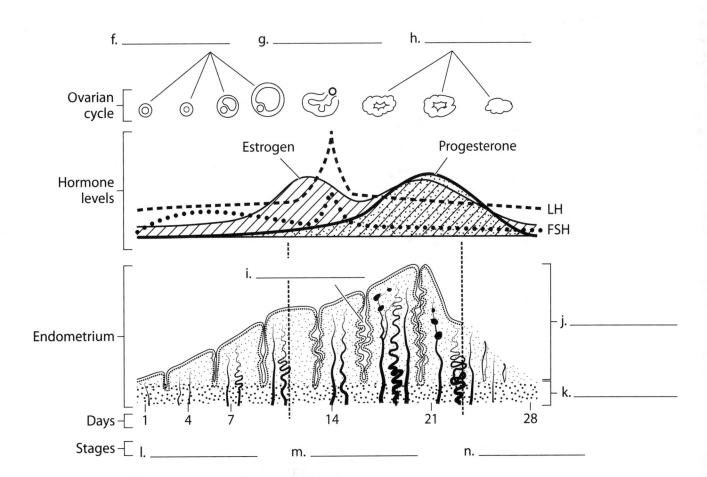

f. _____   g. _____   h. _____

Ovarian cycle

Estrogen   Progesterone

Hormone levels

LH

FSH

i. _____

Endometrium

j. _____

k. _____

Days   1   4   7   14   21   28

Stages   l. _____   m. _____   n. _____

SECTION OF UTERUS AND VAGINA

The **oocyte** is ovulated from the **ovary** and moves into the **uterine tube**. The uterine tube is fringed by small cylindrical structures called **fimbriae**. The **uterus** is a small flask-shaped organ. The uterus has a domed **fundus**, a main **body**, a narrowed **isthmus**, and an inferior **cervix**. The **uterosacral ligament** attaches the uterus to the sacrum. Most of the uterine wall is made of the myometrium, which is a thick layer of smooth muscle. The **vagina** is approximately 10 centimeters in length and is lined with stratified squamous epithelium and smooth muscle. A small ring of mucous membrane called the **hymen** is present in the vagina and is frequently torn during first intercourse. The hymen can rupture prior to intercourse and is not a good indicator of virginity. The vagina has **rugae**, which are folds in the vaginal wall. These stimulate the penis and allow for expansion of the vagina during delivery. Label the **suspensory ligament** and **ovarian ligament** as well as the structures of the uterus, ovary, and vagina.

Color Guide: Color the regions of the uterus, ovary, vagina, and associated structures.

Answer Key

a. Uterine tube
b. Oocyte
c. Uterus
d. Fundus
e. Body
f. Isthmus
g. Cervix
h. Vagina
i. Suspensory ligament
j. Fimbriae
k. Ovary
l. Ovarian ligament
m. Uterosacral ligament
n. Rugae
o. Hymen

LEARNING HINT

The word **fimbriae** is Latin for "fringe." This structure forms a fringe around the uterine tube.

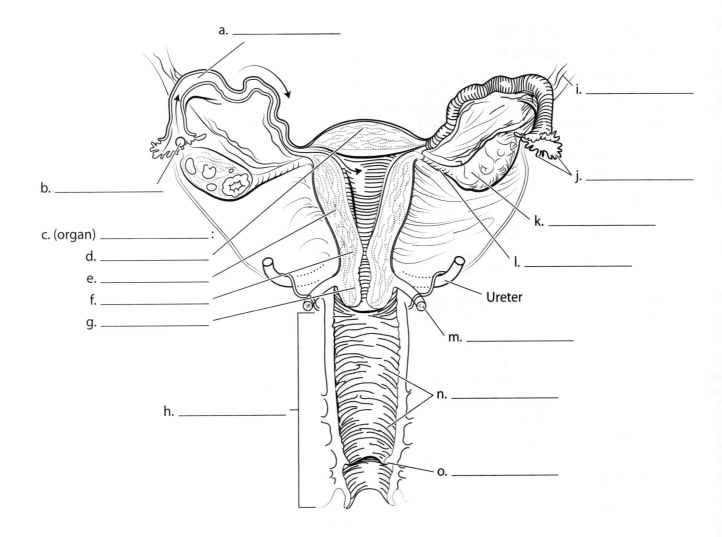

a. _____

b. _____

c. (organ) _____ :

d. _____

e. _____

f. _____

g. _____

h. _____

i. _____

j. _____

k. _____

l. _____

Ureter

m. _____

n. _____

o. _____

FEMALE BREAST AND
EXTERNAL GENITALIA

The **mammary glands** are located in the breast.
They produce milk when a woman is lactating and
lead to **lactiferous ducts**. These ducts take milk to the
lactiferous sinuses, which drain into the nipple. Because
breast cancer is a significant cause of mortality in women,
the lymph drainage of the breast is important. Primary
tumors may originate in the breast tissue and then migrate
by **lymphatic vessels** to the **axillary lymph nodes**. This is
one of the main ways that breast cancer spreads. A small
series of **parasternal lymph nodes** takes a small portion
of the lymph back to the cardiovascular system.

The floor of the pelvis is known as the perineum and
can be divided into a **urogenital triangle** and an **anal
triangle**. The anal triangle contains the **anus**, and
the urogenital triangle houses the **vaginal orifice**, the
urethral orifice, and the **clitoris**. The **mons pubis** is the
most anterior part of the external genitalia, and posterior
to that is the **prepuce**. This structure envelops the **clitoris**.
The **labia majora** and the **labia minora** encircle the
vaginal orifice. The vagina is lubricated internally by some
glands during arousal and intercourse as well as from the
greater vestibular glands located laterally and posteriorly
to the vaginal orifice. Label the structures of the female
breast and the external genitalia.

Color Guide: Use different colors for the structures of the
breast and for the external genitalia.

Answer Key

a. Axillary lymph nodes
b. Lymphatic vessels
c. Parasternal lymph nodes
d. Lactiferous sinuses
e. Lactiferous ducts
f. Urogenital triangle
g. Anal triangle
h. Mons pubis
i. Prepuce
j. Clitoris
k. Labia minora
l. Labia majora
m. Urethral orifice
n. Vaginal orifice
o. Anus

a. _____

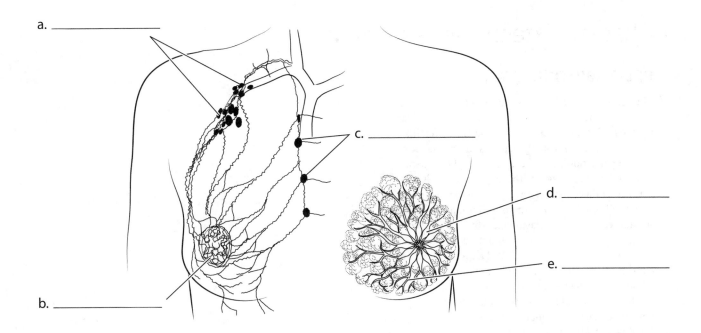

c. _____

d. _____

e. _____

b. _____

Pubic symphysis

h. _____

i. _____

j. _____

k. _____

f. _____

l. _____

Ischial tuberosity

m. _____

n. _____

g. _____

o. _____

Coccyx

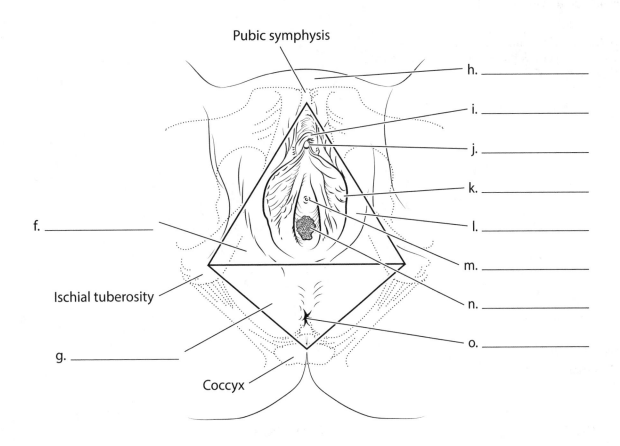

Chapter Sixteen: **Development**

PRE-EMBRYONIC STAGE

The process of development begins with the union of the sperm and oocyte. After **ovulation**, the secondary oocyte moves down the uterine tube and, if **fertilization** occurs by sperm, it usually happens in the uterine tube. Once fertilization occurs, the oocyte and the sperm unite to become a **zygote**. The zygote divides during this **pre-embryonic stage** and forms a **two-cell stage**. These cells go through numerous divisions and are called **blastomeres**. The two blastomeres divide and become four cells, and this process continues until a cluster of cells (16 to 32 of them) is formed called a **morula**. As division continues, this cluster becomes a hollow ball of cells called a **blastocyst**. The hollow cavity of the blastocyst is called the **blastocele**, and most of the wall of the blastocyst consists of a layer of simple squamous epithelia called the **trophoblast**. One part of the wall consists of an inner cell mass known as the **embryoblast**. Some of these cells will develop into the embryo. Label the structures in the pre-embryonic stage of development.

Color Guide: Color in the various stages in different colors, and use one color for the trophoblast and another for the embryoblast.

Answer Key

a. Ovulation
b. Fertilization
c. Two-cell stage
d. Morula
e. Blastocyst
f. Zygote
g. Blastomere
h. Trophoblast
i. Embryoblast
j. Blastocele

LEARNING HINT

The term **blast** is Greek for a "sprout," while **morula** is Latin for "blackberry," as this cluster of cells looks like that fruit.

b. _____

c. _____

g. _____

d. _____

f. _____

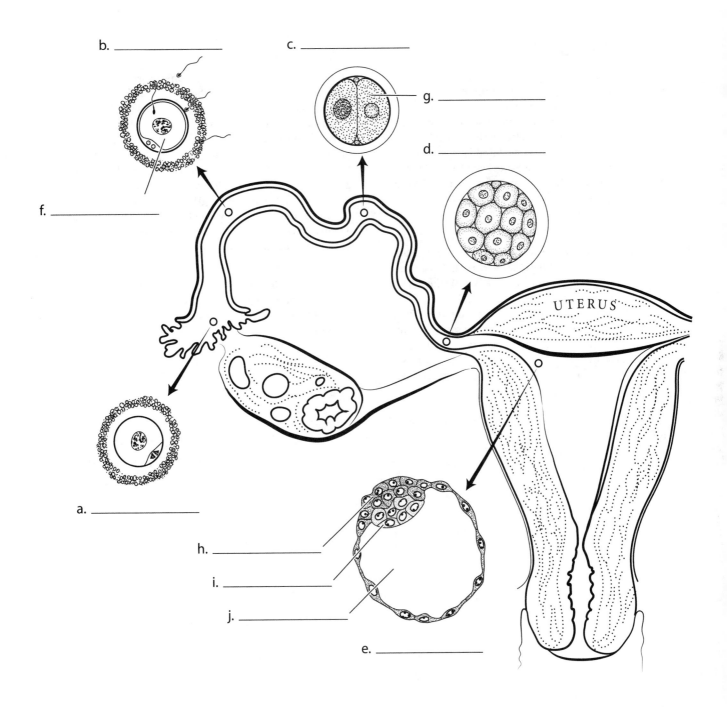

a. _____

h. _____

i. _____

j. _____

e. _____

UTERUS

EMBRYONIC STAGE

The blastocyst is the stage of development in which implantation in the uterus occurs. Implantation is the embedding of the blastocyst in the endometrium of the mother. Once this occurs, a hollow space develops in the embryoblast called the **amniotic cavity**. At this time, the embryoblast is divided into a **bilaminar germ disk** with two primitive tissues called the **epiblast** and the **hypoblast**. The **primitive streak** forms along the anterior/posterior axis of the embryo and becomes a region of growth in the early stage of development.

From this stage, three primary germ layers form. These are the **endoderm**, **ectoderm**, and **mesoderm**. The structure is now referred to as a **trilaminar germ disk** (meaning a developmental structure with three layers). The development of the **notochord** begins, and this structure will make up the center part (nucleosus pulposus) of the intervertebral disks in the adult. The **yolk sac** also forms during this period. Once the germ layers are formed, the pre-embryonic stage ends, and the developing tissue is known as an embryo. The embryonic stage begins about day 16 after fertilization and lasts until about the eighth week of pregnancy. During the embryonic stage, the major organs of the body are initiated in a process called organogenesis.

During the first part of the embryonic phase, the ectoderm begins to fold in on itself and becomes a **neural groove**. This will develop into the nervous system of the body. Other derivatives of the ectoderm are the epidermis and some of the facial bones and muscles. The mesoderm gives rise to most of the bones and muscles of the body, the dermis, and the circulatory system. The endodermis gives rise to the linings of the gastrointestinal tract and respiratory system and some glands. As development continues, the neural groove folds in on itself and becomes a **neural tube**, and the formation of the **gut** takes place. Label the structures in the embryonic phase.

Color Guide: Use blue colors for the ectoderm and derivatives of the ectoderm such as the neural tissue. Use red for the mesoderm, and color the endoderm in yellow.

Answer Key

a. Epiblast
b. Hypoblast
c. Ectoderm
d. Mesoderm
e. Endoderm
f. Amniotic cavity
g. Bilaminar germ disk
h. Primitive streak
i. Notochord
j. Trilaminar germ disk
k. Neural groove
l. Yolk sac
m. Neural tube
n. Gut

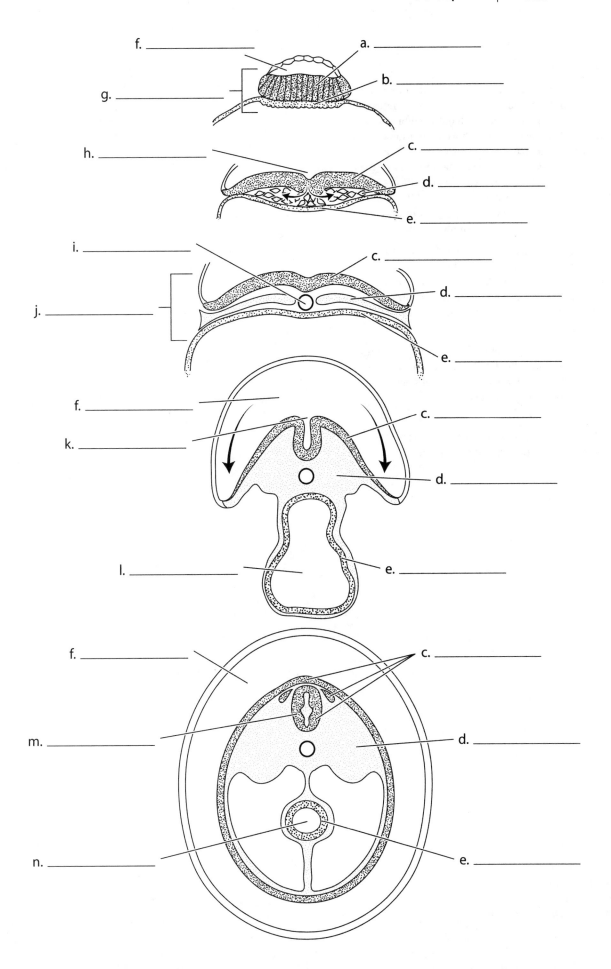

f. _____   a. _____

g. _____   b. _____

h. _____   c. _____

d. _____

e. _____

i. _____   c. _____

j. _____   d. _____

e. _____

f. _____   c. _____

k. _____   d. _____

l. _____   e. _____

f. _____   c. _____

m. _____   d. _____

n. _____   e. _____

FETAL STAGE

At the eighth week after fertilization, the organs are formed, and the embryo has now become a **fetus**. Prior to the fetal stage, the outer wall of the **embryo** develops into a membrane called the **chorion**, and some of this membrane is joined with the maternal vasculature forming the **placenta**. Between the chorion and the embryo is the **chorionic cavity**. This cavity disappears by the eighth week. A membrane called the **amnion** folds around the embryo forming the **amniotic cavity**, and this cavity is filled with amniotic fluid.

The stages of development can be divided into the **pre-embryo** (from fertilization to two weeks), the **embryo** (up to eight weeks after fertilization), and the final stage, the **fetus** (after eight weeks). The **conceptus** is the term used for the developing cells and tissues from the pre-embryo through the fetus.

Before delivery of the fetus, the amniotic sac ruptures releasing amniotic fluid, the uterus contracts expelling the fetus from the uterus, and the final stage occurs when the placenta is released.

Color Guide: Use colors of your choosing for the structures that are seen in development.

Answer Key

a. Amniotic cavity
b. Embryo
c. Chorion
d. Chorionic cavity
e. Placenta
f. Fetus
g. Amnion

Embryonic stage

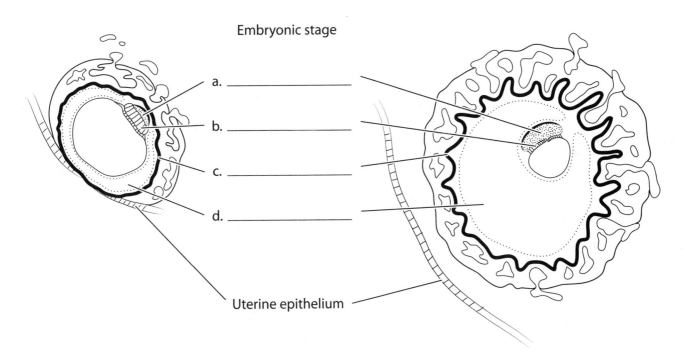

a. _____

b. _____

c. _____

d. _____

Uterine epithelium

Fetal stage

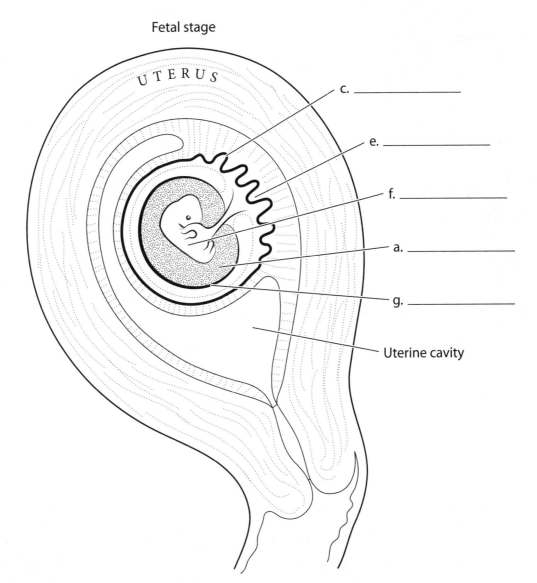

UTERUS

c. _____

e. _____

f. _____

a. _____

g. _____

Uterine cavity

Index

pathway of air, 272–273
pectoral girdle, 44–45, 64–65
pectoralis major, 10–11, 16–17, 104–105
pedal, 16–17
pedicles, 58–59
pelvic arteries, 228–229
pelvic brim, 76–77
pelvic cavity, 20–21
pelvic curvature, 54–55
pelvic girdle, 44–45, 64–65
pelvis, 78–79, 306–307, 310–311
penis, 302–303, 306–307
pepsinogen, 284–285
pericardial cavity, 20–21, 208–209
perilymph, 178–179
perineum, 316–317
periodontal ligaments, 86–87, 280–281
peripheral nervous system, 110–111
peripheral proteins, 22–23
peritubular capillaries, 300–301
permanent teeth, 280–281
peroneal artery, 222–223
peroxisomes, 22–23
perpendicular plate of the ethmoid bone, 50–51, 52–53, 260–261
petrous part of the temporal bone, 52–53
phagocytic vesicles, 22–23
phalanges, 64–65, 74–75, 80–81, 84–85
phalanx, 90–91
pharyngeal tonsils, 246–247
pharynx, 256–257
phosphate molecules, 22–23
phospholipid bilayer, 22–23
photoreceptor layer, 172–173
phrenic nerves, 146–147
pia mater, 142–143
pilosebaceous unit, 42–43
pineal gland, 126–127, 182–183, 184–185
pinna, 174–175
pisiform, 74–75
pituitary, 184–185, 186–187
pituitary fossa, 50–51
pituitary gland, 52–53, 124–125, 126–127, 128–129, 182–183, 184–185
pivot joints, 92–93
placenta, 240–241, 322–333
plantar veins, 236–237
plasma, 36–37, 202–203
plasma cells, 254–255
plasma membrane, 22–23
platelets, 36–37, 202–203
pleura, 20–21, 256–257
pleural cavity, 20–21, 270–271
pleurisy, 20–21
plexus
 brachial, 144–145, 148–149
cervical, 144–145, 146–147
choroid, 136–137
lumbar, 144–145, 150–151
lumbosacral, 144–145
pampiniform, 304–305
sacral, 144–145, 152–153
pollex, 74–75
pons, 124–125, 126–127, 140–141
popliteal, 18–19
popliteal artery, 222–223
popliteal vein, 236–237
portal system, 238–239
portal triad, 290–291
postcentral gyrus, 120–121, 122–123
posterior (position), 2–3
posterior cavity, 170–171
posterior chamber, 170–171
posterior duct, 176–177
posterior junction, 46–47
posterior muscles, 106–107
postganglionic neurons, 158–159
postovulatory, 312–313
postsynaptic neuron, 116–117
precentral gyrus, 120–121, 122–123, 132–133
pre-embryonic stage, 318–319, 322–323
preganglionic neurons, 158–159
premolars, 280–281
preovulatory, 312–313
prepuce, 306–307, 316–317
presynaptic neuron, 116–117
primitive streak, 320–321
principal cells, 190–191
process(es)
 acromion, 68–69
 articular, 58–59, 60–61, 92–93
 clinoid, 52–53
 condylar, 96–97
 coracoid, 66–67, 68--69
 coronoid, 46–47, 72–73, 96–97
 frontal, 260–261
 mastoid, 46–47, 52–53, 104–105
 odontoid, 56–57
 olecranon, 72–73
 palatine, 48–49
 spinous, 56–57, 58–59
 styloid, 46–47, 48–49, 52–53, 72–73
 supracondylar, 70–71
 terminal, 66–67
 transverse, 58–59
 xiphoid, 62–63
 zygomatic, 46–47, 52–53
progesterone, 182–183, 196–197
prolactin, 186–187
proliferative, 312–313
pronation, 102–103
prosencephalon, 118–119
prostate, 306–307
prostate gland, 302–303, 304–305
prostatic urethra, 306–307
proximal (position), 2–3
proximal base, 74–75
proximal convoluted tubule, 300–301
proximal phalanx, 90–91
pseudostratified ciliated columnar epithelium, 24–25, 262–263
pseudounipolar neurons, 116–117
pterygoid plates, 48–49, 52–53
pubic symphysis, 76–77
pubis, 76–77
pudendal artery, 228–229
pudendal nerve, 152–153
pulmonary artery, 200–201, 206–207, 272–273
pulmonary capillary bed, 200–201
pulmonary circulation, 200–201
pulmonary semilunar valve, 208–209, 210–211
pulmonary trunk, 198–199, 204–205, 208–209, 240–241
pulmonary veins, 200–201, 206–207, 272–273
pulp cavity, 280–281
pupil, 166–167
Purkinje fibers, 210–211
pyloric canal, 284–285
pyloric region, 284–285
pyloric sphincter, 284–285
pylorus, 284–285

Q

quadrant regions, 8–9
quadrate lobe, 290–291
quadriceps femoris, 104–105, 150–151

R

radial artery, 214–215, 220–221
radial nerve, 148–149
radial notch, 72–73
radial tuberosity, 72–73
radial veins, 230–231, 234–235
radius, 64–65, 92–93, 94–95
ramus, 46–47
rectal artery, 226–227, 228–229
rectouterine pouch, 310–311
rectum, 274–275, 288–289
rectus abdominis, 104–105
red blood cells, 36–37, 202–203, 272–273
red pulp, 248–249
regions, of the abdomen, 8–9
renal arteries, 224–225, 294–295, 296–297
renal capsule, 296–297
renal columns, 296–297
renal corpuscle, 300–301
renal cortex, 296–297
renal medulla, 296–297
renal pelvis, 296–297

superior (position), 2–3
superior articular facets, 56–57, 58–59
superior articular process, 58–59, 60–61, 92–93
superior atria, 200–201
superior border, 66–67
superior colliculi, 126–127
superior gluteal nerves, 152–153
superior iliac spine, 78–79
superior lobe, 270–271
superior mesenteric artery, 224–225, 226–227
superior mesenteric vein, 238–239
superior nasal conchae, 52–53
superior oblique muscle, 140–141, 168–169
superior pubic ramus, 78–79
superior rectus, 168–169
superior vena cava, 198–199, 200–201, 206–207, 208–209, 230–231, 232–233, 240–241
supination, 102–103
supporting cells, 164–165
supracondylar ridges, 70–71
supraspinous fossa, 66–67
suprasternal notch, 62–63
sural, 18–19
surfactant, 272–273
surgical neck, 70–71
suspensory ligaments, 170–171, 310–311, 314–315
sustenocytes, 306–307
suture, 86–87
sweat glands, 28–29, 40–41
"swimmer's muscle," 106–107
sympathetic chain ganglia, 156–157
sympathetic division, 156–157
symphysis, 88–89
symphysis pubis, 306–307
synapses, 112–113
synaptic cleft, 116–117
synaptic vesicles, 116–117
synarthroses, 86–87
synchondrosis, 88–89
syndesmosis, 86–87
synovial cavity, 90–91
synovial joint, 90–91, 92–93
synovial membranes, 90–91
synovial sheath, 90–91
systemic capillary bed, 200–201
systemic circulation, 200–201
system(s)
 arterial, 200–201
 autonomic nervous, 110–111, 156–157, 158–159
 cardiovascular, 14–15, 198–199, 200–201, 202–203, 204–211
 central nervous, 10–11, 110–111
 digestive system, 12–13, 38–39, 274–275

endocrine, 12–13, 182–183, 182–197
female reproductive, 308–309
hepatic portal, 238–239
integumentary, 12–13, 38–39, 40–41
limbic, 130–131
lymph, 242–243, 244–245
male reproductive, 302–303
muscular, 10–11, 104–105
nervous, 10–11, 110–111
reproductive, 14–15, 38–39, 302–303, 308–309
respiratory, 12–13, 256–257
skeletal, 10–11, 44–45
somatic nervous, 110–111, 112–113

T
T cells, 202–203, 254–255
tactile corpuscles, 160–161
talus, 84–85
tarsals, 80–81, 84–85
taste buds, 162–163
taste pores, 162–163
tectorial membrane, 180–181
teeth, 46–47, 276–277, 280–281
temporal bone, 44–45, 46–47, 50–51, 52–53, 96–97
temporal lobe, 120–121, 124–125, 180–181
temporomandibular joint, 96–97
tendon flexor digitorum profundus muscle, 90–91
tendon flexor digitorum superficialis, 90–91
tendon insertion flexor digitorum profundus, 90–91
tendon sheath, 90–91
teniae coli, 288–289
terminal bouton, 116–117
terminal nerves, 144–145
testes, 14–15, 182–183, 196–197, 302–303, 304–305
testicular artery, 304–305
testosterone, 182–183, 302–303
thalamus, 126–127, 128–129
thermoreceptors, 160–161
third ventricle, 128–129, 134–135, 136–137
thoracic aorta, 214–215, 216–217, 224–225
thoracic artery, 220–221, 224–225
thoracic cavity, 20–21, 270–271
thoracic curvature, 54–55
thoracic duct, 242–243, 244–245
thoracic nerves, 144–145
thoracic vertebra, 54–55, 58–59, 68–69
thoracolumbar division, 156–157
throat, 140–141
thrombocytes, 202–203
thymus, 244–245

thyroid cartilage, 258–259, 264–265, 266–267
thyroid gland, 12–13, 182–183, 188–189
thyroid stimulating hormone (TSH), 186–187
tibal veins, 236–237
tibia, 80–81, 82–83, 86–87
tibial arteries, 222–223
tibial artery, 214–215, 222–223
tibial collateral ligament, 100–101
tibial condyle, 82–83
tibial crest, 82–83
tibial nerve, 152–153
tibial tuberosity, 82–83
tibial veins, 236–237
tibialis anterior muscle, 104–105
tibiofemoral joint, 100–101
tibiofibular ligament, 86–87
tissues, 6–7
tongue, 132–133, 140–141, 162–163, 246–247, 276–277
tonsillar ring, 246–247
tonsils, 246–247
tooth, 86–87
trabeculae carneae, 208–209
trachea, 12–13, 256–257, 258–259, 264–265, 266–267, 268–269
trachea splits, 272–273
tracheal rings, 268–269
trachealis muscle, 268–269
transitional epithelium, 26–27, 298–299
transverse colon, 288–289
transverse costal facets, 58–59
transverse foramina, 56–57, 58–59
transverse lines, 60–61
transverse processes, 58–59
transverse section, 4–5
transverse tibiofibular ligament, 86–87
trapezium, 74–75, 94–95
trapezius muscles, 106–107
trapezoid, 74–75
triceps brachii, 106–107
tricuspid valve, 208–209, 210–211
trigeminal nerve, 140–141
trigone, 298–299
trilaminar germ disk, 320–321
triquetrum, 74–75
trochanter, 80–81
trochlea, 70–71, 140–141
trochlear nerve, 140–141
trochlear notch, 72–73
trophoblast, 318–319
true pelvis, 76–77
tubercle, 62–63, 70–71
tuberosity of the ulna, 72–73
tunica, 212–213
tunica adventitia, 212–213